T0257571

Understanding Peptic Ulcer Disease

Understanding Peptic Ulcer Disease

Edited by **Jessica Brown**

New Jersey

Published by Foster Academics,
61 Van Reypen Street,
Jersey City, NJ 07306, USA
www.fosteracademics.com

Understanding Peptic Ulcer Disease
Edited by Jessica Brown

International Standard Book Number: 978-1-63242-419-8 (Hardback)

Contents

Preface

Peptic ulcer disease is one of the most common chronic infections amongst humans. In spite of centuries of study, this ailment still bothers a lot of people, especially those in third world countries. This book consists of current information on peptic ulcer disease, contributed by distinguished researchers from various countries around the world. It discusses topics like the cause of the disease, clinical care and alternative medicine.

This book unites the global concepts and researches in an organized manner for a comprehensive understanding of the subject. It is a ripe text for all researchers, students, scientists or anyone else who is interested in acquiring a better knowledge of this dynamic field.

I extend my sincere thanks to the contributors for such eloquent research chapters. Finally, I thank my family for being a source of support and help.

Editor

Part 1

Clinical Management of Peptic Ulcer Patients

Perforated Duodenal Ulcer in High Risk Patients

Aly Saber

Port-Fouad general hospital,
Port-Fouad, Port-Said,
Egypt

1. Introduction

Peptic ulcer disease remains one of the most prevalent disease of the gastrointestinal tract with annual incidence ranging from 0.1% to 0.3% in western countries. There are well-known two major precipitating factors: Helicobacter pylori infection and the use of non-steroidal anti-inflammatory drugs (NSAIDs) and the ulcer incidence increases with age for both duodenal and gastric ulcers.

Peptic ulcer disease (PUD) is considered as a mucosal functional derangements due to intraluminal aggressive factors and defects in endogenous defense mechanisms affecting the mucosa and extend through the muscularis mucosa. Some of these functional defects may be caused by the presence of H pylori colonization of the antral mucosa and antral mucosal metaplasia of the proximal duodenum. In vivo and in vitro data support this concept, particularly with reference to the mechanisms of Helicobacter pylori-induced aberrations in gastric and duodenal mucosal function. Standard medical therapy for peptic ulcer disease includes antisecretory medications as well as antibiotics designed to eradicate H pylori colonization.

Complications of peptic ulcer disease are bleeding, perforation and obstruction. These complications can occur in patients with peptic ulcers of any etiology. Perforation occurs in about 5% to 10% of patients with active ulcer disease. Duodenal, antral and gastric body ulcers account for 60%, 20% and 20% of perforations, respectively, of peptic ulcers. Open and laparoscopic abdominal exploration are always indicated in gastroduodenal perforation. Hemodynamic instability, signs of peritonitis and free extravasation of contrast material on upper gastrointestinal tract contrast studies make the decision for operation more urgent and imperative. But, the advent of proton pump inhibitors and Helicobacter pylori eradication in the management of chronic peptic ulcer disease has reduced the operative treatment of this condition to its complications. Perforated duodenal ulcer remains a major life threatening complication of chronic peptic ulcer disease.

The incidence of peptic ulcer disease in normal populations has declined over the past few years following a more streamlined pharmacological intervention. This can be attributed to the efficiency of histamine 2 (H2) blockers and proton pump inhibitors. Additionally, the diagnosis and eradication of Helicobacter pylori infection, now known to be a major factor in the pathogenesis of peptic ulcer disease, has almost eliminated the role of surgery in the elective management of peptic ulcer disease. However, the incidence of perforated duodenal ulcers has either remained the same or has been increasing with the resultant increase in the incidence of emergency surgery. Although the use of potent H2 blockers and proton pump inhibitors has caused a marked decline in the incidence of peptic ulcer perforation, no such decline has been seen in the eradication of H. pylori infection.

Patients with perforated duodenal ulcers include those with acute ulcers, such as patients on nonsteroidal anti-inflammatory drugs (NSAIDs) and those with chronic ulcer disease who are refractory to or noncompliant with medical treatment. Another contributing factor to the increased incidence of perforation of duodenal ulcer is the decrease in elective anti-ulcer surgery. Patients presenting with an acute abdomen suggestive of a perforated duodenal ulcer are generally between 40 and 60 years of age although the number of patients over the age of 60 has been gradually increasing. Approximately 50% to 60% of these patients have a history of peptic ulcer disease, while a smaller number have a history of use of NSAIDs. Now, It's settled that H. pylori infection and NSAID use are two independent risk factors associated with perforated duodenal ulcers, and the lack of duodenitis in NSAID users as compared with those with H. pylori infection suggests a differing pathogenesis.

The frequency of perforated peptic ulcer is decreasing among the overall population but it is becoming more frequent among old people. The higher mortality rate in the old population, justifies the search of prognostic factors specific for the elderly.

2. High risk elderly patients

"High risk" surgical patients
Age > 60
Congestive cardiac failure
Ischaemic heart disease
Cardiac arrhythmia
Hypertension
COPD
Pulmonary embolus
Chronic renal insufficiency
Diabetes mellitus with end-organ damage
Long term steroid therapy
Chronic liver disease
Cerebrovascular disease
Peripheral vascular disease

Table 1. Showed patients with high risk of post operative death.

Risk is a term that is understood differently by different individuals depending on expectation and previous experience. The term "high risk surgical patient" is poorly defined. The term should refer to the group of patients, who were considered to be at high risk of post operative death, and were included in studies of pre-operative "optimization" to a pre-determined oxygen delivery [table 1]. From a practical point of view 'high risk' can probably be defined in two different ways: the first is relevant to an individual and suggests that the risk to an individual is higher than for a population; the second compares the risk of the procedure in question with the risk of surgical procedures as a whole. Furthermore, many investigators suggest that surgical patients for whom the probable mortality is greater than 20% should be considered 'extremely high-risk' patients. There are two main components in identification of high risk for surgery. The first relates to the type of surgery and the second to the cardiopulmonary functional capacity of the patient. There are methods that can be used to assess risk in various patient groups and in the author's opinion , the two most useful scoring systems in surgical risk assessment remain the American Society of Anesthesiologists (ASA) score and the patients' clinical criteria. Both of these assessments are simple to use and do not require additional resources. Surgical risk, in turn, has two components: the extent and the duration of the procedure both can cause an increase in postoperative oxygen demand and an increase in cardiac output or an increase in oxygen extraction. The classification of surgical interference is done in accordance with the extension and/or complexity of the procedure, with one or several of the mentioned characteristics:

S1. Minor Surgery: minimal extension, local anesthesia, ambulatory.

S2. Major Simple Surgery: performed on one organ or system, without any other added procedure

S3. Major Complex Surgery: performed on one organ or system, with other procedure or procedures related with the scheduled one, potential important bleeding, perhaps with some surgical problem that can be solved.

S4. Major Multiple Surgery: on several organs or systems, important bleeding, potential perioperative complications, it needs special preparation

S5. "Rescue" surgery, danger of death

The second item is the functional capacity of the patient that determines his ability to support the postoperative demand of increased oxygen consumption and therefore of cardiac output. Myocardial ischemia only becomes part of this equation if the ischemia limits ventricular function and cardiac output.

The definition of "elderly" is controversial and the traditional demographic definitions include those patients exceeding 65 years of age as the functional deterioration is more frequently apparent beyond the age of 70 years. For the elderly, one should categorize age-related pre-existing chronic illness; age related functional physical decline, or preoperative risk status. The most important surgeon responsibility is to decide whether to operate or not when the patient is of high surgical risk. The decision-making process is complex in elderly surgical candidates. Among the currently available risk assessment tools, American Society of Anesthesiologists (ASA) scoring system despite does not measure operative risk, rather it assesses the degree of sickness or physical state prior to anesthesia and surgery. The assessment of cardiac risk is addressed by the Cardiac Risk Index (CRI) in noncardiac surgery and the risks of postoperative respiratory complications are age over 70; perioperative bronchodilator use; abnormal chest x-ray; and high ASA grade.

The Acute Physiological and Chronic Health Evaluation (APACHE) is the best known physiological scoring system. It is based on twelve physiological variables and is currently being used in general and surgical intensive care patients.   Age is an independent risk factor built into above mentioned risk prediction tools; ASA, Cardiac Risk Index (CRI) and APACHE. Preoperative Assessment of medication use is highest in elderly persons who require multiple medications to treat their complex set of medical problems. Medications necessary for managing medical conditions can put elderly individuals at risk of medication-induced problems such as adverse drug effects, drug-drug interactions, or drug toxicities. The greater the number of medications taken, the greater the risk of a clinically serious drug-drug interaction and the adverse drug reactions experienced by elderly patients often tend to be more severe than those experienced by younger patients. The reduced organ reserve capacity of elderly persons contributes to this as every organ system loses reserve capacity with age.

3. Epidemiology of perforated PUD

Although there is a decreasing incidence , perforated duodenal ulcer remains a serious condition which generally requires surgical intervention, and is associated with a high mortality rate especially among the elderly. The frequency of perforated peptic ulcer is decreasing among the overall population but it is becoming more frequent among old people. The higher mortality rate in the old population, justifies the search of prognostic factors specific for the elderly. The high mortality from perforated peptic ulcer underlines the importance of risk stratification. Over the past decades, important changes have occurred in the epidemiology of peptic ulcer disease. The discovery of Helicobacter pylori in the early 1980s as a major cause of peptic ulcer disease had a significant impact on the treatment of ulcer disease. The significance of the discovery led to the award of the 2005 Nobel Prize in Medicine to Robin Warren and Barry Marshall [figure 1]. H pylori eradication therapy was proven to cure patients with previous chronic, recurrent ulcer disease.

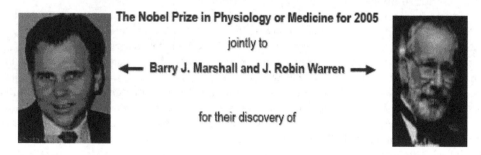

The Nobel Prize in Physiology or Medicine for 2005

jointly to

⟵ Barry J. Marshall and J. Robin Warren ⟶

for their discovery of

"the bacterium *Helicobacter pylori* and its role in gastritis and

peptic ulcer disease"

Fig. 1. Nobel Prize winners in Medicine and Physiology at the 2005

Peptic ulcer complications have a high mortality, especially in elderly patients and it is therefore important to understand the epidemiology of this disease in order to investigate if complications can be prevented. Despite new efficient drugs to treat peptic ulcer disease and increasing knowledge about its aetiology, the incidence of peptic ulcer complications, i.e. perforation and bleeding, have been reported by several groups to be unchanged. Further research into the epidemiology of H pylori infection showed that the prevalence of this bacterium was decreasing over time in recent decades, presumably as a result of improvements in living conditions. The overall decline of peptic ulcer disease is likely to be due to a combination of factors including the introduction of acid suppressive medication, a decreasing prevalence of H pylori in subsequent birth cohorts and the development of eradication treatment for H pylori-positive ulcer patients, which prevents chronic relapsing ulcer disease. The introduction of newer NSAIDs and a tendency for the prescription of lower doses of acetylsalicylic acid for patients with cardiovascular disease may also have contributed to the changing epidemiology of ulcer disease.

With the decreased incidence of ulcer disease, the incidence of ulcer complications may have been affected as well. But most studies showed that the incidence of the most important complication, ulcer bleeding, remained stable notwithstanding the decreasing incidence of peptic ulcers.

The introduction of an endoscopy database allowed for closer investigation of the incidence and epidemiology of gastric and duodenal ulcers, complication rates and classifications. Mortality after perforated and bleeding peptic ulcer increases. An increased burden of comorbidity among elderly patients did not explain the association between advanced age and increased mortality, with the strongest association observed among patients with no history of hospital-diagnosed comorbidity.

Studies on the incidence of perforated duodenal ulcer are limited and data are largely based on findings observed over two decades ago. The epidemiological data on duodenal ulcer perforation was obtained mainly from medical records registry units all over the world for patients admitted with ulcer perforation. The incidence of perforated duodenal ulcer disease increases with advanced age and this increase has been attributed to the high frequency of risk factors for PUD among elderly patients, e.g., Helicobacter pylori colonization or use of non-steroidal anti-inflammatory drugs. Perforated peptic ulcer has an overall reported mortality of 5%–25%, rising to as high as 50% with age. Being closely related to advanced age, increased burden of comorbidity may partially explain the higher mortality among elderly patients.

Several studies support the notion that NSAID is a risk factor not only in uncomplicated peptic ulcer disease, but also in regard to perforated ulcers. The higher risk was maintained during treatment and disappeared after treatment termination. The added risk is dose-dependent and also includes low-dose acetyl salicylic acid. According to a study by Sorensen et al from 2000 the risk increase further when low-dose ASA is combined with NSAID. Proton pump inhibitors (PPI) have become one of the most sold drugs in the world and are nowadays also available over the counter in Sweden. It is a well known fact that PPI protect against peptic ulcer complications in NSAID users. Interestingly the introduction of PPI was almost simultaneous with the beginning of a falling incidence in peptic ulcer complications. H pylori is an important pathogenic factor in peptic ulcer disease, although studies that investigate the connection between H pylori and peptic ulcer complications are somewhat divergent. Helicobacter Pylori is, without a doubt, connected to peptic ulcer disease and its complications , perforation and bleeding, however, other factors such as NSAID and smoking are of great importance as well [figure 2]. Smoking is a another important risk factor for peptic ulcer perforation. smoking more than fifteen cigarettes daily increased the risk of peptic ulcer perforation 3,5 times. The prevalence of smoking has declined during the last twenty years in most western countries, especially in men, which could perhaps account for fewer ulcer complications.

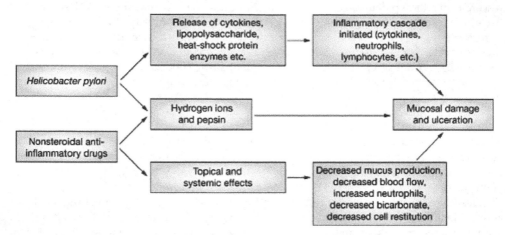

Fig. 2. The synergistic and independent effects of Helicobacter pylori and nonsteroidal anti-inflammatory drugs on gastric mucosal damage.

4. Pathophysiology of perforated peptic ulcer

The duodenal mucosa resists damage from the effect of aggressive factors, such as gastric acid and the proteolytic enzyme pepsin, with the help of several protective factors, such as a mucous layer, bicarbonate secretion, and protective prostaglandins. The epithelial cells of the stomach and duodenum secrete mucus in response to irritation of the epithelial lining and as a result of cholinergic stimulation. A portion of the gastric and duodenal mucus exists in the form of a gel layer, which is impermeable to acid and pepsin. Other gastric and duodenal cells secrete bicarbonate, which aids in buffering acid that lies near the mucosa. Prostaglandins E (PGE) have an important protective role by increasing the production of both bicarbonate and the mucous layer. When an alteration occurs in the aggressive and/or protective factors, a duodenal ulcer occurs such that the balance is in favor of gastric acid and pepsin. Any process that increases gastric acidity (eg, individuals with increased maximal and basal acid output), decreases prostaglandin production (eg, NSAIDs), or interferes with the mucous layer (eg, H pylori infection) can cause such an imbalance and lead to peptic ulcer disease.

Full understanding of the pathophysiology and pathogenesis of duodenal ulcers requires a brief discussion of the two major etiologies: NSAID use and H pylori infection. NSAIDs are pathogenic through their inhibition of the cyclooxygenase-1 (COX-1) pathway, which normally produces protective prostaglandins. These prostaglandins are protective because they augment both bicarbonate and mucous production, as mentioned above. However, perhaps more important, prostaglandins augment mucosal blood flow, and their inhibition leads to impairment of blood flow, leaving the mucosa vulnerable to damage. Infection with H pylori is likely pathogenic by means of a variety of indirect mechanisms as the organism does not generally colonize the duodenum. H pylori infection leads to an inflammatory state in which high levels of tumor necrosis factor-alpha (TNF-alpha) and other cytokines are produced and in turn stimulate gastric acid production directly by increasing gastrin release from G cells and inhibit somatostatin production by antral D cells. This leads to a net increase in gastric acid secretion, which leads to an increased acid load in the duodenum, overwhelming the mucosal defense. Duodenal acid exposure can lead to gastric metaplasia, whereby the duodenal mucosa can take on characteristics of gastric mucosa. H pylori can then colonize the duodenal mucosa and adhere to cells. This adherence leads to a variety of second-messenger signals, which invoke an immunologic response against those cells causing mucosal damage by host neutrophils and other inflammatory cells. H pylori also affects the gastric and duodenal mucous layer, because this organism produces proteases that degrade the protective mucous layer. Moreover, H pylori infection decreases the production of epidermal growth factor, which normally promotes healing of gastric and duodenal mucosa. H pylori produces proteins that may serve as chemotactic factors for neutrophils and monocytes, which act as proinflammatory cells. H pylori also affects the gastric and duodenal mucous layer, because these organisms produce proteases that degrade the protective mucous layer. H pylori does not lead to the development of gastric and duodenal ulcers through alteration of the bacterial flora. In most cases of perforation, gastric and duodenal content leaks into the peritoneum. This content includes gastric and duodenal secretions, bile, ingested food, and swallowed bacteria. The leakage results in peritonitis, with an increased risk of infection and abscess formation. There are three clinical phases in the process of PPU can be distinguished:

Phase 1: Chemical peritonitis/contamination. The perforation causes a chemical peritonitis. Acid sterilizes the gastroduodenal content; it is only when gastric acid is reduced by treatment or disease (gastric cancer) that bacteria and fungi are present in the stomach and duodenum.

Phase 2: Intermediate stage. After 6–12 h many patients obtain some relief of pain. This is probably due to the dilution of the irritating gastroduodenal contents by ensuing peritoneal exudates.

Phase 3: Intra-abdominal infection. After 12–24 h intra-abdominal infection supervenes Subsequent third-spacing of fluid in the peritoneal cavity due to perforation and peritonitis leads to inadequate circulatory volume, hypotension, and decreased urine output. In more severe cases, shock may develop. Abdominal distension as a result of peritonitis and subsequent ileus may interfere with diaphragmatic movement, impairing expansion of the lung bases. Eventually, atelectasis develops, which may compromise oxygenation of the blood, particularly in patients with coexisting lung disease.

5. Prognostic factors

The continuing problem with perforated duodenal ulcer stands in contrast to the fall in admissions for uncomplicated duodenal ulcers noted since the 1970's and largely attributed to the introduction of H 2 antagonists. The high incidence of complications necessitates the identification of factors associated with the morbidity and mortality of patients undergoing surgery for perforated peptic ulcer. The patient population with perforation tends to be elderly ; mean age 60–70, chronically ill and those patients often taking ulcerogenic medication. Mortality rate after surgery for perforated duodenal ulcer is much more higher in the elderly that reach up to 50%. This can be explained by the occurrence of concomitant medical diseases but also by difficulties in making the right diagnosis resulting in a delay of >24 hours. The longstanding perforation more than 24 hours together with major medical illness and preoperative shock collectively predicted the outcome in patients with perforated duodenal ulcer as [table 2].

RISK FACTORS	SCORE
1.Numbers of hrs since ulcer perforation	
24hrs or less	0
More than 24 hrs	1
2.Pre operative systolic BP (mm of Hg)	
100 or more	0
Less than 100	1
3.Any one or more systemic illness	
Absent	0
Present	1

Table 2. Boey score-risk factor to predict mortality

The mortality rate increased progressively with increasing numbers of risk factors: 0%, 10%, 45.5%, and 100% in patients with none, one, two, and all three risk factors of Boey, respectively. Definitive surgery can be done safely in good-risk patients. Simple closure is preferable in those patients with uncomplicated perforations if any risk factor is present. Truncal vagotomy and drainage may be required if there is coexisting bleeding or stenosis. Nonoperative treatment deserves re-evaluation in patients with all three risk factors because of their uniformly dismal outcome after operation.

6. Clinical course of PDU in elderly

Studies have shown that nearly half of patients presenting with complicated peptic ulcer disease (PUD), have no history of the disease. On endoscopy, unsuspected ulcers have been found in people who were taking nonsteroidal anti-inflammatory drugs (NSAIDs). Two courses of the disease were observed: the first is defined by acute disease of less than 24 hours' duration preceding surgery. Classic patients with perforated peptic ulcer disease usually present with a sudden onset of severe sharp abdominal pain that may be generalized pain or epigastric urging these patients assuming a fetal position. Abdominal examination findings are usually consistent with generalized tenderness, rebound tenderness, guarding, and rigidity. However, the degree of peritoneal findings is strongly influenced by a number of factors, including the size of perforation, amount of bacterial and gastric contents contaminating the abdominal cavity, time between perforation and presentation, and spontaneous sealing of perforation. Accordingly, the second course of perforation is of longer duration, starting with various abdominal complaints and presenting more severely only after the first 24 hours. Patients belonging to the second course may also demonstrate signs and symptoms of septic shock, such as tachycardia, hypotension, and anuria, but these indicators of shock may be absent in elderly patients or in those with other systemic illness. In recent years, patients presenting with perforated duodenal ulcers have tended to be elderly and chronically ill and taking one or more ulcerogenic drugs. Several studies have shown the mean age of such patients to be more than 60 years. In elderly patients, signs and symptoms may be minimal. In patients over age 60 with perforated ulcer, more than 80 % had only mild abdominal pain. Other reported symptoms were dyspepsia, anorexia, nausea, and vomiting. Severe abdominal pain was present in only less than 20 % of patients. Duration of symptoms is usually protracted and delayed. Although minority of those patients had no abdominal findings, most had abdominal tenderness, with up to two thirds having classic signs of peritonitis.. There is a changing scene with perforated peptic ulcer. The older age of presentation, the increased association with non-steroidal anti-inflammatory drugs, associated increased debility, and resulting higher mortality in the elderly, are causing a rethink in management protocols.

7. Management protocol

There are two main accepted regimen of treatment of perforated duodenal ulcer; non-operative and surgical treatment. Non-operative treatment should be rendered in perforated peptic ulcers only when the patient shows definite signs of improvement both symptomatically and clinically, and there is a definite "walling off" of the ulceration, or when the patient's condition is too poor to permit operation. With good operative risk, patients should be prepared for surgery of ulcer-definitive procedure of the surgeon's choice; for example vagotomy and pyloroplasty or antrectomy. Purulent peritonitis would dictate only secure closure of the perforation [table 2].

7.1 Nonoperative treatment

The introduction of novel peptic ulcer drugs, such as H2 receptor blockers and proton pump inhibitors, caused a prompt decline in elective operations for peptic ulcer disease in recent times. On the other hand, surgery for peptic ulcer complications, such as perforations has not changed. Effective medical management of peptic ulcer disease has reduced the incidence of gastric outlet obstruction as a complication, but perforation especially in the elderly remains unchanged and is, in fact, on the increase. There is a changing trend in emergency surgery for perforated duodenal ulcer from definitive anti ulcer surgery to simple closure followed by Helicobacter pylori eradication. Surgical emergency due to a perforated peptic ulcer – whether treated laparoscopically or by open repair – is associated with a significant postoperative morbidity and mortality. Therefore, risk-stratification of these subjects provides surgeons with an important tool to plan the management. The dominant treatment of perforated duodenal ulcer in the first half of the 20th century was surgical closure. In most perforated duodenal ulcers that were successfully surgically closed, the perforation was a harbinger of subsequent major morbidity from peptic ulceration. This was in the form of re-perforation, hemorrhage, obstruction, or intractability. The major concern against simple closure is the possible risk of future serious complications of relapse. Some authors claim that prognosis is not related to the surgical procedure itself and the current policy is not to perform definitive ulcer surgery in cases of PPU. A simple procedure should be the one of choice for an emergency operation and extensive procedures should be reserved only in selected patients despite good results are obtained with simple procedures.

Several facts support an alternative to the currently accepted therapy of the perforated duodenal ulcer, that is, immediate surgical closure of the perforation with or without an ulcer-definitive procedure. The following facts are included:

1. Most ulcers are associated with infection with H pylori, including ulcers that perforate.
2. Almost all ulcers associated with H pylori can be healed with combined medical therapy; ie, antibiotics and proton-pump inhibitors or H2 blockers. The rate of relapse is very low and re-infection is rare.
3. The administration of H2 blockers and proton-pump inhibitors and elimination of NSAIDs are now essential components of medical therapy. Such therapy has favorably affected the natural history of duodenal ulcers, including those that perforate.
4. Approximately half of duodenal ulcers that perforate will have self-sealed when first seen by the physician.
5. The perforation of a duodenal ulcer that has sealed spontaneously can be treated nonoperatively with low morbidity, including releakage and abdominal abscess.
6. Death due to peritonitis reflects protracted leakage and secondary bacterial contamination.
7. Major associated disease is a significant risk factor for death following perforation of a duodenal ulcer.

7.1.1 Principles of conservative treatment
Principles of conservative treatment include nasogastric suction, pain control, antiulcer medication, and antibiotics. Nonsurgical treatment has been recognized for a long time. The first major series was published by Taylor nearly 50 years ago; it reported a mortality rate of 11% in the nonsurgical treatment group, compared to 20% in the surgical group. Since then, because of improvements in operative and postoperative care, the mortality rate with surgical treatment of perforated peptic ulcer has decreased to about 5%. Failure of conservative treatment is generally defined as development of septic shock, multiple organ failure or intra-abdominal abscess. Conservative treatment failure exposes patients to the risk of delayed surgical closure with mortality rates between up to 50% , depending on the timing of secondary surgery. While conservative treatment was first proposed to patients not eligible for surgery, some few investigators have tried this approach in rather fit patients but in fact these studies have reported high mortality compared to the results achieved by surgical repair in elderly or medically frail patients. The systematic introduction of PPI use and HP eradication seems to have favorably influenced the results of conservative therapy through reduction of mortality.

7.1.2 Failure of conservative treatment
Definition of prognostic factors for conservative treatment has been a concern for all investigators. The presence of shock at admission is a major criterion for conservative treatment failure and implies that, even in a moribund patient. The presence of haemodynamic instability militates in favor of prompt surgery. The presence of shock being one of the Boey criteria, has a strong correlation of mortality.

7.2 Surgical Therapy
Surgery is recommended in patients who present with hemodynamic instability, signs of peritonitis and free extravasation of contrast on upper gastrointestinal contrast studies. If

contamination of the upper abdomen is minimal and the patient is stable, a definitive ulcer procedure can be performed. For a perforated duodenal ulcer, this may include a highly selective vagotomy, a truncal vagotomy and pyloroplasty, or vagotomy and antrectomy.

7.2.1 Preoperative preparation

Fluid resuscitation should be initiated as soon as the diagnosis is made. Essential steps include insertion of a nasogastric tube to decompress the stomach and a Foley catheter to monitor urine output. Intravenous infusion of fluids is begun, and broad-spectrum antibiotics are administered. In select cases, insertion of a central venous line for accurate fluid resuscitation and monitoring. As soon as the patient has been adequately resuscitated, emergent exploratory laparotomy should be performed.

7.2.2 Surgical procedures

a. Laparoscopic Surgery

The traditional management of a perforated duodenal ulcer is closure with omental patch and a thorough abdominal lavage. More recently this has been shown to be able to performed using a laparoscope. The only proven advantage of the laparoscopic technique appears to be decreased postoperative pain. Operating times are longer compared to open techniques and hospital time appears to be similar to conventional treatment.

b. Immediate Definitive Surgery

Attempts have been made to improve upon the results of simple closure and lavage in response to the large number of patients more than 25% continue to have symptoms attributable to their ulcer diathesis after surgery. Since the 1940's the concept of immediate definitive ulcer surgery has been raised but debated amongst surgeons. There is good evidence that, in the emergency situation, highly selective vagotomy combined with simple omental patch closure of the perforation, in patients without the risk factors, is just as effective as that performed in the elective setting with less mortality and ulcer recurrence rate. Truncal vagotomy with drainage has its advocates as an expedient operation familiar to most surgeons. Immediate definitive ulcer surgery has not gained widespread popularity as it is associated with a higher mortality than simple closure in patients at risk of suffering from complications of surgery. Many agree that an appropriate approach is to select only those with a chronic history of ulcer disease for more than 3 months and without preoperative risk factors for immediate definitive surgery. A major difficulty is defining preoperatively the patients with chronic ulcer history as many ulcers showed silent history, many patients are too unwell to give a reliable history of their disease and finally, perforations occurs as the first manifestation of the ulcer diathesis.

7.3 Percutaneous peritoneal drainage

The higher mortality rate in the old population, justifies the search of prognostic factors specific for the elderly in whom the difficult management was attributed to their concomitant diseases. The criteria of Taylor's method in selected cases were diagnosis of perforation in less than 12 hours, with stable hemodynamic condition and age not exceeding 70 years. Emergency abdominal operations are commonly performed and carry high morbidity and mortality risk, particularly in elderly patients due to presence of coexisting cardiopulmonary disease, late admission and presence of peritonitis. So, in high risk elderly patients with perforated duodenal ulcer and established peritonitis, pus should be drained with the least invasive maneuver. Transnasogastric placement of a drainage catheter through the perforated ulcer was said to be as successful as definitive therapy. High-risk peptic ulcer perforation patients can be managed by putting in an intra-abdominal drain supported by conservative treatment with reduced death rate and patients improvements.

7.3.1 Operative technique

In conjunction with conservative measures, percutaneous peritoneal drainage was performed under local anaesthesia through a 3- cm long skin incision at the level of right anterior superior iliac spine and the lateral edge of the rectus muscle. The incision spitted the external oblique aponeurosis, internal oblique and transversus abdominus along the direction of their fibers. Upon interning the peritoneal cavity, the index finger was swiped in all direction to allow protection and good drainage. A wide bored percutaneous intra-abdominal drain.

8. Aims and concerns

Type of surgery	Morbidity	Total no. (%)
Simple closure (n = 29)	a. Pulmonary embolism (1)	8 (27.5)
	b. Septicemia (4)	
	c. Respiratory failure (1)	
	d. Wound infection (1)	
Closure + Acid reduction procedure (n = 8)	a. Stomal obstruction (1)	3 (37.5)
	b. Post operative anastamotic leak with septicemia (1)	
	c. Gastric fistula (1)	
Gastric resection (n = 17)	a. Wound infection (1)	6 (35.2)
	b. Duodenal blow out (1)	
	c. Respiratory failure (4)	

Table 3. Morbidity related to type of surgery.

Perforated peptic ulcer disease continues to inflict high morbidity and mortality. Although patients can be stratified according to their surgical risk, optimal management has yet to be described. The accepted therapeutic options in patients with perforated peptic ulcer are simple closure or immediate definitive operation. The non-operative management of perforated peptic ulcer has previously been shown to be both safe and effective although it remains controversial. Taylor's conservative treatment, originally proposed for the treatment of choice in perforated acute peptic ulcer in 1951. Today it is reserved for patients considered to be too ill to stand the stress of surgery or in situations where immediate surgery is unavailable. Minimal surgical intervention (percutaneous peritoneal drainage) can significantly lower the mortality rate among a selected group of critically ill, poor risk patients with perforated peptic ulcer disease.

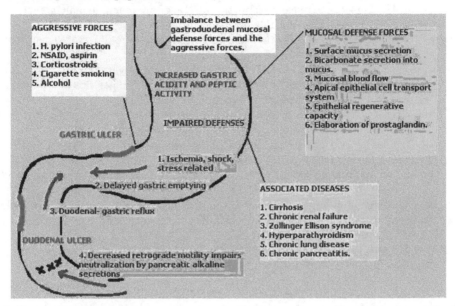

Fig. 3. Shows the imbalance between aggressive factors and protective factors in peptic ulcer disease.

9. References

[1] Karangelis D, Tagarakis GI, Karathanos C, Bouliaris K, Baddour AJ, Giaglaras A. Synchronous perforation of a duodenal and gastric ulcer: a case report. J Med Case Reports. 2010 Aug 18;4:272.

[2] Lui FY, Davis KA. Gastroduodenal perforation: maximal or minimal intervention?. Scand J Surg. 2010;99(2):73-7. Review.) Nuhu A, Kassama Y. Experience with acute perforated duodenal ulcer in a West African population. Niger J Med. 2008 Oct-Dec;17(4):403-6.

[3] Uccheddu A, Floris G, Altana ML, Pisanu A, Cois A, Farci SL. Surgery for perforated peptic ulcer in the elderly. Evaluation of factors nfluencing prognosis. Hepatogastroenterology. 2003 Nov-Dec;50(54):1956-8.

[4] Noguiera C, Silva AS, Santos JN, Silva AG, Ferreira J, Matos E, Vilaça H. Perforated peptic ulcer: main factors of morbidity and mortality. World J Surg. 2003 Jul;27(7):782-7.

[5] Canoy, D.S. Hart, A.R. , Todd, C.J. Epidemiology of duodenal ulcer perforation: A study on hospital admissions in Norfolk, United Kingdom. Digestive and Liver Disease. Can J Gastroenterol. 2009 Sep;23(9):604-8.

[6] Michael H , Anders E , Jonas R , Thomas Z. Decreasing incidence of peptic ulcer complications after the introduction of the proton pump inhibitors, a study of the Swedish population from 1974–2002 , BMC Gastroenterology, 2009, Apr. 9 (1),.25-

[7] Girbes AR. The high-risk surgical patient and the role of preoperative management. Neth J Med. 2000 Sep;57(3):98-105. Review.

[8] Yuan Y, Padol IT, Hunt RH. Peptic ulcer disease today. Nat Clin Pract Gastroenterol Hepatol. 2006 Feb;3(2):80-9.

[9] Konturek SJ, Konturek PC, Konturek JW, Plonka M, Czesnikiewicz-Guzik M, Brzozowski T, Bielanski W. Helicobacter pylori and its involvement in gastritis and peptic ulcer formation. J Physiol Pharmacol. 2006 Sep;57 Suppl 3:29-50.

[10] Sarath Chandra S, Kumar SS. Definitive or conservative surgery for perforated gastric ulcer?--An unresolved problem. Int J Surg. 2009 Apr;7(2):136-9. Epub 2008 Dec 25.

[11] Saber A, Ellabban GM, Gad MA. An unusual presentation of anteriorly perforated duodenal ulcer: a case report. Case Study Case Rep. 2011; 1(2): 53 - 60.

[12] Saber A. Pneumatosis intestinalis with complete remission: a case report. Cases J. 2009; 29: 7079.

[13] Saber A. Uncommon presentation of perforated duodenal ulcer: A report of three different cases. The 26th Annual Summer Meeting of the Egyptian Society of Surgeons, Alexandria, Egypt. October, 2008.

[14] Saber A. Uncommon presentation of perforated duodenal ulcer: A report of three different cases. Surg Chronicles 2011; 16(1):42-45.

2

Management of Acute Gastric Ulcer Bleeding

Christo van Rensburg and Monique Marais
Stellenbosch University
South Africa

1. Introduction

Acute gastric ulcer bleeding frequently presents as a gastrointestinal emergency. It has important implications for healthcare costs worldwide. Negative consequences include rebleeding and death usually caused by the functional worsening of concomitant medical conditions, precipitated by the acute bleeding incident. Advances in medical practice in recent decades have influenced the aetiology and management of upper gastrointestinal bleeding (UGIB), but their impact on the incidence and mortality is unclear.

2. Epidemiology

At one time peptic ulcer disease accounted for 50–70% of acute non-variceal UGIB (Barkun et al., 2004). Approximately 80% of these ulcers stop bleeding spontaneously. Gastric ulcer is more frequently the source of UGIB (55% versus 37%); compared to duodenal ulcer (Enestvedt et al., 2008). The current practice to use proton pump inhibitors as ulcer prophylaxis and eradication of *Helicobacter pylori*, has led to a worldwide decrease in the incidence of bleeding from peptic ulcer. However, this seems applicable only to patients younger than 70 years of age (Lanas et al., 2005; Loperfido et al., 2009; Targownik et al., 2006). Recent population-based estimates have suggested that the incidence is about 60 per 100,000 of the population (Lassen et al., 2006), with the incidences related to the use of aspirin and non-steroidal anti-inflammatory drugs on the increase (Ohmann et al., 2005). The mortality associated with peptic ulcer bleeding remains high at 5 to 10% (Lim et al., 2006). The estimated direct medical costs annually incurred in the United States for the in-hospital care of patients with peptic ulcer bleeding amounts to a total of more than $2 billion (Viviane et al., 2008).

3. Pathophysiology

3.1 Risk factors

There are four major risk factors for bleeding peptic ulcers namely *Helicobacter pylori* infection, non-steroidal anti-inflammatory drugs (NSAIDs), stress and gastric acid (Hunt et al., 1995; Hallas et al., 1995). Reduction or elimination of these risk factors lessens ulcer recurrence and rebleeding rates (Graham et al., 1993; Tytgat 1995).

3.1.1 *Helicobacter pylori*

Compared to non-bleeding duodenal ulcers (70–90%), *Helicobacter pylori* plays a lesser role in the aetiology of bleeding and gastric ulcers (Maury et al., 2004). However, it is important to exclude *Helicobacter pylori* as a factor in the aetiology.

Helicobacter pylori eradication should be attempted in all peptic ulcer patients diagnosed with the infection to prevent ulcer recurrence and rebleeding (Hopkins et al., 1996). In Hopkin's report of 19 published studies, the recurrence rates in cured versus uncured *Helicobacter pylori* infection was 6% versus 67% for duodenal ulcer, and 4% versus 59% for gastric ulcer. Various regimens that usually combine one or two antibiotics plus an anti-secretory agent have eradication rates that vary between 80% and 90% (Walsh et al., 1995).

3.1.2 Non-steroidal anti-inflammatory drugs

NSAIDs, including aspirin, frequently cause gastrointestinal ulceration (Lanas et al., 2005; Scheiman 1994). NSAID-induced injury results from both local effects and systemic prostaglandin inhibition effected by blocking cyclooxygenase-1. The majority of these ulcers are asymptomatic and uncomplicated. However, elderly patients with a prior history of bleeding ulcer disease are at increased risk for recurrent ulcer and complications (Hansen et al., 1996; Smalley et al., 1995). NSAIDs are also implicated as critical in the non-healing of ulcers (Lanas et al., 1995). Aspirin in dosages as low as 75 mg daily transfer an increased risk of ulcers and bleeding (Lim et al., 2004).

Combining corticosteroids with NSAIDs doubles the risk of ulcer complications whilst the risk of gastrointestinal bleeding is increased ten fold (Piper et al., 1991). Cyclooxygenase-2 inhibitors reduce the risk of ulcer bleeding only when not combined with aspirin therapy. Of concern, is the increase in incidence of myocardial infarction and cerebrovascular accidents in patients taking selective cyclooxygenase-2 inhibitors. The combination of *Helicobacter pylori* infection and NSAID use may increase the risk of ulcer bleeding; however, the need for eradication of *Helicobacter pylori* in patients who are taking NSAIDs remains controversial. (al-Assi et al., 1996).

3.1.3 Stress-related ulcers

The incidence of stress-related ulcers in intensive care units (ICU) is approximately 0.67. This form of ulceration tends to occur in severely ill patients and is almost certainly triggered by ischaemia due to a combination of decreased mucosal protection and reduced mucosal blood flow (Cooper et al., 1999). It is a frequent cause of acute UGIB in patients who are hospitalized for life-threatening non-bleeding illnesses (Navab et al., 1995). The risk of stress ulcer-related bleeding is increased in patients with respiratory failure and those with a bleeding disorder (Cook et al., 1994). Also, the mortality is higher in patients that present with a UGIB after hospitalization compared to those primarily admitted with UGIB (Zimmerman et al. 1994).

Primary ulcer prophylaxis with anti-secretory agents such as H_2–receptor antagonists or proton pumps inhibitors (PPIs) decreases the risk of stress-related mucosal damage and UGIB in high-risk patients (Cook et al., 1996). Achlorhydria associated with prophylactic acid inhibition effects bacterial growth in the stomach and possible ventilator-associated pneumonia in ICU patients. Furthermore, stress-related ulcers tend to have high rebleeding rates and are not as amenable to endoscopic therapy as patients that present to the hospital with bleeding peptic ulcer (Jensen et al., 1988).

3.1.4 Gastric acid

Gastric acid and pepsin are essential cofactors in the pathogenesis of peptic ulcer (Peterson et al., 1995). Factors such as *Helicobacter pylori*, NSAIDs, or physiologic stress impair the mucosal integrity leading to increased cell membrane permeability and back diffusion of hydrogen ions, resulting in intramural acidosis, cell death, and ulceration. Hyperacidity as is prevalent in patients with Zollinger-Ellison syndrome, is rarely the sole cause of peptic ulceration. However, control of gastric acidity is considered an essential therapeutic manoeuvre in patients with active UGIB.

4. Acute management (Figure 1)

Patients with acute gastric ulcer bleeding frequently present with haematemesis (vomiting of red blood that is suggestive of active bleeding or vomiting of coffee-ground material indicative of older non-active bleeding) and/or melaena (black tarry stools which suggests passage of old blood, usually from an upper gastrointestinal source). Haematochezia (the passage of red blood per rectum) can occasionally be due to massive UGIB as suggested by a hypotensive or shocked patient. Patients who presents with haematemesis and melaena generally have more severe bleeding than those who present with melaena only. Immediate evaluation and appropriate resuscitation are critical as these can reduce mortality in acute UGIB (Baradarian et al., 2004).

4.1 Resuscitation and stabilization

As first priority, the haemodynamic stability (pulse and blood pressure, including orthostatic changes) and the need for fluid replacement must initially be assessed at presentation of a patient with UGIB. A full blood count, urea, electrolytes, creatinine, international normalized ratio (INR), blood type and cross-match should be obtained. If indicated, volume resuscitation should be initiated with crystalloids and blood products in all patients with haemodynamic instability or active bleeding (manifested by haematemesis, bright red blood per nasogastric tube, or haematochezia). Patients with a resting tachycardia ≥ 100 beats per minute, a systolic blood pressure < 100 mmHg, orthostatic hypotension (an increase in the pulse rate ≥ 20 beats per minute or drop in blood pressure of ≥ 20 mmHg on standing), a decrease in haematocrit of ≤ 6%, or transfusion requirement over two units of packed red blood cells) should be admitted to an intensive care unit for resuscitation. The haemoglobin in high-risk patients should be maintained above 10 g/dL, whereas a haemoglobin ≥ 7 g/dL is acceptable in young and otherwise healthy individuals. Patients with active bleeding and a bleeding disorder should be transfused with plasma and platelets if the INR ≥1.5 and the platelets ≤ 50 000/μL respectively.

The vital signs (blood pressure, ECG monitoring, and pulse oximetry), clotting profile and urinary output should be closely monitored. If indicated, elective endotracheal intubation in patients with respiratory failure and decreased consciousness may facilitate endoscopy and decrease the risk of aspiration. Patients older than 60 years, with chest pain or a history of heart disease should also be evaluated for myocardial infarction with electrocardiograms and serial troponin measurements. Nasogastric (NG) tube placement to aspirate and characterize gastric contents can be useful to determine if large amounts of red blood, coffee - grounds, or non-bloody fluid are present. Patients with definite haematemesis do not need an NG tube for diagnostic purposes, but may need one to clear gastric contents before endoscopy and to minimize the risk of aspiration. Approximately 15% of patients without bloody or coffee-ground material in nasogastric aspirates are found to have high-risk lesions on endoscopy (Aljebreen et al., 2004).

Clinical and laboratory findings are useful to risk-stratify patients (Table 1). The Blatchford score or the clinical Rockall score have been validated as clinical tools in the risk assessment (Blatchford et al., 2000; Rockhall et al., 1996). Poor prognostic factors for bleeding peptic ulcers include the following: age >60 years, comorbid medical illness, orthostatic hypotension, bleeding disorder, bleeding onset in the hospital, multiple blood transfusions and red blood in the NG tube.

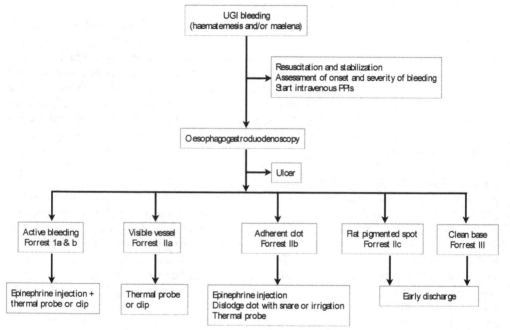

Fig. 1. Approach to upper gastrointestinal (UGI) bleeding. PPIs, proton pump inhibitors.

4.2 Diagnostic endoscopy

Its high sensitivity and specificity in identifying and localizing bleeding lesions, makes upper endoscopy the diagnostic modality of choice for acute UGIB. Early endoscopy within 24 hours of presentation, aids risk stratification of patients and reduces the need for hospitalization. However, it may also expose additional cases of active bleeding and hence increases the use of therapeutic endoscopy. No evidence exists that very early endoscopy (within a few hours of presentation) can reduce risk of rebleeding or improve survival (Tsoi et al., 2009).

A large channel therapeutic upper endoscope should be used to allow for rapid removal of blood from the stomach and to utilize larger endoscopic hemostasis accessories. Well-trained assistants who are familiar with endoscopic hemostasis devices are critical to successful endoscopic hemostasis. At times it may be worth delaying a procedure in order to utilize assistants who are competent at using accessories in emergency situations. Forrest described an endoscopic classification system that is commonly used (Figure 2). At index endoscopy the prevalence of ulcers with stigmata of recent haemorrhage, defined as Forrest I, IIa and IIb generally accounts for one third and Forrest IIc or III for the remainder (Lau et al., 1998) (Figure 2). An adherent clot is defined as a lesion that is red, maroon, or black and amorphous in texture which cannot be dislodged by suction or forceful water irrigation) (grade IIb). Low-risk lesions include flat, pigmented spots (grade IIc) and clean-base ulcers (grade III) (Figure 3). The inter-observer variation in diagnosing these endoscopic stigmata is low to moderate. At index endoscopy, high-risk lesions with rebleeding rates from 22% to 55% are seen in one–third to one–half of all patients.

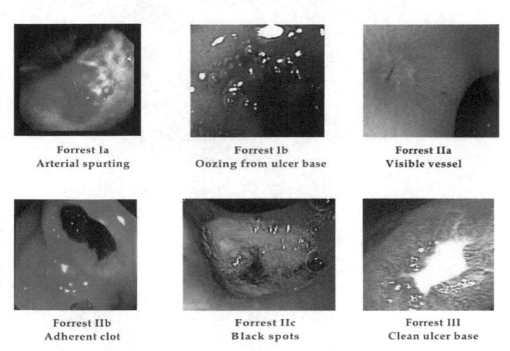

Forrest Ia	Forrest Ib	Forrest IIa
Arterial spurting	Oozing from ulcer base	Visible vessel

Forrest IIb	Forrest IIc	Forrest III
Adherent clot	Black spots	Clean ulcer base

Fig. 2. Endoscopic grading according to Forrest classification

4.2.1 Preparation for emergency esophagogastroduodenoscopy

A large-bore orogastric or NG tube with gastric lavage (use tap water at room temperature) is useful to improve visualization of the gastric fundus on endoscopy; however, this practice has not predictably improved the outcome (Lee et al., 2004). Intravenous erythromycin, as a motilin receptor agonist, promotes gastric motility and substantially improves visualization of the gastric mucosa at index endoscopy. However, erythromycin does not substantially improve the diagnostic yield of endoscopy or the outcome of acute peptic ulcer bleeding. A single 250–mg dose of erythromycin 30–60 minutes before endoscopy should be considered (Carbonell et al., 2006).

Empiric intravenous PPI treatment can be initiated prior to endoscopy in patients that presents with severe UGIB. Several studies and meta-analyses have shown that this practice significantly reduces the proportion of patients with stigmata of recent bleeding at index endoscopy and therefore the need for endoscopic therapy. However, there is no evidence that PPI treatment affects clinically important consequences, namely mortality, rebleeding or need for surgery (Sreedharan et al., 2010).

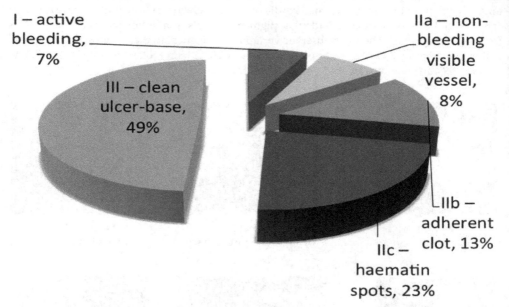

Fig. 2. Stigmata of bleeding prevalence according to the Forrest classification

4.2.2 Stratification of the rebleeding risk

Rebleeding the vital risk factor for mortality increases the rate 5 times compared to patients in whom the bleeding has spontaneously stopped (Church et al., 1999; Forrest et al., 1974). Predictive models evolved to identify high-risk patients for rebleeding and those for early hospital discharge or outpatient care.

The Rockall scoring system is probably the most widely known risk-stratification tool for UGIB. This represents an accurate and validated predictor of rebleeding and death, achieving better results in the prediction of mortality (Rockall et al., 1996). The clinical Rockall score (i.e. the score before endoscopy) is calculated solely on the basis of clinical variables at the time of presentation. For the complete Rockall score the clinical and endoscopic stigmata to predict the risks of rebleeding and death are added; the scale ranges from 0 to 11 points, with higher scores indicating greater risk.

The clinical Rockall and Blatchford scores share mutual features that include the patient's hemodynamic status and comorbid illnesses. These might reduce the need for urgent endoscopic evaluation in patients deemed at low risk. In addition to clinical and laboratory features, endoscopic stigmata can be used to risk-stratify patients that present with acute gastric ulcer bleeding (Table 1).

The endoscopic stigmata of bleeding gastric ulcers provide excellent predictability of the likelihood of rebleeding based on the Forrest classification, which ranges from Ia to III. The risk for rebleeding varies from 55 – 22% in gastric ulcers if left endoscopically untreated

(Laine & Peterson, 1994; Lau et al., 1998). The highest risk is in those with active arterial bleeding (grade I), a non-bleeding visible vessel (grade IIa) and an adherent clot (grade IIb). Additional data are needed to confirm the possible improvement in risk stratification provided by the use of endoscopic Doppler ultrasonography applied directly to the ulcer stigmata.

A. Blatchford Score – At Presentation	Score	B. Rockall Initial Score /7 – Criteria (before gastroscopy)		Score
Systolic Blood Pressure				
• 100 – 109 mmHg	1	Age (years)	• < 60	0
• 90 – 99 mmHg	2		• 60 – 79	1
• <90 mmHg	3		• ≥ 80	2
Blood urea nitrogen		Shock	• "No shock" = (SBP ≥100 mmHg, Pulse <100 /min)	0
• 6.5 – 7.9 mmol/L	2		• "Tachycardia" = (SBP ≥100 mmHg, Pulse ≥100 /min)	1
• 8.0 – 9.9 mmol/L	3		• "Hypotension" = (SBP <100 mmHg)	2
• 10.0 – 24.9 mmol/L	4			
• ≥25 mmol/L	6	Co-morbidity	• No major co-morbidity	0
Haemoglobin for men			• Cardiac failure, IHD or any major co-morbidity	2
• 12.0 – 12.9 g/dL	1		• Renal or liver failure, disseminated malignancy	3
• 10.0 – 11.9 g/dL	3			
• <10.0 g/dL	6	Rockall Full Score /11 – Additional Criteria (after gastroscopy)		
Haemoglobin for women				
• 10.0 – 11.9 g/dL	1	Diagnosis	• Mallory–Weiss tear, no lesion seen, no SRH	0
• <10.0 g/dL	6		• All other diagnosis	1
Other presentation variables			• Malignancy of upper GI tract	2
• Pulse >100/minute	1			
• Maelena	1	Major stigmata	• None – clean ulcer base, flat pigmented spot	0
• Syncope	2	of recent	• Blood in upper GI tract, active bleeding, visible	2
• Hepatic disease	2	haemorrhage	vessel, clot	
• Cardiac failure	2			

Table 1. Risk–stratification tools for UGIB

4.3 Therapeutic endoscopy

Gastric ulcers with a high risk of rebleeding should be treated endoscopically at the initial endoscopy. Since the late 1980s, endoscopic haemostatic therapy has been widely accepted as the first-line therapy for UGIB. Many well–conducted, randomized controlled trials, meta-analyses, and consensus conferences have confirmed the efficacy of endoscopic therapy in this setting (Sacks HS et al. 1990; Cook DJ et al., 1992). These data supported a reduction in recurrent bleeding, the need for urgent surgery, and mortality in patients with high–risk stigmata (Barkun et al., 2003; Adler et al., 2004). However, most of these studies were conducted before the widespread use of PPIs, and predominantly used injection therapy, bipolar-probe coagulation therapy, or a combination of injection and coagulation therapy.

In general, for the highest-risk lesions of active bleeding or non-bleeding visible vessels, endoscopic haemostasis alone will decrease the rebleeding rate to approximately 20–25%. The adjunctive use of PPIs decreases this rate even further. Endoscopic therapy can be broadly categorized into injection therapy, thermal coagulation, and mechanical haemostasis. As no single method of endoscopic thermal coagulation therapy is necessarily superior. Therefore, a familiar haemostatic technique applicable to the identified ulcer stigmata should be used.

4.3.1 Injection therapy

Injection therapy is the most commonly used treatment worldwide, mainly because it is widely available, easy to perform, safe and inexpensive. A disposable needle is used to inject a solution (1:10,000) of diluted adrenaline in normal saline. This mainly has a tamponade-effect induced by the volume of solution injected (15–25 ml being a standard dose). Although solutions of agents other than adrenaline (such as polidocanol, saline and even dextrose) may have a similar effect, none proofed superior in achieving haemostasis. The injection of sclerosant (including absolute alcohol) should be avoided as extensive and uncontrolled tissue necrosis of the ulcer base can lead to perforation and related complications. Adrenaline injection as definite haemostatic therapy is not recommended for the risk of rebleeding, but it should be followed either by contact thermal therapy or a second injectable agent (e.g. fibrin glue) to avoid further bleeding, the need for surgery and mortality in bleeding peptic ulcer (Vergara et al., 2007). This practice reduces the risk of perforation and subsequent thermal burn damage that might complicate endoscopic therapy.

4.3.2 Thermal devices
Thermal devices are the mainstay of endoscopic haemostasis and can be divided into contact (heater probe, monopolar and bipolar electrocoagulation) and noncontact types (laser treatment, argon plasma coagulation [APC]). Although no single method of endoscopic thermal coagulation therapy is superior, electrocoagulation with bipolar contact probes is more commonly used. Haemostasis of the underlying vessel is achieved when heat is generated during contact of these probes with the bleeding lesion. Thermal contact probes can seal arteries up to 2 mm. The risks of thermal probes include perforation and inducing more bleeding. While the haemostatic effects of contact probes are well established by clinical trials, the use of APC in the treatment of peptic ulcer bleeding has only recently been reported. In a randomised, controlled study comparing APC with heater probe coagulation, the former proofed equally safe and effective (Chau et al., 2003). No significant differences were detected in terms of initial haemostasis at index endoscopy, frequency of recurrent bleeding, requirement for emergency surgery, number of units of blood transfused, length of hospital stay, and mortality rate.

4.3.3 Mechanical devices
Mechanical devices in the form of haemoclips for endoscopic haemostasis in bleeding gastric ulcer disease have gained popularity in recent years. In a landmark study by Cipolleta and colleagues, they compared haemoclips with heater probe thermocoagulation (Cipolletta et al., 2001). The successful application of haemoclips led to a significantly decline in recurrent bleeding (1.8% versus 21%). Deployment of haemoclips on fibrotic ulcer floors may proof problematic, especially when used tangentially, or with the endoscope retroflexed. The difficulty of successful application in these situations may limit the efficacy of haemoclips. These technical problems might be overcome with improvements in future design.

4.4 Control of active bleeding or high-risk lesions
Despite many endoscopists favouring dual endoscopic therapy in patients with severe peptic ulcer bleeding, there is currently no definite recommendation in this regard. In actively bleeding ulcers, an injection can diminish or even stop bleeding; allowing a clear view of the bleeding vessel that in turn facilitates accurate thermal coagulation. Theoretically, the cessation of blood flow prevents dissipation of thermal energy, thereby minimizing tissue injury.

In a systematic review and meta-analysis dual endoscopic therapy proved significantly superior to injection therapy alone. However, it had no advantage over thermal or mechanical monotherapy to improve the outcome of patients with high-risk peptic ulcer bleeding (Marmo et al. 2007). When combining injected substances with thermal coagulation in bleeding peptic ulcer disease, there is a significant risk of complications such as perforation and gastric wall necrosis. Successful application of haemoclips is comparable to thermocoagulation (Sung et al. 2007).

4.5 Managing an ulcer with an adherent clot
In the event of an ulcer with an overlying clot, attempting to remove the clot by targeted washing is critical. Endoscopic removal of the clot by washing or cold snare has been demonstrated to be effective in reducing the recurrence of bleeding (Bini et al., 2003). The findings under the clot (e.g. bleeding vessel, visible vessel, flat spot, clean base) help determine the therapy needed and improve efficacy by allowing treatment to be applied directly to the vessel. A combination of injection with heater probe or bipolar coaptive coagulation is often used and has been shown to be more effective in patients with active bleeding. Vigorous washing of the clot formed after therapy is useful to determine the adequacy of coagulation.

4.6 Treatment of persistent or recurrent bleeding after initial haemostasis
Despite the effectiveness of endoscopic haemostasis, rebleeding occurs in 10–25% of cases, irrespective of the method of treatment. A second attempt at endoscopic control is warranted. Some experts have concerns about the perils of a second endoscopy, which may result in delayed surgery, perforation, and increased morbidity and mortality. Combining techniques is sensible when re-treating the ulcer site as the first attempt at endoscopic therapy might have produced necrosis and weakening of the intestinal wall. By using injection as the first step the thickness of the submucosal layer is increased, thus providing some margin of safety.

4.7 Second-look endoscopy
A planned, second-look endoscopy within 24 hours after initial endoscopic therapy is not recommended on the basis of existing evidence (Barkun et al. 2003; Adler et al. 2004). Even though it proofed to be efficacious in two meta-analyses that second–look endoscopy with heater probe coagulation reduces the risk of recurrent bleeding, it had no overall effect on mortality or the need for surgery (Marmo et al. 2003; Tsoi et al. 2009). Also, this approach may not be cost-effective when profound acid inhibition is achieved by high-dose intravenous PPIs (Spiegel et al. 2003). Second–look endoscopy may be considered in patients who are categorized as high risk for rebleeding (shock at presentation, fresh blood in the stomach, endoscopic stigmata of active bleeding, large ulcers and high lesser curvature gastric ulcers) if adjunctive high–dose intravenous PPI was not commenced. Similarly, if at the time of index endoscopy clots obscured the endoscopic view or the efficacy of the primary endoscopic haemostasis is doubtful, second-look endoscopy may be indicated (Chiu & Sung, 2010).

4.8 *Helicobacter pylori* testing
As one of the main etiological risk factors, all patients with acute bleeding gastric ulcers should be tested for *Helicobacter pylori* infection. Confirmatory testing for *Helicobacter pylori*

in the setting of acute ulcer bleeding may be false negative. Biopsy-based methods, such as rapid urease test, histology, and culture, have a low sensitivity, but a high specificity, in patients with UGIB. The accuracy of ^{13}C-urea breath test remains very high under these circumstances. Stool antigen test is less accurate in UGIB. Although serology seems not to be influenced by UGIB, it cannot be recommended as the initial diagnostic test for *Helicobacter pylori* infection in this setting (Gisbert et al., 2006). Treatment of *Helicobacter pylori* infection is more effective than anti–secretory non-eradicating therapy (with or without long-term maintenance anti-secretory therapy) in preventing recurrent bleeding from peptic ulcer (Gisbert et al., 2004). Therefore, if this infection is not initially detected, it is important to repeat the evaluation subsequently to confirm the initial result. The economic impact of this strategy, especially in young ulcer patients, must be emphasized.

5. Pharmacotherapy

Proton pump inhibitors initiated after endoscopic haemostasis of bleeding peptic ulcer significantly reduced rebleeding compared with placebo or H_2–receptor antagonists (Sung et al., 2009; van Rensburg et al., 2009). The initiation of PPIs before endoscopy significantly decreases the proportion of patients with stigmata of a recent bleed (e.g. visible vessel) and a need for endoscopic haemostasis, but does not reduce mortality, rebleeding, or surgery risks compared with H_2–receptor antagonists or placebo (Dorward et al 2006; Lau et al., 2007). The effects of PPIs are more pronounced in Asian compared with non–Asian populations. There is no role for H_2–receptor antagonist, somatostatin, or octreotide in the treatment of acute bleeding gastric ulcer.

The rationale for using acid inhibition in peptic ulcer disease is based on the observation that the stability of a blood clot is reduced in an acidic environment. Acid impairs platelet aggregation and causes disaggregation. Clot lysis is accelerated predominately by acid-stimulated pepsin. Furthermore, it may impair the integrity of the mucus-bicarbonate-barrier. Thus a pH greater than 6 is necessary for platelet aggregation while clot lysis occurs when the pH drops below 6.

5.1 Role of H_2–receptor antagonists and somatostatin (octreotide)

There are no convincing data to support the use of H_2–receptor antagonists as these drugs do not reliably or consistently increase gastric pH to 6 irrespective of the route of administration (Julapalli & Graham, 2005). These drugs had minimal efficay in clinical trials and the development of tolerance is a problem.

Somatostatin and its analogue, octreotide, inhibit both acid and pepsin secretion and reduce gastroduodenal mucosal blood flow. However, these drugs are not routinely recommended in patients with peptic ulcer bleeding, since contemporary randomized, controlled trials have shown little or no benefit attributable to them, either alone or in combination with an H_2–receptor antagonist. Furthermore, there are no strong data to support the adjunctive use of these drugs after endoscopic therapy for ulcer bleeding. (Arabi et al., 2006).

5.2 Role of proton pump inhibitors

Proton pump inhibitors can increase the intra-gastric pH > 6.0 for 84 – 99% of the day (Lin et al., 1998). Tolerance has not been reported and continuous infusion is superior to intermittent bolus administration (Brunner et al., 1996). Pantoprazole given as an initial 80-

mg bolus injection, followed by 8 mg/h continuous infusion, seems to be the adequate treatment in patients with a high risk of rebleeding. Compared to an initial 80 mg–bolus injection, followed by 6-mg/h continuous insion, it demonstrated a lower inter-individual variability of intra-gastric pH and the pH was ≥ 6 for a greater percentage of time (van Rensburg et al. 2003). About five percent of patients with peptic ulcer bleeding responded poorly to intravenous omeprazole with rebleeding rates higher in patients with a mean intra-gastric pH of less than 6 (Hsieh et al., 2004).

PPIs in bleeding peptic ulcer have shown to reduce the rebleeding rate and the need for surgery, but not mortality whether the patients had an attempt at endoscopic haemostasis or not. PPI therapy for ulcer bleeding proofed more efficacious in Asia than elsewhere. This may be due to an enhanced pharmacodynamic effect of PPIs in Asian patients (Leontiadis et al., 2005). The use of high-dose PPIs (80-mg bolus, followed by 8-mg/h as continuous infusion for 72 hours) has been widely studied and used. However, the most effective schedule of proton pump PPI administration following endoscopic haemostasis of bleeding ulcers remains uncertain. It has been shown in a systemic review and meta-analysis that compared with low-dose PPIs, high-dose PPIs do not further reduce the 30–day rates of rebleeding, surgical intervention, or mortality after endoscopic treatment in patients with bleeding peptic ulcer (Wang et al., 2010).

5.2.1 Proton pump inhibitors – clinical effectiveness and cost-effectiveness

Potent acid-suppressing PPIs do not induce tachyphylaxis and have had favorable clinical results. Recent meta-analyses showed that the use of proton-pump inhibitors significantly decreased the risk of ulcer rebleeding (odds ratio, 0.40; 95% confidence interval [CI], 0.24 to 0.67), the need for urgent surgery (odds ratio, 0.50; 95% CI, 0.33 to 0.76), and the risk of death (odds ratio, 0.53; 95% CI, 0.31 to 0.91), (Bardou et al., 2005; Leontiadis et al., 2006) findings that have also been confirmed in a "real-world" setting (Barkun et al., 2004). In ulcer bleeding, PPIs reduce rebleeding and the need for surgery and repeated endoscopic treatment. PPIs improve mortality among patients at highest risk i.e. patients with active bleeding or a non-bleeding visible vessel (Leontiadis et al., 2007) compared with placebo or H_2–receptor antagonists. PPI treatment initiated prior to endoscopy in UGIB significantly reduces the proportion of patients with stigmata of recent bleeding at index endoscopy but does not reduce mortality, re-bleeding or the need for surgery. The strategy of giving oral PPI before and after endoscopy, with endoscopic haemostatic treatment for those with major stigmata of recent haemorrhage, is likely to be the most cost-effective.

Treatment of *Helicobacter pylori* infection was found to be more effective than anti-secretory therapy in preventing recurrent bleeding from peptic ulcer. *Helicobacter pylori* eradication alone or eradication followed by misoprostol (with switch to PPI, if misoprostol is not tolerated) are the two most cost-effective strategies for preventing bleeding ulcers among *Helicobacter pylori*-infected NSAID users, although the data cannot exclude PPIs also being cost-effective. Further large randomised controlled trials are needed to address areas such as PPI administration prior to endoscopic diagnosis, different doses and administration of PPIs, as well as the primary and secondary prevention of UGIB (Leontiadis et al., 2007).

6. Interventional radiology

Angiography with transcatheter embolization provides a non-operative method to identify and control bleeding when the endoscopic approach fails. Although the technical success rate can be as high as 90–100%, the clinical success rate varies from 50–83% (Cheung et al., 2009). Embolization might not stop the bleeding permanently.

7. Surgery

The role of surgery in acute peptic ulcer bleeding has markedly changed over the past two decades. The widespread use of endoscopic treatment has reduced the number of patients requiring surgery. Therefore, the need for routine early surgical consultation in all patients presenting with acute UGIB is now obviated (Gralnek et al., 2008).

Emergency surgery should not be delayed, even if the patient is in haemodynamic shock, as this may lead to mortality (Schoenberg, 2001). Failure to stop bleeding with endoscopic haemostasis and/or interventional radiology is the most important and definite indication. The surgical procedures under these circumstances should be limited to achieve haemostasis. The widespread use of PPIs obviated further surgical procedures to reduce acid secretion. Rebleeding tends to necessitate emergency surgery in approximately 60% of cases with an increase in morbidity and mortality (Schoenberg et al.; 2001). The reported mortality rates after emergency surgery range from 2 – 36%.

Whether to consider endoscopic retreatment or surgery for bleeding after initial endoscopic control is controversial (Cheung et al., 2009). A second attempt at endoscopic haemostasis is often effective (Cheung et al., 2009), with fewer complications avoiding some surgery without increasing mortality (Lau et al., 1999). Therefore, most patients with evidence of rebleeding can be offered a second attempt at endoscopic haemostasis. This is often effective, may result in fewer complications than surgery, and is the current recommended management approach.

Available data suggest that early elective surgery for selected high-risk patients with bleeding peptic ulcer might decrease the overall mortality rate. It is a reasonable approach in ulcers measuring ≥2 cm or patients with hypotension at rebleeding that independently predicts endoscopic retreatment failure (Lau et al., 1999). Early elective surgery in patients presenting with arterial bleeding or a visible vessel of ≥2 mm is superior to endoscopic retreatment and has a relatively low overall mortality rate of 5% (Imhof et al., 1998 & 2003). Additional indications for early elective surgery include age >65 years, previous admission for ulcer plication, blood transfusion of more than 6 units in the first 24 hours and rebleeding within 48 hours (Bender et al., 1994; Mueller et al., 1994). This approach is associated with a low 30–day mortality rate as low as 7%.

8. Conclusion and recommendations

Peptic ulcer bleeding, the most common cause for UGIB, is best managed using a multidisciplinary approach. The initial clinical evaluation involves an assessment of haemodynamic stability and the necessity for fluid replacement. Combined with early endoscopic findings (within the first 24 hours), patients can effectively be risk–stratified for recurrent ulcer bleeding and managed accordingly. Those patients with active arterial bleeding or a visible vessel in the ulcer base should receive combined endoscopic therapy (that is, injection and thermal coagulation) as standard of care.

Despite a lack of concrete evidence of high-dose PPIs being more effective than non–high-dose PPIs, an 80–mg bolus followed by 8–mg/h as continuous infusion for 72 hours should be commenced as this is the only method of administration that reliably achieves the desired high intra-gastric target–pH. Optimal management of bleeding peptic ulcer with an adherent clot should probably include an attempt at endoscopic removal, where after the same treatment to reduce the risk of recurrent bleeding should be affected. In the event of rebleeding after initial successful endoscopic haemostasis repeat–endoscopic therapy should be performed rather than surgery with generally a similar outcome with fewer complications.

For refractory bleeding, transcatheter angiography is equally effective as surgery and should be considered particularly in patients at high surgical risk. Second–look endoscopy should not routinely be performed considering the limited reduction in rebleeding rate and the questionable cost-effectiveness as profound acid inhibition is achieved with current medical treatment. Critical issues are detecting and eradicating *Helicobacter pylori* infection and the resuming NSAIDs or anti-platelet agents when clinically indicated with co-administration of gastro protective agents.

9. References

al-Assi, M.; Genta, R. & Karttunen, T. (1996) Ulcer site and complications: relation to Helicobacter pylori infection and NSAID use. Endoscopy. Vol.28, No.2, (February 1996), pp. 229-33.

Adamopoulos, A.; Efstathiou, S. & Tsioulos, D. (2003). Acute upper gastrointestinal bleeding: comparison between recent users and nonusers of nonsteroidal anti-inflammatory drugs. Endoscopy, Vol.35, No.4, (April 2003), pp. 327-32.

Adler, D; Leighton, J. & Davila, R. (2004) ASGE guideline: The role of endoscopy in acute non-variceal upper-GI hemorrhage. Gastrointest Endosc. Vol.60, No.4 (December 2004), pp. 497-504.

Aljebreen, A.; Fallone, C. & Barkun, A. (2004). Nasogastric aspirate predicts high-risk endoscopic lesions in patients with acute upper-GI bleeding. Gastrointest Endosc. Vol.59, No.2, (February 2004), pp. 172-8.

Arabi, Y.; Al Knawy, B. & Barkun, A. (2006). Pro/con debate: octreotide has an important role in the treatment of gastrointestinal bleeding of unknown origin? Crit Care. Vol.10, No.4, (2006), pp. 218, Review.

Baradarian, R.; Ramdhaney, S. & Chapalamadugu, R. (2004) Early intensive resuscitation of patients with upper gastrointestinal bleeding decreases mortality. Am J Gastroenterol., Vol.99, No.4, (2004 Apr), pp. 619-22.

Bardou, M.; Toubouti, Y. & Benhaberou-Brun, D. Meta-analysis: proton-pump inhibition in high-risk patients with acute peptic ulcer bleeding. Aliment Pharmacol Ther. Vol.15, No.21, (March 2005), pp. 677-86.

Barkun, A.; Sabbah, S. & Enns, R. (2004). The Canadian Registry on Nonvariceal Upper Gastrointestinal Bleeding and Endoscopy (RUGBE): endoscopic hemostasis and proton pump inhibition are associated with improved outcomes in a real-life setting. Am J Gastroenterol, Vol.99, No.7, (July 2004), pp.1238–46.

Bender, J.; Bouwman, D. & Weaver, D. Bleeding gastroduodenal ulcers: improved outcome from a unified surgical approach. Am. Surg., Vol.60, No.5, (May 1994), pp. 313–15.

Bini, E. & Cohen J. (2003). Endoscopic treatment compared with medical therapy for the prevention of recurrent ulcer hemorrhage in patients with adherent clots. Gastrointest Endosc. Vol.58, No.5, (November 2003), pp. 707-14.

Brunner, G. (2006). Proton-pump inhibitors are the treatment of choice in acid-related disease. Eur J Gastroenterol Hepatol. Vol.8, Suppl 1, (October 1996), pp. S9-13

Carbonell, N.; Pauwels, A. & Serfaty, L. Erythromycin infusion prior to endoscopy for acute upper gastrointestinal bleeding: a randomized, controlled, double-blind trial. Am J Gastroenterol., Vol.101, No.6, (June 2006), pp. 1211-5.

Chau, C.; Siu, W. & Law, B. (2003). Randomized controlled trial comparing epinephrine injection plus heat probe coagulation versus epinephrine injection plus argon plasma coagulation for bleeding peptic ulcers. Gastrointest Endosc, Vol.57, No.4, (April 2003), pp. 455-461.

Cheung, F. & Lau, J. (2009). Management of massive peptic ulcer bleeding. Gastroenterol. Clin. North Am., Vol.38, No.2, (June 2009), pp. 231–43.

Chiu, P. & Sung, J. (2010). High Risk Ulcer Bleeding: When Is Second-Look Endoscopy Recommended? Clin Gastroenterol Hepatol., Vol.8, No.8, (August 2010), pp. 651–654.

Church, N. & Palmer, K. (1999). Diagnostic and therapeutic endoscopy. Curr Opin Gastroenterol., Vol.15, No.6., (November 1999), pp. 504-8.

Cipolletta, L.; Bianco, M. & Marmo, R. (2001). Endoclips versus heater probe in preventing early recurrent bleeding from peptic ulcer: a prospective and randomized trial. Gastrointest Endosc, Vol.53, No.2, (February 2001), pp. 147-151.

Cook, D.; Fuller, H. & Guyatt, G. (1994). Risk factors for gastrointestinal bleeding in critically ill patients. Canadian Critical Care Trials Group. N Engl J Med. Vol.330, No.6, (February 1994), pp. 377-81.

Cook, D.; Reeve, B. & Guyatt, G. (1996). Stress ulcer prophylaxis in critically ill patients. Resolving discordant meta-analyses. JAMA., Vol.275, No.4, (January 1996), pp. 308-14.

Cook, D.; Guyatt, G. & Salena, B. (1992). Endoscopic therapy for acute non-variceal upper gastrointestinal hemorrhage -- a meta-analysis. Gastroenterology (January 1992) Vol.102, No.1, pp. 139-148.

Cooper, G.; Chak, A. & Way, L. (1999). Early endoscopy in upper gastrointestinal hemorrhage: associations with recurrent bleeding, surgery, and length of hospital stay. Gastrointest Endosc., Vol.49, No.2, pp. 145-52.

Dorward, S.; Sreedharan, A. & Leontiadis, G. (2006). Proton pump inhibitor treatment initiated prior to endoscopic diagnosis in upper gastrointestinal bleeding. Cochrane Database Syst Rev., Vol.18, No.4, (October 2006), CD005415.

Enestvedt, B.; Gralnek, I. & Mattek, N. (2008). An evaluation of endoscopic indications and findings related to nonvariceal upper-GI hemorrhage in a large multicenter consortium. Gastrointest Endosc , Vol.67, No.3, (March 2008), pp. 422-9.

Forrest, J.; Finlayson, N. & Shearman, D. (1974). Endoscopy in gastrointestinal bleeding. Lancet , Vol.2, No.7877 (August 1974), pp. 394-7.

Gisbert, J. & Abraira, V. (2006). Accuracy of Helicobacter pylori diagnostic tests in patients with bleeding peptic ulcer: a systematic review and meta-analysis. Am J Gastroenterol., Vol.101, No.4, (April 2006), pp. 848-63. Epub 2006 Feb 22. Review.

Gisbert, J.; Khorrami, S. & Carballo, F. (2004). H.pylori eradication therapy vs. antisecretory non-eradication therapy (with orwithout long-term maintenance antisecretory therapy) for the prevention ofrecurrent bleeding from peptic ulcer. Cochrane Database Syst Rev., No.2, CD004062.

Graham, D.; Hepps, K. & Ramirez, F. (1993). Treatment of Helicobacter pylori reduces the rate of rebleeding in peptic ulcer disease. Scand J Gastroenterol., Vol.28, No.11, (November 1993), pp. 939-42.

Gralnek, I, Barkun, A. & Bardou, M. (2008). Management of acute bleeding from a peptic ulcer. N. Engl. J. Med., Vol.359, No.9, (August 2008), pp. 928-37.

Hallas, J.; Lauritsen, J. & Villadsen, H. (1995). Nonsteroidal anti-inflammatory drugs and upper gastrointestinal bleeding, identifying high-risk groups by excess risk estimates. Scand J Gastroenterol., Vol.30, No.5, (May 1995), pp. 438-44.

Hsieh, Y.; Lin, H. & Tseng, G. (2004). Poor responders to intravenous omeprazole in patients with peptic ulcer bleeding. Hepatogastroenterology, Vol.51, No.55, (January 2004), pp. 316-9.

Hepps, K.; Ramirez, F. & Lew, G. (1993). Treatment of Helicobacter pylori reduces the rate of rebleeding in peptic ulcer disease. Scand J Gastroenterol., Vol.28, No.11, (November 1993), pp. 939-42.

Hopkins, R.; Girardi, L. & Turney, E. (1996). Relationship between Helicobacter pylori eradication and reduced duodenal and gastric ulcer recurrence: a review. Gastroenterology, Vol.110, No.4, (April 1996), pp. 1244-52.

Hunt, R.; Malfertheiner, P. & Yeomans, N. (1995). Critical issues in the pathophysiology and management of peptic ulcer disease. Eur J Gastroenterol Hepatol., Vol.7, No.7, (July 1995), pp. 685-99. Review.

Imhof, M.; Ohmann, C. & Röher, H. (2003). DUESUC study group. Endoscopic versus operative treatment in high-risk ulcer bleeding patients – results of a randomised study. Langenbecks Arch. Surg. Vol.387, No.9-10, (January 2003), pp. 327–36.

Imhof, M.; Schröders, C. & Ohmann, C. (1998). Impact of early operation on the mortality from bleeding peptic ulcer - ten years' experience. Dig. Surg., Vol.15, No.4, (1998), pp. 308–14.

Jensen, D. (1998). Economic assessment of peptic ulcer disease treatments. Scand J Gastroenterol Suppl., Vol.30, No.8, (October 1998), pp. 214-24.

Julapalli, V. & Graham, D. (2005). Appropriate use of intravenous proton pump inhibitors in the management of bleeding peptic ulcer. Dig Dis Sci., Vol.50, No.7, (July 2005), pp. 1185-93.

Lanas, A.; Perez-Aisa, M. & Feu, F. (2005)A nationwide study of mortality associated with hospital admission due to severe gastrointestinal events and those associated with nonsteroidal antiinflammatory drug use. Am J Gastroenterol, Vol.100, No.8, (August 2005), pp. 1685–93.

Lanas, A. ; Nerín, J. & Esteva, F. (1995). Non-steroidal anti-inflammatory drugs and prostaglandin effects on pepsinogen secretion by dispersed human peptic cells. Gut, Vol.36, No.5, (May 1995), pp. 657-63.

Lassen, A.; Hallas, J. & Schaffalitzky deMuckadell OB. (2006). Complicated and uncomplicated peptic ulcers in a Danish county 1993-2002: a population-based cohort study. Am J Gastroenterol , Vol.101, No.5. (May 2006), pp. 945-53.

Laine, L. & Peterson, W. (1994). Bleeding peptic ulcer. N Engl J Med, Vol.331, No.11, (September 1994), pp. 717–27. Review.

Lau, J.; Sung, J. & Lee, K. (2000). Effect of intravenous omeprazole on recurrent bleeding after endoscopic treatment of bleeding peptic ulcers . N Engl J Med, Vol.343, No.5, (August 2000), pp. 310 – 16.

Lau, J.; Leung, W. & Wu, J. (2007). Omeprazole before endoscopy in patients with gastrointestinal bleeding. N Engl J Med., Vol.356, No.16, (April 2007), pp. 1631-40.

Lee, S. & Kearney, D. (2004). A randomized controlled trial of gastric lavage prior to endoscopy for acute upper gastrointestinal bleeding. J Clin Gastroenterol, Vol.38, No.10, (November 2004), pp. 861-5.

Leontiadis, G.; Sharma, V. & Howden, W. (2006). Proton pump inhibitor treatment for acute peptic ulcer bleeding. Cochrane Database Syst Rev., No.1 (January 2006), CD002094.

Leontiadis, G.; Sharma, V. & Howden, W. (2005). Systematic review and meta-analysis: proton-pump inhibitor treatment for ulcer bleeding reduces transfusion requirements and hospital stay--results from the Cochrane Collaboration. Aliment Pharmacol Ther., Vol.22, No.3, (August 2005), pp. 169-74.

Leontiadis, G.; Sharma, V. & Howden, W. (2005). Systematic review and meta-analysis: enhanced efficacy of proton-pump inhibitor therapy for peptic ulcer bleeding in Asia--a post hoc analysis from the Cochrane Collaboration. Aliment Pharmacol Ther., Vol.21, No.9, (May 2005), pp.1055-61.

Leontiadis, G.; Sreedharan, A & Dorward, S. (2007). Systematic reviews of the clinical effectiveness and cost-effectiveness of proton. Health Technol Assess, Vol.11, No.51, (December 2007), pp. iii-iv, 1-164.

Lim, C. & Chalmers, D. (2004). Upper gastrointestinal haemorrhage. Postgrad Med J., Vol.80, No.946, (August 2004), pp. 492, 494.

Lim, C. & Heatley, R. (2005). Prospective study of acute gastrointestinal bleeding attributable to anti-inflammatory drug ingestion in the Yorkshire region of the United Kingdom. Postgrad Med J, Vol.81, No.954, (April 2005), pp. 252-4; 4.

Laporte, J.; Ibáñez, L & Vidal, X. (2004). Upper gastrointestinal bleeding associated with the use of NSAIDs: newer versus older agents. Drug Saf, Vol.27, No.6, (2004), pp. 411-20.

Lim, C.; Vani, D. & Shah, S. (2006). The outcome of suspected upper gastrointestinal bleeding with 24-hour access to upper gastrointestinal endoscopy: a prospective cohort study. Endoscopy, Vol.38, No.6, (June 2006), pp. 581-5.

Lin, H.; Lo, W. & Lee, F. (1998). A prospective randomized comparative trial showing that omeprazole prevents rebleeding in patients with bleeding peptic ulcer after successful endoscopic therapy. Arch Intern Med., Vol.158, No.1, (January 1998), pp. 54-8.

Lin, H.; Lo, W. & Perng, C. (2004). YH. Helicobacter pylori stool antigen test in patients with bleeding peptic ulcers. Helicobacter, Vol.9, No.6, (December 2004), pp. 663-8.

Loperfido, S.; Baldo, V. & Piovesana, E. (2009). Changing trends in acute upper-GI bleeding: a population-based study. Gastrointest Endosc., Vol.70, No.2, (August 2009), pp. 212-24.

Marmo, R.; Rotondano, G. & Piscopo, R. (2007). Dual therapy versus monotherapy in the endoscopic treatment of high-risk bleeding ulcers: a meta-analysis of controlled trials. Am J Gastroenterol., Vol.102, No.2, pp. 279-89.

Maury, E.; Tankovic, J. & Ebel, A. (2005). An observational study of upper gastrointestinal bleeding in intensive careunits: is Helicobacter pylori the culprit? Crit Care Med, Vol.33, No.7, (July 2005), pp. 1513-8.

Mueller, X.; Rothenbuehler, J. & Amery, A. (1994). Outcome of peptic ulcer hemorrhage treated according to a defined approach. World J. Surg., Vol.18, No.3, (May 1994), pp. 406-9.

Navab, F. & Steingrub, J. (1995). Stress ulcer: is routine prophylaxis necessary? Am J Gastroenterol, Vol.90, No.5, (May 1995), pp. 708-12. Review.

Ohmann, C.; Imhof, M. & Ruppert, C. (2005). Time-trends in the epidemiology of pepticulcer bleeding. Scand J Gastroenterol, Vol.40, No.8, (August 2005), pp. 914-20.

Peterson WL. (1995). The role of acid in upper gastrointestinal haemorrhage due to ulcer and stress-related mucosal damage. Aliment Pharmacol Ther., Vol.9, Suppl.1, (1995), pp. 43-6.

Piper, J.; Ray, W. & Daugherty, J. (1991). Corticosteroid use and peptic ulcer disease: role of nonsteroidal anti-inflammatory drugs. Ann Intern Med, Vol.114, No.9, (May 1), pp. 735-40.

Rockall, T.; Logan, R. & Devlin, H. (1996). Northfield TC. Selection of patients for early discharge or outpatient care after acute upper gastrointestinal haemorrhage. National Audit of Acute Upper Gastrointestinal Haemorrhage. Lancet, Vol.347, No.9009, (April 27), pp. 1138-40.

Sacks, H.; Chalmers, T. & Blum, A. (1990). Endoscopic hemostasis: an effective therapy for bleeding peptic ulcers. JAMA, Vol.264, No.4, (July 1990), pp. 494-9.

Schoenberg MH. Surgical therapy for peptic ulcer and nonvariceal bleeding. Langenbecks Arch. Surg. 2001; 386 (2): 98-103

Scheiman, J. (1994). NSAID-induced peptic ulcer disease: a critical review of pathogenesis and management. Dig Dis., Vol.12, No.4, (July 1994), pp. 210-22. Review.

Shorr, R.; Ray, W. & Daugherty, J. (1993). Concurrent use of nonsteroidal anti-inflammatory drugs and oral anticoagulants places elderly persons at high risk for hemorrhagic peptic ulcer disease. Arch Intern Med., Vol.153, No.14, (July 1993), pp. 1665-70.

Smalley, W.; Ray, W. & Daugherty, J. (1995). Nonsteroidal anti-inflammatory drugs and the incidence of hospitalizations for peptic ulcer disease in elderly persons. Am J Epidemiol., Vol.141, No.6, (March 1995), pp. 539-45.

Spiegel, B.; Ofman, J. & Woods, K. (2003). Minimizing recurrent peptic ulcer hemorrhage after endoscopic hemostasis: the cost-effectiveness of competing strategies. Am J Gastroenterol., Vol.98, No.1, (January 2003), pp. 86-97.

Sreedharan, A.; Martin, J. &, Leontiadis, G. (2010). Proton pump inhibitor treatment initiated prior to endoscopicdiagnosis in upper gastrointestinal bleeding. Cochrane Database Syst Rev., Vol.7, No.7, (July 2010), CD005415.

Sung, J.; Tsoi, K, & Lai, L. (2007). Endoscopic clipping versus injection and thermo-coagulation in the treatment of non-variceal upper gastrointestinal bleeding: a meta-analysis. Gut., Vol.56. No.10, (October 2007), 1364-73.

Sung, J.; Barkun, A. & Kuipers, E. (2009) Peptic Ulcer Bleed Study Group. Intravenous esomeprazole for prevention of recurrent peptic ulcer bleeding: a randomized trial. Ann Intern Med., Vol.150, No.7, (April 2007), pp. 455-64.

Targownik, L. & Nabalamba, A. (2006). Trends in management and outcomes of acute nonvariceal upper gastrointestinal bleeding:1993-2003. Clin Gastroenterol Hepatol, Vol.52, No.9, (December 2006), pp. 1459-66. [Erratum, Clin GastroenterolHepatol, Vol.5, No.6, (March 2007), pp. 403.

Tsoi, K.; Chan, H. & Chiu, P. (2010). Second look endoscopy with thermal coagulation or injections for peptic ulcer bleeding: a meta-analysis. J Gastroenterol Hepatol., Vol.25, No.1, (January 2010), pp. 8–13. Review.

Tytgat, G. (1995). Peptic ulcer and Helicobacter pylori: eradication and relapse. Scand J Gastroenterol. Suppl., Vol.210, (1995), pp. 70-2.

van Rensburg, C.; Barkun, A. & Bornman, P. (2009). Clinical trial: intravenous pantoprazole vs. ranitidine for the prevention of peptic ulcer rebleeding: a multicentre, multinational, randomized trial. Aliment Pharmacol Ther., Vol.29, No.5, (March 2009), pp. 497-507.

van Rensburg, C.; Hartmann, M. & Thorpe, A. (2003). Intragastric pH during continuous infusion with pantoprazole in patients with bleeding peptic ulcer. Am J Gastroenterol., Vol.98, No.12, (December 2003), pp. 2635-41.

Vergara, M.; Calvet, X. & Gisbert, J. (2007). Epinephrine injection versus epinephrine injection and a second endoscopic method in high risk bleeding ulcers. Cochrane Database Syst Rev., Vol.18, No.2, (April 2007), CD005584.

Viviane, A. & Alan, B. (2008). Estimates of costs of hospital stay for variceal and non-variceal upper gastrointestinal bleeding in the United States. Value Health, Vol.11, No.1, (January 2008), pp. 1–3.

Walsh, J. & Peterson, W. (1995). The treatment of Helicobacter pylori infection in the management of peptic ulcer disease. N Eng J Med, Vol.333, No.15, (October 1995), pp. 984–91. Review.

Wang, C.; Ma, M. & Chou, H. (210). High-dose vs non-high-dose proton pump inhibitors after endoscopic treatment in patients with bleeding peptic ulcer: a systematic review and meta-analysis of randomized controlled trials. Arch Intern Med., Vol.170, No.9, (May 2010), pp. 751–8.

Zimmerman, J.; Meroz, Y. & Siguencia, J. (1994). Upper gastrointestinal hemorrhage. Comparison of the causes and prognosis in primary and secondary bleeders. Scand J Gastroenterol., Vol.29, No.9, (September 1994), pp. 795–8.

3

Helicobacter pylori Infection in Elderly Patients

Nathalie Salles
Pôle de Gérontologie Clinique
Hôpital Xavier Arnozan
France

1. Introduction

Epidemiological studies report an increased rate of gastrointestinal diseases in subjects older than 65 years, and these diseases constitute one of the most frequent indications for medical consultation in this population (Pilotto, 2004). Oesophageal and gastroduodenal diseases, especially *Helicobacter pylori* (*H. pylori*) infection, are frequent in this population since they account for 40% of the total digestive pathologies in the elderly. Even if data in the literature report an increased prevalence of *H. pylori* infection in the elderly, clinical interest remains low. Only 56% of elderly patients hospitalized for peptic ulcers in the United States were tested for *H. pylori* infection, among whom only 73% were then treated (Ofman et al., 2000). However, studies report an increased rate of peptic ulcer disease (PUD) complications and mortality in older patients (1 per million in young adults aged 20 years to 200 per million after 70 years) (Younger&Duggan, 2002). This alarming finding has stimulated further studies on the pathophysiological and clinical aspects of *H. pylori* infection in the geriatric population. Indeed, recent data reported that *H. pylori* chronic infection plays a role in gastric aging, appetite regulation, and possibly extra-digestive diseases such as Alzheimer disease in the elderly.

2. Epidemiology in the elderly

The principal reservoir for *H. pylori* infection appears to be the human stomach, especially the antrum (Megraud, 2003). In developing countries, the oro-fecal route as well as the oro-oral route coexists because of poor socioeconomic and hygienic conditions (Nurgalieva et al., 2002). In developed countries, the oro-fecal transmission has gradually disappeared, leaving the oro-oral route, which is secondary to vomiting and gastro-oesophageal reflux (Megraud, 2003). Even if socioeconomic progress has led to a decrease in the incidence of the infection in developed countries, the prevalence of *H. pylori* infection still remains high in people born at the beginning of the 20eth century. In fact, Gause-Nilsson *et al.* (Gause-Nilsson et al., 1998) reported that when cohorts of 70 year old subjects born in 1901-1902 and 1922 were compared, the latter cohort showed a significantly lower *H. pylori* positive serology. This difference in *H. pylori* prevalence may reflect changes in socioeconomic conditions. Epidemiologic studies on elderly people, with a mean age of approximately 70 years, reported a prevalence of nearly 60 percent in asymptomatic subjects (Pilotto et al.,

1996; Regev et al., 1999) and more than 70 percent among the most elderly patients with gastrointestinal diseases (Pilotto, 2001; Pilotto&Salles, 2002). Other studies reported a high prevalence of *H. pylori* infection in the most elderly population, especially in institutionalized old people, with a prevalence ranging from 70 to 85 percent (Regev, Fraser, Braun, Maoz, Leibovici&Niv, 1999). These results can be explained by the mode of transmission of *H. pylori* (oro-fecal or oro-oral), taking into account the promiscuity and living conditions in an institution. Regev *et al.* showed that living in an institution increased the risk of *H. pylori* infection, the prevalence of the infection being positively correlated with the duration of stay (Regev et al., 1999). Nevertheless, even if prevalence increases with age, the prevalence curve appears to be flat and tends to decrease after 85 years (Pilotto&Salles, 2002; Salles-Montaudon et al., 2002). Thus, Neri *et al.* showed that *H. pylori* infection passed from 70 to 50 percent after 90 years (Neri et al., 1996). Two hypotheses can explain this trend. The first hypothesis is an underestimation of *H. pylori* infection, because of frequent chronic atrophic gastritis and frequent current or previous use of antisecretory and antibiotic treatments in this frail population. In a previous work, we showed a lower prevalence of *H. pylori* infection (47.7%) than expected in hospitalized elderly people, which can be explained on one hand by the higher polymedication with repetitive antibiotherapies and on the other hand by more frequent gastric atrophic lesions which offers a less favorable ground for *H. pylori* (Salles-Montaudon et al. 2002). The second hypothesis is a premature death of *H. pylori* infected subjects due to various comorbidities, e.g., gastric cancer, peptic ulcer diseases (PUD) and possibly other diseases such as cardiovascular diseases. Based on the data from the PAQUID Cohort study ("Personnes Agées Quid?" which was designed to enrol and follow-up elderly subjects randomly selected in the South-Western France4), we recently evaluated the impact of *H. pylori* infection on the mortality rate in a population of subjects older than 65 years. The follow-up of 605 subjects over 15 years, after adjustment for age, gender, and cardiovascular comorbidity, showed that an *H. pylori* infection was not a risk factor for mortality (HR=1.2, 95% CI [0.94; 1.52]) (Salles et al.).

3. *H. pylori* infection and peptic ulcer disease

The elderly are particularly susceptible to peptic ulcer disease (PUD) and complications due to their higher *H. pylori* prevalence and use of non-steroidal anti-inflammatory drugs (NSAIDs) (Bhala&Newton, 2005; Chow et al., 1998; Jones&Hawkey, 2001). Even if it is well known that the incidence of gastric ulcers increases in elderly people, little is known about gastric mucosal healing alterations during ageing. Newton et al. reported that gastric ageing induces gastric frailty, characterized by a reduction in protective factors, i.e., mucus layer, prostaglandin levels, mucosal growth, and gastric blood flow, and a higher susceptibility to aggressive factors, i.e., NSAID and H. pylori infection (Newton, 2004). Age-related changes could occur as a result of increased exposure to exogenous factors, alterations in the secretion of endogenous aggressive factors, or changes in the production or repair of the mucus bicarbonate layer, the primary barrier against acid and pepsin digestion. The increased risk of severe complications in this population (haemorrhage, gastric perforation) is likely to mask important early symptomatic signs which make PUD treatment difficult in the elderly (Kemppainen et al., 1997). Most of the studies suggested that ulcer pain is less common in this age group. Indeed, the diagnosis of PUD is usually delayed, because symptoms are not easily detected in this population. Typical pain is often absent; only one third of people older than 60 years experience painful symptoms (Seinela&Ahvenainen,

2000). In geriatric practice, anorexia and malnutrition frequently represent alarm symptoms and lead to gastroduodenal endoscopy. Endoscopic exploration, which is most of the time well tolerated in elderly patients, allows a diagnosis in more than 50 percent of the cases (Van Kouwen et al., 2003). Another contributing factor to PUD in the elderly is a high usage of NSAIDs and/or aspirin. Pilotto et al. showed that NSAID use independently increases the risk of peptic ulcer and ulcer bleeding. This risk increases with age in a linear manner, and increases further in the event of comorbidities and polymedication which are common in this population (Pilotto et al., 2003). *H. pylori* infection also independently increases the risk of PUD in the elderly. Clinical studies reported that approximately 50 to 70 percent of elderly peptic ulcer patients are *H. pylori* positive (Pilotto, 2001). The short- and long-term studies performed on elderly patients demonstrated that treatment of *H. pylori* infection in patients with peptic ulcer resulted in ulcer healing in over 95 percent of the patients and significantly improved clinical outcomes, including a decrease in recurrence (Pilotto&Salles, 2002). With regard to the respective responsibility of the two risk factors previously mentioned (AINS, *H. pylori*) in PUD, studies confirmed that both independently and significantly increase the risk of PUD and ulcer bleeding.

4. *H. pylori* infection and gastric aging

The ageing stomach is usually described in terms of the occurrence of gastric atrophic lesions. Thus, a wide range of studies reported an increased prevalence of atrophic gastritis in elderly patients, with rates ranging between 50 to 70% in patients over eighty (Sachs et al., 2003; Younger&Duggan, 2002). Only a few studies provided results on intrinsic gastric ageing and most were animal studies. In contrast, most of the literature reported the strong role played by chronic H. pylori infection in the occurrence of atrophic gastric lesions. The discovery of H. pylori chronic infection has cast a doubt on the reality of the physiological gastric ageing process which is now considered as a process of "pathological gastric ageing". Since the discovery of the strong role of this chronic gastric infection in the development of a gastric atrophy and PUD, we actually consider that most of the observed changes in the stomach that appear during ageing are, in fact, the result of environmental causes, such as chronic infection, nutritional, and pharmacological factors. These environmental factors may participate in inducing gastric frailty with impaired mucosal defence.

4.1 Chronic atrophic gastritis

A series of studies, mainly from Japan, has focused on the long-term effects of *H. pylori* infection and its role in the development of the histological changes that occur with ageing, i.e., atrophic gastritis (Salles, 2007). In a large multicenter trial, authors reported that both atrophic gastritis and intestinal metaplasia were strongly associated with *H. pylori* infection and not with ageing *per se* (Asaka et al., 2001). Interventional prospective studies reported that *H. pylori* eradication induces a significant reduction of inflammatory and atrophic gastric lesions (Ito et al., 2002; Kokkola et al., 2002). Kokkola et al. reported that advanced atrophic gastritis may improve and heal after *H. pylori* eradication in elderly subjects (Kokkola et al., 2002). They followed prospectively 22 elderly men (55–69 years of age) with *H. pylori* infection and atrophic corpus gastritis. During a 7.5-year period prior to eradication therapy, no significant changes were observed in the mean atrophy and IM scores. However, after *H. pylori* eradication, a significant improvement occurred in the mean histological Sydney system score of inflammation (from 2.2 to 0.5), atrophy (from 2.2 to 1.2) and IM (from 1.6 to 1.1). These findings are in agreement with the results of another study carried out in 132 subjects aged from 34 to 68 years (mean age 50 years) with multifocal (nonautoimmune) atrophic gastritis. Six years after cure of *H. pylori* infection, a significant improvement in antral atrophy was detected in subjects who received anti-*H. pylori* treatment, the effect being greater among those who were free of infection at the end of the trial (Ruiz et al., 2001). Since the response to treatment was similar in patients of different ages, we may assume that the cure of *H. pylori* infection is as recommended in elderly patients with gastric mucosal modifications as it is for young and adult patients. During gastric ageing, histological modifications are frequently observed leading to physiological gastric disturbances. Thus, a high prevalence of chronic atrophic gastritis is frequently observed in the gastric mucosa of elderly people (Ofman et al., 2000; Pilotto, 2004). These histological lesions lead to hypochlorhydria with a risk of bacterial overgrowth in the proximal digestive tract and intestinal malabsorption.

4.2 Gastric acid secretion

Between 1920 and 1980, many studies reported a significant reduction in gastric acid secretion with age. The majority of these studies was retrospective and did not take into account the presence of possible gastric atrophic lesions (Salles, 2007). More recent studies including elderly patients showed that there is no change in acid secretion with age, whereas others even showed an increase in acid secretion. Those studies that demonstrate hyposecretion in elderly patients offer chronic H. pylori infection and atrophic gastritis of the oxyntic mucosa as a reasonable explanation. Shih et al. found that gastric acid secretion does not change with age (Shih et al., 2003). Feldman et al. studied gastric acid secretion in elderly patients and found that basal acid output and peak acid output did not correlate with age (Feldman&Cryer, 1998). Similarly, Lijima et al., reported that gastric acid secretion was well preserved irrespective of ageing, however it seemed to increase with ageing in the H. pylori-negative subjects (Iijima et al., 2004). The decline in gastric acid secretion in H. pylori-positive patients depends on both an increasing prevalence of fundic atrophic gastritis and inflammatory cytokines, i.e., interleukin (IL) IL-1β and TNF-α, which are known to inhibit parietal cells. The mechanism promoting the increase in acid secretion with ageing is unknown. However, since the alteration of acid secretion by the inflammation of oxyntic mucosa can be ignored in the H. pylori-free stomach, two main possibilities could be considered: one is an increase in the total parietal cell mass with age, and the second is an increase in the reactivity of parietal cells. Because the previous studies failed to find any change in parietal cell mass with ageing, the second possibility is more likely.

4.2.1 Gastrointestinal bacterial overgrowth

Only a few clinical studies investigated the prevalence of gastrointestinal bacterial overgrowth in older healthy people, and most of the results showed that bacterial overgrowth occurs rarely during the normal process of gastric ageing, but is rather an iatrogenic process (antisecretory drugs) in the elderly. Mitsui *et al.* performed a study (Mitsui et al., 2006) and included healthy and disabled older people, aged over 70 years. They reported no bacterial overgrowth among healthy patients, but only in disabled or frail older people. Parlesak *et al.* also performed a study in older adults using a hydrogen breath test (Parlesak et al., 2003) and reported a 15.6% prevalence of small bowel bacterial overgrowth. They showed that PPI treatments played a role in increasing the prevalence of positive breath tests in older adults, which was associated with lower body weight, lower body mass index, lower plasma albumin concentration, and higher prevalence of diarrhea. The pH of gastric acid and bacterial counts in the stomach showed a close correlation. In normal subjects the gastric pH is usually below pH 4, a critical level for protection against enteric pathogens, and the stomach is virtually sterile. At a pH of 4–5 bacteria from the saliva are present in the stomach. A pH greater than 5 allows bacterial, viral and protozoan pathogens to survive and enteric bacteria can be found in the stomach. Other drugs which decrease acid production are anticholinergic drugs and tricyclic antidepressant drugs. In geriatrics, malnutrition is one of the clinical consequences of bacterial overgrowth, and antibiotic treatment may lead to the improvement of the anthropometric parameters of these patients (Lewis et al., 1999).

4.2.2 Vitamin B12 deficiency

Cobalamin or vitamin B12 deficiency is common in elderly patients (Dali-Youcef&Andres, 2009). The Framingham study demonstrated a prevalence of 12% among elderly people living in the community. Other studies focusing on elderly sick and malnourished people living in institutions have suggested a higher prevalence of 30–40%. The main causes of cobalamin deficiency include food-cobalamin malabsorption, pernicious anaemia, and insufficient nutritional vitamin B12. Dietary causes of deficiency are limited to elderly people who are already malnourished with lower albumin level, such as frail elderly patients with severe co morbidities (Salles-Montaudon et al., 2003). First described by Carmel in 1995, food-cobalamin malabsorption is frequent in elderly people, and is characterized by the inability of the body to release cobalamin from food or intestinal transport proteins, particularly in the presence of hypochlorhydria, where the absorption of 'unbound' cobalamin is normal (Carmel et al., 2003). Food-cobalamin malabsorption is caused primarily by chronic atrophic gastritis. In fact, Andres et al, reported in a recent meta-analysis, that cobalamin deficiency, other than those caused by nutritional deficiency, can be treated by oral administration of vitamin B12 in the form of cyanocobalamin (free cobalamin) (Andres et al., 2009). An evidence-based analysis by the *Vitamin B12 Cochrane Group* also supports the efficacy of oral cobalamin therapy. In this analysis, serum vitamin B12 levels increased significantly in patients receiving either oral vitamin B12 alone or patients receiving both oral and intramuscular treatment (Vidal-Alaball et al., 2005). Other factors that contribute to food-cobalamin malabsorption in elderly people include chronic carriage of *H. pylori* and intestinal microbial proliferation, situations in which cobalamin deficiency can be corrected by antibiotic treatment, long-term ingestion of antiacids such as H2-receptor antagonists and PPI, and biguanides (metformin) (Dali-Youcef&Andres, 2009). Sipponen et al, reported normalization of vitamin B12 levels after *H. pylori* eradication (Sipponen et al., 2003).

5. *H. pylori* infection and gastric cancer

Gastric carcinoma and gastric MALT lymphoma have been causally associated with *H. pylori*, and the bacterium has been categorized as a group I carcinogen by the International Agency for Research on Cancer (IARC). The incidence of gastric cancer increases with age worldwide. However, the association between *H. pylori* infection and gastric cancer might have been underestimated due to possible clearance of the infection in the course of disease development, especially among older patients who generally have more severe mucosal atrophy and intestinal metaplasia in the stomach. Recently, a new analytical investigation to minimize a potential underestimation of the association of *H. pylori* with gastric cancer was performed on Western populations [60]. Applying various more stringent exclusion criteria to minimize a potential bias from this source increased the odds ratio (95% confidence interval) of non-cardia gastric cancer from 3.7 to 18.3 for any *H. pylori* infection, and from 5.7 to 28.4 for cagA-positive *H. pylori* infection (Brenner et al., 2004). A possible mechanism to explain the link between *H. pylori* infection and gastric carcinoma is inflammation which increases the risk of mutations. Many of the mediators and byproducts of inflammation are mitogenic and mutagenic. Release of pro-inflammatory cytokines, reactive oxygen species and upregulation of Cox-2 all contribute to an intragastric environment conducive to neoplastic transformation. The mechanisms involve direct DNA damage, inhibition of apoptosis, subversion of immunity, and stimulation of angiogenesis. In addition, chronic inflammation in the gastrointestinal tract is also known to affect proliferation, adhesion and cellular transformation. There is also evidence of a direct carcinogenic effect of *H. pylori* per se on the gastric mucosa. As mentioned before, the type 4 secretion system encoded by the cag PAI allows the bacterium to inject molecules into the epithelial cells. The CagA protein is one of them. It acts on numerous cell effectors disturbing cell physiology leading to several proneoplastic processes, e.g. activation of growth factor receptors, increased proliferation, evasion of apoptosis, sustained angiogenesis and cell dissociation, and tissue invasion.

6. Impact of *H. pylori* infection on appetite regulation

The results showed that the expression of leptin and ghrelin peptides decreased both in the presence of an *H. pylori* infection and in the presence of atrophic gastritis lesions. The possible role of *H. pylori* infection in the regulation of appetite in the elderly is an interesting new research topic. Studies reported that *H. pylori* eradication appeared to improve certain nutritional parameters, i.e., body mass index (BMI), and albumin (Azuma et al., 2002; Fujiwara et al., 2002). Kamada et al. recently showed a significant increase in the BMI after *H. pylori* eradication among patients suffering from gastric ulcers, with a parallel increase in triglyceride and cholesterol levels (Kamada et al., 2005). In geriatric practice, anorexia and weight loss are often the only symptoms of PUD and are signs warranting endoscopic exploration. It is also crucial to investigate *H. pylori* infection in such cases. Studies performed on adults indicate that inflammatory cytokines may cause anorexia by inducing variations in circulating gastrointestinal hormones, neuropeptides, and NO, all of which can alter food intake (Chapman, 2004; Morley, 2001). Recently, we showed that chronic inflammation in the gastric mucosa affects the expression of gastric satiety inducible peptides such as leptin and ghrelin (Salles et al., 2006). Recent evidence suggests that, in humans and rats, leptin is secreted not only from adipose tissue but also from the gut (Bado et al., 1998). Studies indicate that gastric inflammation induced by *H. pylori* infection raises gastric leptin expression which then induces satiety and lower BMI (Azuma et al., 2001; Konturek et al., 2001). Ghrelin is a newly discovered peptide which is produced mainly in the stomach and is involved in the control of food intake and energy homeostasis in both humans and rodents (Kojima et al., 1999). In a recent study, authors reported that a cure of *H. pylori* infection increased plasma ghrelin, which in turn led to an increased appetite and weight gain (Nwokolo et al., 2003). Consequently, chronic gastric inflammation may induce variations in the expression of both leptin and ghrelin and may play a role in the pathophysiology of anorexia in elderly patients. In a study on frail elderly patients over 80 years old, we showed that the presence of *H. pylori* chronic gastritis induced a decrease in both leptin and ghrelin gastric production; this finding may, in fact, be due to the high prevalence of atrophic lesions observed in this particular population (Salles et al., 2006). Furthermore, the presence of *H. pylori* chronic gastritis was negatively correlated to the caloric ratio and the body mass index of these aged patients. The decrease in plasmatic and gastric levels of the strong orexigen, ghrelin, could explain the lack of appetite and the malnutrition of aged people who have chronic gastritis lesions due to *H. pylori*

7. *H. pylori* infection and Alzheimer's disease

The risk factors identified for dementia are often inaccessible to intervention (age, gender, genetic). New hypotheses have recently been suggested, such as the possible relationship between *H. pylori* infection and dementia via inflammatory mechanisms, both pro-oxidant and carential. Indeed, in addition to two case-control studies pointing out an association between *H. pylori* infection and Alzheimer disease (Kountouras et al., 2006; Malaguarnera et al., 2004), an interventional study has shown that *H. pylori* eradication positively influences Alzheimer disease manifestations, especially cognitive decline (Kountouras et al., 2009). Preliminary results of a cohort study conducted in our laboratory concluded that *H. pylori* infection was a significant risk factor for developing Alzheimer disease. One of the hypothesis is that *H. pylori* infection could act as a trigger in the genesis or in the accumulation of Alzheimer disease lesions via cerebral hypoperfusion due to atherosclerosis, or via an exacerbation of neuroinflammation.

8. Diagnosis of H. pylori infection in the elderly

Diagnosis of *H. pylori* infection remains difficult in elderly patients because of the characteristics of this population.

8.1 Non-invasive methods
The advantage of these methods is that they are global tests, i.e., *H. pylori* can be detected even if the patchy distribution of the bacteria, when gastric atrophy is present, precludes their histological detection.

8.1.1 Serology
Generally speaking, *H. pylori* immunoglobulin G (IgG) antibodies appear 2 to 3 weeks following infection, and slowly decrease after *H. pylori* eradication. In adulthood, the performance of serology (ELISA) shows 85 to 95 percent sensitivity and 80 to 95 percent specificity (Granberg et al., 1993). Even if most of the epidemiologic studies included serology to detect *H. pylori* infection in the elderly, data concerning the performance of this test remain contradictory for this population. Some authors consider that there is a risk of over-estimating infection in the elderly when using serology, because antibodies remain present for months or even years after *H. pylori* eradication (Kosunen et al., 1992). Indeed, in this population, the prevalence of *H. pylori* infection is significantly higher when detected by serology than by histology. Studies reported that in *H. pylori* positive patients with atrophic body gastritis, after eradication therapy, the time delay concerning the decrease in *H. pylori* IgG did not always correlate with the reduction in gastric inflammation (Kosunen et al.,

1992). This suggests that, in patients with atrophic body gastritis, serology alone may not be valid for assessing the efficacy of eradication treatment. Liston et al. showed that nearly one third of their study patients had positive serology without signs of active *H. pylori* infection (Liston et al., 1996). In addition, other authors reported that serology may not be useful in determining successful eradication post-therapy in the elderly, because of a great heterogeneity in the decrease in IgG antibody titer (6 months or more) (Kosunen et al., 1992). On the contrary, some authors consider that serology may underestimate the infection in the elderly. This could be explained by a possible lack of antibody response due to a frequent immunodeficiency diagnosed in frail elderly people. In fact, immunodeficiency may be the consequence of protein malnutrition which occurs in more than 30 percent of the elderly population (Burns, 2004; Salles-Montaudon et al., 2002). The infection could also be underestimated because of the characteristics of this elderly population, often hospitalized and treated with antibiotics for recurrent urinary tract or pulmonary infections which can induce false negative results.

Immunoblot (Western blot) is another serologic method useful in the elderly, for the detection of antibodies directed against particular antigenic proteins of *H. pylori* (CagA, VacA, urease A and B). Pilotto et al. showed that the presence of a CagA positive *H. pylori* infection was independently correlated with atrophic gastritis and intestinal metaplasia in the elderly (Monteiro et al., 2002; Pilotto et al., 1998).

8.1.2 13Carbon-Urea Breath Test

The [13]carbon-urea breath test (^{13}C-UBT) has an excellent diagnostic performance including the post-therapy determination of successful *H. pylori* eradication. The principal disadvantage of this method is the need for specific equipment which associates gas chromatography and mass spectrometry. In the elderly, this test has the advantage of being easily performed with a minimum of cooperation from the patient, and it is very well tolerated. Pilotto et al. demonstrated the excellent performance of this test on elderly patients, with a diagnostic accuracy of 97.9%. They found it useful even for patients with severe cognitive impairment (Pilotto et al., 2000). In a recent study performed on hospitalized patients older than 85 years, we reported that almost one-third of the *H. pylori*-positive patients would have remained undetected without this test, including treated patients (PPIs and antibiotics), or patients with chronic corpus atrophic gastritis [16]. Some studies reported the risk of an overestimation of *H. pylori* infection when using this test on the elderly. This could be explained by a hypochlorhydria due to gastric atrophy, which allows gastric colonization by urease-producing bacteria present in the mouth, oropharynx, and small intestine and decreases the specificity of the test (Chen et al., 2000). Certain situations can, to the contrary, involve an underestimation of *H. pylori* diagnosis in older subjects. Among these various cases, a past gastric resection may decrease the amount of urea present in the stomach, leading to an insufficient *H. pylori* detection.

8.1.3 Stool test

One of the formats of this test is a microwell-based immunoassay (HpSA), which detects *H. pylori* antigens present in human stools (Vaira et al., 1999). This test has a good diagnostic performance and can be easily carried out in routine. The test's lower sensitivity in the elderly can be explained by the higher frequency of chronic constipation in this group. Indeed, the passage of the bacteria into the colon may be prolonged, leading to a degradation of *H. pylori* antigens and jeopardizing their detection. This has been shown experimentally in stools spiked with *H. pylori*. Moreover, studies have shown that PPI treatment decreases the accuracy of HpSA by increasing the gastric pH and suppressing *H. pylori* colonization (Monteiro et al., 2001). The HpSA test also presents the disadvantage of being more difficult to carry out in this very old population, mainly for practical reasons, in dependent or demented older subjects (Salles-Montaudon et al., 2002).

8.2 Invasive methods
Most of the time, older patients have diagnostic indications for upper gastrointestinal endoscopy, i.e., chronic anemia, dysphagia, epigastralgia, etc. Biopsy sampling per endoscopy permits the detection of *H. pylori* infection by urease test, histological analysis, culture or PCR.

8.2.1 Biopsy urease test
There are several tests available based on the the urease activity of *H. pylori* present in biopsy specimens, among which are the CLO test® and the PyloriTek®. In the elderly, studies reported a lower sensitivity of these tests (57%) compared to histology or serology (Abdalla et al., 1998). As stated previously, the lower sensitivity can be explained by multiple treatments for various infections, and frequent gastric atrophic lesions which may induce a hostile environment for the bacterium.

8.2.2 Histology
In the elderly, the performance of this test increased when biopsy specimens were taken from two areas of the stomach, i.e., the antrum and the body. Indeed, chronic gastric atrophy may induce gastric hypochlorhydria which may in turn reduce *H. pylori* colonization in the antrum. In the elderly, a histological analysis should not be the only diagnostic method for *H. pylori* infection, because of its lower sensitivity as previously stated.
Nevertheless, this method presents the advantage of evaluating the morphological parameters of the gastric mucosa, using the Sydney System classification suggested in 1990 by Price et al. (Price, 1991). The revised classification made in 1994 in Houston is now widely accepted (Genta&Dixon, 1995). These criteria are studied and quantified as either mild, moderate or severe: activity, inflammation, atrophy, intestinal metaplasia, and the presence of *H. pylori* infection. Given the increased incidence of malignancy in the elderly population, histology has become mandatory.

8.2.3 Culture
Microbiological examination of biopsy specimens is considered as the reference technique. Culture provides unique information which is helpful in the management of *H. pylori* infection, in particular the strain's susceptibility to antimicrobial agents (Mégraud, 1996). Concerning all of the "invasive methods", they may underestimate *H. pylori* infection in the elderly because of the frequent antibiotic and PPI treatments, and also the high prevalence of chronic atrophy lesions.

8.2.4 Molecular methods
Molecular diagnosis of *H. pylori* infection presents a real interest. PCR detection of *H. pylori* in gastric biopsies offers very sensitive and accurate results in a short time. Many protocols

have been developed for targeting different genes with specific primers for *H. pylori*. Recently, realtime PCR assays were developed allowing simultaneous detection and quantification as well as the determination of antibiotic susceptibility and genotyping of *H. pylori* (Oleastro et al., 2003).

9. Indications for treatment in geriatrics

9.1 Peptic ulcer disease
The short- and long-term studies performed on elderly patients indicate that treatment of *H. pylori* infection in patients with peptic ulcers results in healed ulcers in over 95% of the patients, and significantly improves the clinical outcome, reducing ulcer recurrence, and histological signs of ulcer-associated chronic gastritis activity [13,86]. It is, thus, strongly recommended to test and treat *H. pylori* infection among the elderly presenting peptic ulcers. Pilotto et al. showed that the rate of peptic ulcer relapse in eradicated older patients was 2 percent versus 42 percent in those non-eradicated (Pilotto, 2001).

9.2 Atrophic chronic gastritis
As stated previously, *H. pylori* eradication induces a decrease in the severity of gastric inflammation, atrophy and intestinal metaplasia (Kokkola et al., 2002). The Maastricht 2-2000 Consensus Report recommends treating patients with atrophic gastritis (Malfertheiner et al., 2002).

9.3 Non-ulcer dyspepsia
The effectiveness of *H. pylori* eradication in patients with non-ulcer dyspepsia is still a matter of debate. A study carried out on a geriatric population showed a significant improvement in symptoms of functional dyspepsia in 70% of the patients two months after eradication (Pilotto et al., 1999). However, the long-term benefit was not studied.

9.4 Gastroesophageal reflux disease
The relationship between *H. pylori* infection and the clinical evolution of gastroesophageal reflux disease has not yet been clarified in elderly subjects (Kountouras et al., 2004; Kountouras et al., 2006). In a study carried out on elderly patients with esophagitis, Pilotto et al. reported that healing of esophagitis after a 2 month treatment with PPIs was similar in *H. pylori*-positive and *H. pylori*-negative patients (Pilotto et al., 2002). Moreover, eradication therapy did not accelerate the clinical response to short-term PPI therapy among these patients. *H. pylori* eradication is thus not recommended for elderly patients with gastroesophageal reflux disease.

9.5 Use of non-steroidal anti-inflammatory drugs
It is now established that most peptic ulcers are caused by *H. pylori* or NSAIDs. Studies showed that *H. pylori* eradication is not sufficient in preventing ulcer bleeding in high-risk NSAID users (Chan et al., 2002; Lai et al., 2003; Pilotto et al., 2000a). It does not enhance the healing of peptic ulcer in patients taking antisecretory therapy who continue to take NSAIDs. However, PPI was superior to the eradication of *H. pylori* in preventing recurring bleeding in patients who are taking NSAIDs.
Among patients with *H. pylori* infection and a history of upper gastrointestinal bleeding who are taking low-dose aspirin, the eradication of *H. pylori* is equivalent to treatment with

omeprazole in preventing recurrent bleeding (Chan et al., 2001). In conclusion, there is no clear proof which supports the systematic eradication of *H. pylori* in elderly patients treated with short- or long-term aspirin and/or NSAID drugs.

10. *H. pylori* eradication in geriatrics

Many clinical trials demonstrated that PPI-based triple therapies for 1 week, as recommended by the Maastricht 2-2000 Consensus Report, were highly effective in the elderly population (Pilotto&Malfertheiner, 2002). *H. pylori* eradication is more effective in elderly people compared to younger individuals. Studies performed on elderly patients also showed that a reduction in the PPI dosage, i.e. omeprazole (20 mg) and pantoprazole (40 mg), from twice daily to once daily did not influence the cure rates of triple therapies consisting of either PPI plus clarithromycin (250 mg b.i.d.) and metronidazole (500 mg b.i.d.), or PPI plus clarithromycin (250 mg b.i.d.) and amoxicillin (1 g b.i.d.) (Pilotto et al., 2001; Pilotto&Malfertheiner, 2002; Pilotto&Salles, 2002).
Bad compliance, which is frequently observed in elderly subjects, and *H. pylori* resistance to antibiotics, are the major reasons for treatment failure in elderly patients (Pilotto&Salles, 2002). Studies reported that metronidazole resistance decreased with age (OR for patients over 60 years = 0.63, 95% CI = 0.48–0.80) and was higher in females than in males (Pilotto&Salles, 2002). The optimal strategy for second-line therapy associates PPI with amoxicillin and metronidazole or PPI with tetracycline and metronidazole, with a recommendation to increase the duration of treatment (10 to 14 days) as well as the metronidazole doses. Concerning the poor compliance in older patients, the use of structured patient counselling and follow-up may have a significant effect on *H. pylori* cure rates and should be part of therapy management.

11. Conclusion

The strongest prevalence of *H. pylori* infection in the elderly as well as the role of *H. pylori* in the occurrence of gastric lesions, in particular ulcer diseases, gastric precancerous lesions, and gastric cancer, render the diagnosis and the eradication of *H. pylori* capital in this population. However, studies evaluating the prevalence, diagnosis and treatment of this infection are still few concerning this population, especially in frail patients older than 80 years.

12. References

Abdalla, A. M., Sordillo, E. M., Hanzely, Z., Perez-Perez, G. I., Blaser, M. J., et al. (1998)."Insensitivity of the CLOtest for H. pylori, especially in the elderly" *Gastroenterology* 115, 243-244.
Andres, E., Serraj, K., Mecili, M., Ciobanu, E., Vogel, T., et al. (2009)."[Update of oral vitamin B12.]" *Ann Endocrinol (Paris)*.
Asaka, M., Sugiyama, T., Nobuta, A., Kato, M., Takeda, H., et al. (2001)."Atrophic gastritis and intestinal metaplasia in Japan: Results of a large multicenter study" *Helicobacter* 6, 294-299.

Azuma, T., Suto, H., Ito, Y., Muramatsu, A., Ohtani, M., et al. (2002)."Eradication of *Helicobacter pylori* infection induces an increase in body mass index" *Aliment Pharmacol Ther* 16 Suppl 2, 240-244.

Azuma, T., Suto, H., Ito, Y., Ohtani, M., Dojo, M., et al. (2001)."Gastric leptin and *Helicobacter pylori* infection" *Gut* 49, 324-329.

Bado, A., Levasseur, S., Attoub, S., Kermorgant, S., Laigneau, J. P., et al. (1998)."The stomach is a source of leptin" *Nature* 394, 790-793.

Bhala, N., &Newton, J. L. (2005)."Upper gastrointestinal alarms in older people" *Lancet* 366, 982-983.

Brenner, H., Arndt, V., Stegmaier, C., Ziegler, H., &Rothenbacher, D. (2004)."Is Helicobacter pylori infection a necessary condition for noncardia gastric cancer?" *Am J Epidemiol* 159, 252-258.

Burns, E. A. (2004)."Effects of aging on immune function" *J Nutr Health Aging* 8, 9-18.

Carmel, R., Green, R., Rosenblatt, D. S., &Watkins, D. (2003)."Update on cobalamin, folate, and homocysteine" *Hematology (Am Soc Hematol Educ Program)*, 62-81.

Chan, F. K., Chung, S. C., Suen, B. Y., Lee, Y. T., Leung, W. K., et al. (2001)."Preventing recurrent upper gastrointestinal bleeding in patients with Helicobacter pylori infection who are taking low-dose aspirin or naproxen" *N Engl J Med* 344, 967-973.

Chan, F. K., To, K. F., Wu, J. C., Yung, M. Y., Leung, W. K., et al. (2002)."Eradication of Helicobacter pylori and risk of peptic ulcers in patients starting long-term treatment with non-steroidal anti-inflammatory drugs: a randomised trial" *Lancet* 359, 9-13.

Chapman, I. M. (2004)."Endocrinology of anorexia of ageing" *Best Pract Res Clin Endocrinol Metab* 18, 437-452.

Chen, X., Haruma, K., Kamada, T., Mihara, M., Komoto, K., et al. (2000)."Factors that affect results of the 13C urea breath test in Japanese patients" *Helicobacter* 5, 98-103.

Chow, L. W., Gertsch, P., Poon, R. T., &Branicki, F. J. (1998)."Risk factors for rebleeding and death from peptic ulcer in the very elderly" *Br J Surg* 85, 121-124.

Dali-Youcef, N., &Andres, E. (2009)."An update on cobalamin deficiency in adults" *Qjm* 102, 17-28.

Feldman, M., &Cryer, B. (1998)."Effects of age on gastric alkaline and nonparietal fluid secretion in humans" *Gerontology* 44, 222-227.

Fujiwara, Y., Higuchi, K., Arafa, U. A., Uchida, T., Tominaga, K., et al. (2002)."Long-term effect of Helicobacter pylori eradication on quality of life, body mass index, and newly developed diseases in Japanese patients with peptic ulcer disease" *Hepatogastroenterology* 49, 1298-1302.

Gause-Nilsson, I., Gnarpe, H., Gnarpe, J., Lundborg, P., &Steen, B. (1998)."Helicobacter pylori serology in elderly people: a 21-year cohort comparison in 70-year-olds and a 20-year longitudinal population study in 70-90-year-olds" *Age Ageing* 27, 433-436.

Genta, R. M., &Dixon, M. F. (1995)."The Sydney System revisited: the Houston International Gastritis Workshop" *Am J Gastroenterol* 90, 1039-1041.

Granberg, C., Mansikka, A., Lehtonen, O. P., Kujari, H., Grönfors, R., et al. (1993)."Diagnosis of *Helicobacter pylori* infection by using pyloriset EIA-G and EIA-A for detection of serum immunoglobulin G (IgG) and IgA antibodies" *J Clin Microbiol* 31, 1450-1453.

Iijima, K., Ohara, S., Koike, T., Sekine, H., &Shimosegawa, T. (2004)."Gastric acid secretion of normal Japanese subjects in relation to Helicobacter pylori infection, aging, and gender" *Scand J Gastroenterol* 39, 709-716.

Ito, M., Haruma, K., Kamada, T., Mihara, M., Kim, S., et al. (2002)."Helicobacter pylori eradication therapy improves atrophic gastritis and intestinal metaplasia: a 5-year prospective study of patients with atrophic gastritis" *Aliment Pharmacol Ther* 16, 1449-1456.

Jones, J. I., &Hawkey, C. J. (2001)."Physiology and organ-related pathology of the elderly: stomach ulcers" *Best Pract Res Clin Gastroenterol* 15, 943-961.

Kamada, T., Hata, J., Kusunoki, H., Ito, M., Tanaka, S., et al. (2005)."Eradication of *Helicobacter pylori* increases the incidence of hyperlipidaemia and obesity in peptic ulcer patients" *Dig Liver Dis* 37, 39-43.

Kemppainen, H., Raiha, I., &Sourander, L. (1997)."Clinical presentation of peptic ulcer in the elderly" *Gerontology* 43, 283-288.

Kojima, M., Hosoda, H., Date, Y., Nakazato, M., Matsuo, H., et al. (1999)."Ghrelin is a growth-hormone-releasing acylated peptide from stomach" *Nature* 402, 656-660.

Kokkola, A., Sipponen, P., Rautelin, H., Harkonen, M., Kosunen, T. U., et al. (2002)."The effect of Helicobacter pylori eradication on the natural course of atrophic gastritis with dysplasia" *Aliment Pharmacol Ther* 16, 515-520.

Konturek, J. W., Konturek, S. J., Kwiecien, N., Bielanski, W., Pawlik, T., et al. (2001)."Leptin in the control of gastric secretion and gut hormones in humans infected with *Helicobacter pylori*" *Scand J Gastroenterol* 36, 1148-1154.

Kosunen, T. U., Seppala, K., Sarna, S., &Sipponen, P. (1992)."Diagnostic value of decreasing IgG, IgA, and IgM antibody titres after eradication of Helicobacter pylori" *Lancet* 339, 893-895.

Kountouras, J., Boziki, M., Gavalas, E., Zavos, C., Grigoriadis, N., et al. (2009)."Eradication of Helicobacter pylori may be beneficial in the management of Alzheimer's disease" *J Neurol* 256, 758-767.

Kountouras, J., Tsolaki, M., Gavalas, E., Boziki, M., Zavos, C., et al. (2006a)."Relationship between Helicobacter pylori infection and Alzheimer disease" *Neurology* 66, 938-940.

Kountouras, J., Zavos, C., &Chatzopoulos, D. (2004)."H pylori infection and reflux oesophagitis" *Gut* 53, 912.

Kountouras, J., Zavos, C., Chatzopoulos, D., &Katsinelos, P. (2006b)."Helicobacter pylori and gastro-oesophageal reflux disease" *Lancet* 368, 986; author reply 986-987.

Lai, K. C., Lam, S. K., Chu, K. M., Hui, W. M., Kwok, K. F., et al. (2003)."Lansoprazole reduces ulcer relapse after eradication of Helicobacter pylori in nonsteroidal anti-inflammatory drug users--a randomized trial" *Aliment Pharmacol Ther* 18, 829-836.

Lewis, S. J., Potts, L. F., Malhotra, R., &Mountford, R. (1999)."Small bowel bacterial overgrowth in subjects living in residential care homes" *Age Ageing* 28, 181-185.

Liston, R., Pitt, M. A., &Banerjee, A. K. (1996)."IgG ELISA antibodies and detection of Helicobacter pylori in elderly patients" *Lancet* 347, 269.

Malaguarnera, M., Bella, R., Alagona, G., Ferri, R., Carnemolla, A., et al. (2004)."Helicobacter pylori and Alzheimer's disease: a possible link" *Eur J Intern Med* 15, 381-386.

Malfertheiner, P., Megraud, F., O'Morain, C., Hungin, A. P., Jones, R., et al. (2002)."Current concepts in the management of Helicobacter pylori infection--the Maastricht 2-2000 Consensus Report" *Aliment Pharmacol Ther* 16, 167-180.

Megraud, F. (2003)."[When and how does Helicobacter pylori infection occur?]" *Gastroenterol Clin Biol* 27, 374-379.

Mégraud, F. (1996). *In "Helicobacter pylori* - Epidémiologie, pathogénie, diagnostic" (F. Mégraud&H. Lamouliatte, eds.), Vol. 1, pp. 249-266. Elsevier, Paris.

Mitsui, T., Shimaoka, K., Goto, Y., Kagami, H., Kinomoto, H., et al. (2006)."Small bowel bacterial overgrowth is not seen in healthy adults but is in disabled older adults" *Hepatogastroenterology* 53, 82-85.

Monteiro, L., Bergey, B., Gras, N., &Megraud, F. (2002)."Evaluation of the performance of the Helico Blot 2.1 as a tool to investigate the virulence properties of *Helicobacter pylori*" *Clin Microbiol Infect* 8, 676-679.

Monteiro, L., Gras, N., Vidal, R., Cabrita, J., &Megraud, F. (2001)."Detection of Helicobacter pylori DNA in human feces by PCR: DNA stability and removal of inhibitors" *J Microbiol Methods* 45, 89-94.

Morley, J. E. (2001)."Anorexia, sarcopenia, and aging" *Nutrition* 17, 660-663.

Neri, M. C., Lai, L., Bonetti, P., Baldassarri, A. R., Monti, M., et al. (1996)."Prevalence of Helicobacter pylori infection in elderly inpatients and in institutionalized old people: correlation with nutritional status" *Age Ageing* 25, 17-21.

Newton, J. L. (2004)."Changes in upper gastrointestinal physiology with age" *Mech Ageing Dev* 125, 867-870.

Nurgalieva, Z. Z., Malaty, H. M., Graham, D. Y., Almuchambetova, R., Machmudova, A., et al. (2002)."Helicobacter pylori infection in Kazakhstan: effect of water source and household hygiene" *Am J Trop Med Hyg* 67, 201-206.

Nwokolo, C. U., Freshwater, D. A., O'Hare, P., &Randeva, H. S. (2003)."Plasma ghrelin following cure of Helicobacter pylori" *Gut* 52, 637-640.

Ofman, J. J., Etchason, J., Alexander, W., Stevens, B. R., Herrin, J., et al. (2000)."The quality of care for Medicare patients with peptic ulcer disease" *Am J Gastroenterol* 95, 106-113.

Oleastro, M., Ménard, A., Santos, A., Lamouliatte, H., Monteiro, L., et al. (2003)."Real-time PCR assay for rapid and accurate detection of point mutations conferring resistance to clarithromycin in *Helicobacter pylori*" *J Clin Microbiol* 41, 397-402.

Parlesak, A., Klein, B., Schecher, K., Bode, J. C., &Bode, C. (2003)."Prevalence of small bowel bacterial overgrowth and its association with nutrition intake in nonhospitalized older adults" *J Am Geriatr Soc* 51, 768-773.

Pilotto, A. (2001)."Helicobacter pylori-associated peptic ulcer disease in older patients: current management strategies" *Drugs Aging* 18, 487-494.

Pilotto, A. (2004)."Aging and upper gastrointestinal disorders" *Best Pract Res Clin Gastroenterol* 18 Suppl, 73-81.

Pilotto, A., Di Mario, F., Franceschi, M., Leandro, G., Battaglia, G., et al. (2000a)."Pantoprazole versus one-week Helicobacter pylori eradication therapy for the prevention of acute NSAID-related gastroduodenal damage in elderly subjects" *Aliment Pharmacol Ther* 14, 1077-1082.

Pilotto, A., Fabrello, R., Franceschi, M., Scagnelli, M., Soffiati, F., et al. (1996)."Helicobacter pylori infection in asymptomatic elderly subjects living at home or in a nursing home: effects on gastric function and nutritional status" *Age Ageing* 25, 245-249.

Pilotto, A., Franceschi, M., Leandro, G., Bozzola, L., Fortunato, A., et al. (1999)."Efficacy of 7 day lansoprazole-based triple therapy for Helicobacter pylori infection in elderly patients" *J Gastroenterol Hepatol* 14, 468-475.

Pilotto, A., Franceschi, M., Leandro, G., Bozzola, L., Rassu, M., et al. (2001)."Cure of Helicobacter pylori infection in elderly patients: comparison of low versus high doses of clarithromycin in combination with amoxicillin and pantoprazole" *Aliment Pharmacol Ther* 15, 1031-1036.

Pilotto, A., Franceschi, M., Leandro, G., Paris, F., Niro, V., et al. (2003)."The risk of upper gastrointestinal bleeding in elderly users of aspirin and other non-steroidal anti-inflammatory drugs: the role of gastroprotective drugs" *Aging Clin Exp Res* 15, 494-499.

Pilotto, A., Franceschi, M., Leandro, G., Rassu, M., Bozzola, L., et al. (2002)."Influence of Helicobacter pylori infection on severity of oesophagitis and response to therapy in the elderly" *Dig Liver Dis* 34, 328-331.

Pilotto, A., Franceschi, M., Leandro, G., Rassu, M., Zagari, R. M., et al. (2000b)."Noninvasive diagnosis of *Helicobacter pylori* infection in older subjects: Comparison of the C-13-urea breath test with serology" *J Gerontol Ser A Biol Sci Med* 55, M163-M167.

Pilotto, A., &Malfertheiner, P. (2002)."Review article: an approach to Helicobacter pylori infection in the elderly" *Aliment Pharmacol Ther* 16, 683-691.

Pilotto, A., Rassu, M., Bozzola, L., Leandro, G., Franceschi, M., et al. (1998)."Cytotoxin-associated gene A-positive Helicobacter pylori infection in the elderly. Association with gastric atrophy and intestinal metaplasia" *J Clin Gastroenterol* 26, 18-22.

Pilotto, A., &Salles, N. (2002)."*Helicobacter pylori* infection in geriatrics" *Helicobacter* 1, 56-62.

Price, A. B. (1991)."The Sydney System: histological division" *J Gastroenterol Hepatol* 6, 209-222.

Regev, A., Fraser, G. M., Braun, M., Maoz, E., Leibovici, L., et al. (1999)."Seroprevalence of Helicobacter pylori and length of stay in a nursing home" *Helicobacter* 4, 89-93.

Ruiz, B., Garay, J., Correa, P., Fontham, E. T., Bravo, J. C., et al. (2001)."Morphometric evaluation of gastric antral atrophy: improvement after cure of Helicobacter pylori infection" *Am J Gastroenterol* 96, 3281-3287.

Sachs, G., Weeks, D. L., Melchers, K., &Scott, D. R. (2003)."The gastric biology of Helicobacter pylori" *Ann Rev Physiol* 65, 349-369.

Salles, N. (2007)."Basic mechanisms of the aging gastrointestinal tract" *Dig Dis* 25, 112-117.

Salles, N., Letenneur, L., Buissonniere, A., Jehanno, A., Dartigues, J. F., et al. Does Helicobacter pylori affect life expectancy?" *J Am Geriatr Soc* 58, 1607-1609.

Salles, N., Menard, A., Georges, A., Salzmann, M., de Ledinghen, V., et al. (2006)."Effects of Helicobacter pylori infection on gut appetite peptide (leptin, ghrelin) expression in elderly inpatients" *J Gerontol A Biol Sci Med Sci* 61, 1144-1150.

Salles-Montaudon, N., Dertheil, S., Broutet, N., Gras, N., Monteiro, L., et al. (2002)."Detecting Helicobacter pylori infection in hospitalized frail older patients: the challenge" *J Am Geriatr Soc* 50, 1674-1680.

Salles-Montaudon, N., Parrot, F., Balas, D., Bouzigon, E., Rainfray, M., et al. (2003)."Prevalence and mechanisms of hyperhomocysteinemia in elderly hospitalized patients" *J Nutr Health Aging* 7, 111-116.

Seinela, L., &Ahvenainen, J. (2000)."Peptic ulcer in the very old patients" *Gerontology* 46, 271-275.

Shih, G. L., Brensinger, C., Katzka, D. A., &Metz, D. C. (2003)."Influence of age and gender on gastric acid secretion as estimated by integrated acidity in patients referred for 24-hour ambulatory pH monitoring" *Am J Gastroenterol* 98, 1713-1718.

Sipponen, P., Laxen, F., Huotari, K., &Harkonen, M. (2003)."Prevalence of low vitamin B12 and high homocysteine in serum in an elderly male population: association with atrophic gastritis and Helicobacter pylori infection" *Scand J Gastroenterol* 38, 1209-1216.

Vaira, D., Malfertheiner, P., Megraud, F., Axon, A. T., Deltenre, M., et al. (1999)."Diagnosis of Helicobacter pylori infection with a new non-invasive antigen-based assay. HpSA European study group" *Lancet* 354, 30-33.

Van Kouwen, M. C., Drenth, J. P., Verhoeven, H. M., Bos, L. P., &Engels, L. G. (2003)."Upper gastrointestinal endoscopy in patients aged 85 years or more. Results of a feasibility study in a district general hospital" *Arch Gerontol Geriatr* 37, 45-50

Vidal-Alaball, J., Butler, C. C., Cannings-John, R., Goringe, A., Hood, K., et al. (2005)."Oral vitamin B12 versus intramuscular vitamin B12 for vitamin B12 deficiency" *Cochrane Database Syst Rev*, CD004655

Younger, J., &Duggan, A. (2002)."Helicobacter pylori infection in elderly patients" *Lancet* 360, 947; author reply 948

4

Case Study in Optimal Dosing in Duodenal Ulcer

Karl E. Peace

Jiann-Ping Hsu College of Public Health, Georgia Southern University Statesboro
USA

1. Introduction

Duodenal ulcers occur in the duodenum – the upper portion of the small intestine as it leaves the stomach. A duodenal ulcer is characterized by the presence of a well-demarcated break in the mucosa that may extend into the muscularis propria [Thompson et al, 2010]. Cimetidine (C) was the first H_2-Receptor Antagonist to receive regulatory approval (in the late 1970s) for the treatment of duodenal ulcers. When it was being developed it was widely held that duodenal ulcers were caused by excessive gastric acid production. In fact the prevailing medical opinion was *no acid, no ulcer*. Sir James Black and colleagues at SmithKline and French Laboratories are credited with the discovery of C. They discovered that histamine released by the H_2-receptor stimulated the production of gastric acid, and that C by blocking the release of this histamine would suppress both normal and food stimulated gastric acid secretion [Nayak & Ketteringham, 1986]. In a reduced acidic environment, ulcers would be able to heal. The first C regimen approved for the treatment of duodenal ulcers in the United Kingdom was 1000 mg per day, given as: 200 mg at breakfast, lunch and dinner, and 400 mg at bed time, for up to 4 weeks. The first regimen approved in the United States for this indication was 1200 mg per day, given as: 300 mg q.i.d. for up to 4 weeks. Subsequently, other indications were obtained, and dosing regimens modified; for example, 800 mg per day, given as 400 mg bid.

In the mid 1980's, based upon data from gastric acid anti-secretory studies at various doses and frequencies of dosing, there was reason to believe that a single night time (hs) dose of 800 mg of C for up to 4 weeks would be the clinically optimal regimen for treating patients with duodenal ulcers. A large, landmark, dose comparison clinical trial [Dickson et al, 1985; Peace et al, 1985; Valenzuela et al, 1985; Young et al, 1989] was undertaken to confirm the effectiveness of 800 C mg hs in the treatment of duodenal ulcers for up to four weeks. When the author was first consulted by the project physician and regulatory affairs expert, the clinical development plan consisted of two, randomized, double-blind, placebo controlled, pivotal proof of efficacy trials with single nighttime dosing for four weeks:

Trial 1: 800 mg C hs vs. Placebo, and Trial 2: 1200 mg C hs vs. Placebo.

Each trial was to enroll 150 patients per treatment group, for a total of 600 patients. One-hundred-fifty patients per group would provide a power of 95% to detect a 20% difference in cumulative four-week ulcer healing rates between the C and Placebo groups with a 1-

sided, Type I error [Peace, 1991a] of 5%. Since conducting these trials would subject ½ the patients to Placebo, the author recommended amalgamating the two trials into a single trial:

Trial 3: 1200 mg C hs vs. 800 mg C hs vs. 0 mg C hs (Placebo)

with 164 patients per treatment group, for a total of 492 patients. One-hundred sixty-four patients per treatment group would provide a power of 95% to detect a difference of 20% in four week ulcer healing rates between any two of the treatment groups with an experiment wise Type I error of 5% (1.67% per each 1-sided, pair-wise comparison). Not only would this trial require fewer patients and be less expensive to conduct, it would also provide a within trial comparison between C doses, for dose discrimination.

Further savings could be realized by incorporating into the Trial #3 protocol, a planned interim analysis after ½ the patients had been entered and completed. At the interim analysis, the efficacy comparisons: 1200 mg C vs. Placebo, and 800 mg C vs. Placebo would be tested. If both were statistically significant, then the entire study could be stopped – if efficacy of the doses were the only objective. If comparing the doses of C was also of clinical importance, then the Placebo arm could be stopped and the two C arms run to full completion to assess dose discrimination. By conducting Trial #3 (instead of the two separate trials) and incorporating the interim analysis, potential savings of up to 190 patients could be realized. Additional savings would be expected due to less time required to conduct the trial [Peace, 1990, 1991b].

The primary objective in conducting a clinical trial of C in the treatment of duodenal ulcers with a single nighttime dose was to demonstrate that 800 mg C was clinically optimal. We therefore added a 400 mg dose and replaced the 1200 mg dose with a 1600 mg dose (a two-fold increase among consecutive doses) in the final trial protocol, which was IRB approved.

2. Materials and methods

2.1 Objective

Both primary and secondary efficacy objectives were identified in the final protocol. The primary objective addressed ulcer healing. The secondary objective addressed upper gastrointestinal (UGI) pain relief.

The primary objective was to confirm that C given as a single nighttime dose of 800 mg for up to 4 weeks was clinically optimal in healing duodenal ulcers. Clinically optimal meant that 800 mg C was effective (significantly superior to placebo), that 800 mg C was superior to 400 mg C, and that 1600 mg C was not significantly superior to 800 mg C. Symbolically the primary (note p subscript of H) objective derives from three null and alternative hypotheses:

$$H_{p01}: P_{uh800} = P_{uh0}, \quad H_{p02}: P_{uh800} = P_{uh400}, \quad H_{p03}: P_{uh1600} = P_{uh800}$$

$$H_{pa1}: P_{uh800} > P_{uh0}, \quad H_{pa2}: P_{uh800} > P_{uh400}, \quad H_{pa3}: P_{uh1600} \neq P_{uh800}.$$

where P_{uh0}, P_{uh400}, P_{uh800} and P_{uh1600} represent the cumulative ulcer healing (uh) rates by week 4 in the Placebo, 400 mg C, 800 mg C and 1600 mg C treatment groups, respectively, under single nighttime (hs) dosing. Specifically, H_{pa1}, H_{pa2} and H_{p03} comprised the primary study objective.

Symbolically, the secondary (note s subscript of H) objective derives from the three null and alternative hypotheses:

$$H_{s01}: P_{pr800} = P_{pr0}, \quad H_{s02}: P_{pr800} = P_{pr400}, \quad H_{s03}: P_{pr1600} = P_{pr800}$$

$$H_{sa1}: P_{pr800} > P_{pr0}, \quad H_{sa2}: P_{pr800} > P_{pr400}, \quad H_{sa3}: P_{pr1600} \neq P_{pr800}.$$

where P_{pr0}, P_{pr400}, P_{pr800} and P_{pr1600} represent the UGI pain relief (pr) rates in the Placebo, 400 mg C, 800 mg C and 1600 mg C treatment groups, respectively, under single nighttime (hs) dosing. Specifically, H_{sa1}, H_{sa2} and H_{s03} comprised the secondary study objective.

Of the six possible pairwise comparisons among the 4 dose groups, only three comprised the study objective. The other three: 1600 mg C versus 0 mg C, 1600 mg C versus 400 mg C, and 400 mg C versus 0 mg C were not part of the study objective and thus did not exact a Type I error penalty (i.e. the overall Type I error of 5% was 'Bonferonnied' across the three pairwise comparisons comprising the study objective, and not across the 6 possible pairwise comparisons).

2.2 Designing and planning the investigation

The trial was multicenter, stratified, randomized, double-blind and Placebo (0 mg C) controlled. Neither patients, investigators nor their staff knew the identity of the C regimens. As there had been reports [Korman et al, 1981; Korman et al, 1983; Lam & Koo, 1983; Barakat et al, 1984] of the influence of smoking on the healing of duodenal ulcers at the time of protocol development, patients were stratified by smoking status within each center prior to randomization to the treatment groups. Smoking strata were Light Smokers and Heavy Smokers. Patients who smoked at most 9 cigarettes per day comprised the Light Smoker stratum. Patients who smoked at least 10 cigarettes per day comprised the Heavy Smoker stratum.

2.3 Blinded treatment groups

Blinded treatment group medication was packaged using the existing regulatory approved 400 mg C tablet. A 400 mg Placebo tablet was formulated identical to the 400 mg C tablet except that it contained 0 mg C. Blinded trial medication for the four treatment groups was packaged in blister packs for 4 weeks of nightly treatment as identified below:

0 mg C Group:	Four 400 mg Placebo tablets
400 mg C Group:	One C 400 mg tablet + three 400 mg Placebo tablets
800 mg C Group:	Two C 400 mg tablets + two 400 mg Placebo tablets
1600 mg C Group:	Four C 400 mg tablets.

2.4 Sample size determination

The trial was designed to recruit and enter enough patients to complete one-hundred sixty-four (164) per treatment group, for a total of 656 patients. One-hundred sixty-four patients per treatment group would provide a power of 95% to detect a difference of 20% in cumulative four week ulcer healing rates between any two of the treatment groups with an experiment wise Type I error rate of 5% (1.67% per each 1-sided, pair-wise comparison). This number was inflated to account for a 15% drop out rate. A cumulative four week healing rate of 45% among Placebo treated patients [de Craen et al, 1999] in previous trials was used in the sample size determination.

2.5 Entry requirements and assessment schedule

Patients were required at entry to have an endoscopically confirmed duodenal ulcer of size at least 0.3 cm, and either daytime or nighttime UGI pain. After providing informed consent, at the preliminary examination or baseline visit, patients provided a history (including prior use of medications, particularly anti-ulcer ones or antacids), underwent a physical examination, had vital signs measured, provided blood and urine samples for clinical laboratory assessments, in addition to having UGI pain assessed and undergoing endoscopy. Patients were also instructed how to use a daily diary to record the severity of daytime or nighttime UGI pain, as well as to record any adverse experience or concomitant medication use. Diaries and trial medication were dispensed and the patients instructed to return at weeks 1, 2 and 4 of the treatment period for follow-up endoscopy, UGI pain assessment and assessment of other clinical parameters. Antacids were provided to patients for relief of severe pain during the first six days/ nights of therapy only, and were limited to 4 tablets per day of low acid-neutralizing capacity. Table 1 summarizes clinical assessments made throughout the trial.

Follow-up endoscopic evaluation was carried out following strict time windows (Table 1) at week 1 (Days 7-8), week 2 (Days 13-15) and week 4 (Days 26-30). Patients whose ulcers were healed at any follow-up endoscopy were considered trial completers and received no further treatment or endoscopic assessment.

Clinical Parameter	Preliminary Examination[1]	Week 1 (Days 7-8)	Week 2 (Days 13-15)	Week 4 (Days 26-30)
History	Y			
Physical Exam	Y			
Vital Signs	Y	Y	Y	Y
Adv. Events		Y	Y	Y
Con. Meds	Y	Y	Y	Y
Endoscopy	Y	Y	Y	Y
Pain Assessment	Y	Y	Y	Y
Clin. Labs.	Y	Y		Y

[1] After providing Informed Consent

Table 1. Clinical Evaluation Schedule

2.6 Primary and secondary endpoints

The **primary efficacy data** was ulcer healing at week 1, 2 or 4. Ulcer healing was defined as complete reepithelization of the ulcer crater (normal or hyperemic mucosa), documented by endoscopy. The **primary efficacy endpoint** was cumulative ulcer healing at week 4 (healed at week 1 or week 2 or week 4).

Secondary efficacy data were the severity ratings of daytime and nighttime UGI pain recorded by the patient on the daily diary card. The severity of daytime pain was recorded just prior to going to sleep at night. The severity of nighttime pain was recorded upon arising in the morning. At each follow-up visit, the physician would review the diary card and record the most severe rating of daytime and nighttime pain since the previous clinic visit. Daytime and nighttime UGI pain were rated separately according to the following scale:

>0 = None = I had no pain
>1 = Mild = I had some pain, but it didn't bother me much
>2 = Moderate = I had pain that was annoying, but it didn't interrupt my activities
>3 = Severe = I had pain which was so bad I couldn't do my usual activities

For nighttime pain, activities reflected sleep. The **secondary efficacy endpoint** was whether the patient was free of daytime or nighttime pain at weeks 1, 2 or 4.

2.7 Conducting the investigation

When the trial was conducted, there was great pressure to complete it as quickly as possible. This was due in part to Ranitidine's rapid gains into the antiulcer market, of which C had exclusivity for several years. Approximately 60 centers were recruited. The centers were rigorously and frequently monitored for conformity to protocol and federal regulations, in an attempt to minimize violations to protocol and collection of questionable if not unusable data. Roughly half of the sites were monitored by in-house Clinical Monitoring Personnel (CRA = Clinical Research Associates). The remaining sites were monitored by an outside Contract Research Organization (CRO).

A fairly heavy advertisement campaign was initiated to recruit possible trial participants. Ads ran on television and radio and appeared in the print media. In addition circulars were posted in public areas such as supermarket and laundromat bulletin boards. The ads were targeted to adults who had been having UGI or ulcer like pain, but who were otherwise healthy.

Weekly meetings were held during the conduct of the trial to monitor progress and deal with any issues. A proactive approach to clinical data management was taken. Data collection forms (DCFs) were expressed by each clinic to the data management group (or picked up by the CRA) where they were rapidly reviewed for completeness, legibility, entered into the computerized trial database, verified and quality assured. The goal was to provide a quality assured database for statistical analysis in as short a time as possible after each patient completed the protocol.

At the time the duodenal ulcer trial was conducted, there was no commercially available 800 mg C tablet. The commercially available 400 mg C tablet was used. Therefore a blood level trial that demonstrated bioequivalence [Randolph et al, 1986a] between a new 800 mg C tablet formulation (to be marketed) and two-400 mg C commercially available tablets had to be conducted with results available by the completion of the duodenal ulcer trial. Results from these two trials as well as that from specified drug interaction studies provided the primary data to support filing a supplemental new drug application (SNDA) to the FDA for the approval of C as a single 800 mg tablet taken at bedtime for the treatment of duodenal ulcers.

2.8 Statistical analysis methods
2.8.1 Methods

Descriptive and inferential methods were used in presentations and analysis of the trial data using procedures (PROCS) in the Statistical Analysis System (SAS). Both tables and graphs reflecting the number of patients, the mean (percent for dichotomous data) and standard deviation by treatment group and time of assessment were developed.

Inferential analyses, significance tests and confidence intervals, derived from an analysis of variance model containing fixed effects of center, strata and treatment group, with contrasts specified for the pairwise comparisons of interest. P-values for the pairwise comparisons comprising the primary trial objective were used for statistical inference. Confidence intervals were used as the basis of inference for secondary trial objectives and for the three pairwise comparisons not a part of the trial objective.

Since there were many centers and relatively few patients per treatment group per strata per center were expected, 12 blocks reflecting smoking status (2 levels)-by-baseline ulcer size (6 levels) were defined *a priori* (Table 2). An analysis of variance model containing the fixed effects of blocks and treatment was also used to assess the effect of treatment adjusted for blocks.

Gereralizability (poolability) of treatment effects was assessed by running an analysis of variance model with block, treatment group and block-by-treatment interaction. In these analyses the sole interest was the P-value for the interaction term. The blocking factor was smoking status-by-baseline ulcer size as defined in Table 2. A separate analysis that included the factors: smoking status, baseline ulcer size, their interaction, and the interaction of each of these with treatment was also performed.

Light	[0.3]
Light	(0.3; 0.4]
Light	(0.4; 0.5]
Light	(0.5; 1.0)
Light	[1.0]
Light	(1.0; 3.0]
Heavy	[0.3]
Heavy	(0.3; 0.4]
Heavy	(0.4; 0.5]
Heavy	(0.5; 1.0)
Heavy	[1.0]
Heavy	(1.0; 3.0]

Table 2. Smoking Status by Ulcer Size (cm) Blocks

Bivariate plots of the proportion of patients with ulcers remaining unhealed and the proportion of patients with UGI pain (daytime or nighttime) by time of endoscopic evaluation and treatment group were developed. These plots illustrate the rate of ulcer healing and pain relief across the times of endoscopic evaluation.

2.8.2 Interim analysis

Prior to finalizing the protocol, we considered including an interim analysis plan. Incorporating such a plan could result in completing approximately ½ the planned number of patients. More importantly, it could reduce the time from starting the trial to filing the SNDA. The idea was accepted initially, but later rejected by upper management; so the final protocol did not include an interim analysis plan.

However after the trial started, there was a push to conduct an interim analysis. A plan was developed to conduct an interim (mid-study) analysis after ½ the patients had entered. The plan was filed by in-house regulatory affairs personnel with the FDA. Essential features of the plan ensured preservation of the Type I error and safe guarded blindedness among investigators, patients, and in-house personnel. We hired an outside consulting group that generated dummy investigator, patient and treatment group identification. The group also computed the P-values associated with the 3 pairwise comparisons comprising the study objectives and reported them to FDA Biometrics and in-house statistical personnel. The trial was not stopped and ran to completion, eventually enrolling 768 patients. The final results, based upon more than twice the number of patients in the interim analysis, were similar to those of the interim analysis in terms of estimates of treatment effects.

3. Results and discussion

3.1 Interim or mid study analysis results

3.1.1 Numbers of patients and baseline characteristics

Table 3 summarizes the number of patients available for the mid-study, interim analysis. Three hundred and thirty-seven (337) were randomized of which 315 [Peace et al, 1985; Valenzuela et al, 1985] were considered evaluatable [Peace, 1984] for efficacy for at least one follow-up visit. The fact that 17 more patients were assigned to the 1600 mg C group illustrates that slight imbalance across treatment groups can occur in randomized trials consisting of many centers.

Table 4 contains descriptive results of data available at baseline for mid-study analysis patients by C treatment group. The treatment groups appear balanced in terms of demographic characteristics, UGI pain and ulcer size, although the 800 mg C group had patients with the largest ulcers.

	Total	0 mg	400 mg	800 mg	1600 mg
# Randomized	337	76	83	85	93
# Evaluatable					
Week 1	304	67	80	73	84
Week 2	235	46	63	60	66
Week 4	174	41	47	47	39
≥ 1 week	315	71	82	75	87

Table 3. Number of Patients by Treatment Group (Mid Study Analysis)

3.1.2 Distribution of patients according to ulcer size

Table 5 provides the distribution of patients at baseline according to ulcer size. Ten percent (10%) of patients had ulcers of size 0.30 cm; 12.5% had ulcers of size greater than 0.30 but at most 0.40 cm; 17.8% had ulcers of size greater than 0.40 cm but at most 0.50 cm; 27.2% had ulcers of size between 0.50 cm and 1.00 cm; 17.8% had ulcers 1.00 cm in size; and 14.7% had ulcers of size greater than 1.00 cm but at most 3.00 cm.

Table 6 provides the distribution of patients in the Placebo group by baseline ulcer size whose ulcers had healed by 4 weeks. Seventy-one percent (71%) of Placebo patients with ulcers of size 0.30 cm healed; 78% of Placebo patients with ulcers of size greater than 0.30 but at most 0.40 cm healed; 45% of Placebo patients with ulcers of size greater than 0.40 cm but at most 0.50 cm healed; 41% of Placebo patients with ulcers between 0.50 cm and 1.00 cm in size healed; 30% of Placebo patients with ulcers 1.00 cm in size healed; and 25% of Placebo patients with ulcers of size greater than 1.00 cm but at most 3.00 cm healed. Table 6 reflects a strong negative correlation (or trend) between baseline ulcer size and ulcer healing by 4 weeks; i.e. the smaller the ulcer, the greater is ulcer healing by 4 weeks.

Characteristic	Statistic	0 mg	400 mg	800 mg	1600 mg
Age (yr)	Mean	42	40	44	42
Height (in)	Mean	67	67	67	67
Weight (lb)	Mean	169	160	163	160
Sex	Male (N)	50	62	51	55
	Female (N)	26	21	34	38
Race	Caucasian(N)	44	50	58	61
	Black (N)	24	21	18	24
	Other (N)	8	12	9	8
Day Pain	Mean	2.89	3.13	2.91	2.92
Night Pain	Mean	2.68	2.84	2.80	3.05
Ulcer Size(cm)	Mean	0.76	0.71	0.85	0.75
Smoking	Heavy (N)	40	45	45	48
	Light (N)	36	38	40	45

Table 4. Baseline Characteristics (Mid Study Analysis)

Ulcer Size (cm)	% Patients
[0.30]	10.0%
(0.30; 0.40]	12.5%
(0.40; 0.50]	17.8%
(0.50; 1.00)	27.2%
[1.00]	17.8%
(1.00; 3.00]	14.7%

Table 5. Distribution by Ulcer Size - Mid Study Analysis

Ulcer Size (cm)	Healed
[0.30]	71%
(0.30; 0.40]	78%
(0.40; 0.50]	45%
(0.50; 1.00)	41%
[1.00]	30%
(1.00; 3.00]	25%

Table 6. Cumulative 4-week Ulcer Healing Rates: Mid Study Analysis Placebo Patients

3.1.3 Influence of smoking and ulcer size on ulcer healing

Figure 1 provides a summary of the cumulative proportion of patients across all treatment groups with healed duodenal ulcers by week of endoscopy and smoking status. Figure 1 reflects a strong negative correlation between smoking status and ulcer healing; i.e. light smokers have a higher percentage of healed ulcers than do heavy smokers at all weeks of endoscopy.

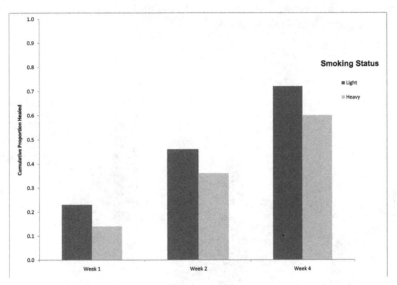

Fig. 1. Cumulative Proportion Healed: Light vs Heavy Smokers, Combined Treatment Groups

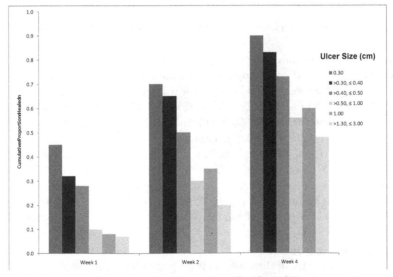

Fig. 2. Cumulative Proportion Healed by Ulcer Size, Combined Treatment Groups

Figure 2 provides a summary of the cumulative proportion of patients across all treatment groups with healed duodenal ulcers by week of endoscopy and baseline ulcer size. Figure 2 reflects a strong negative correlation between ulcer size and ulcer healing; i.e. patients with smaller ulcers have a higher percentage of healed ulcers than do patients with larger ulcers at all weeks of endoscopy. Note that the categories of ulcer size in Figure 2 are those that were defined *a priori*.

The negative correlation between ulcer size and healing is sharpened when collapsing the six ulcer size categories into three (Figure 3).

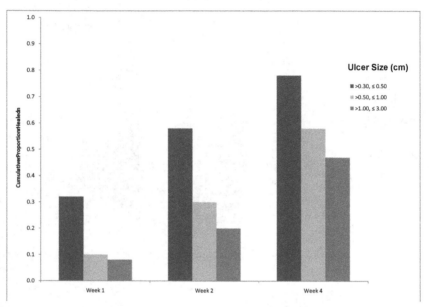

Fig. 3. Cumulative Proportion Healed by Ulcer Size, Combined Treatment Groups

3.1.4 Cumulative ulcer healing

The cumulative duodenal ulcer healing rates are summarized [Peace et al, 1985; Valenzuela et al, 1985] in Figure 4 by week of endoscopy and treatment group. The healing rates were: 19%, 18%, 16% and 21% at week 1; 29%, 37%, 38% and 49% at week 2; and 41%, 62%, 72% and 74%; for the Placebo, 400 mg C, 800 mg C and 1600 mg C groups respectively. At week 4: 800 mg C was effective (P = 0.0002) as compared to Placebo; 800 mg C was marginally superior to 400 mg C (P = 0.1283); and 1600 mg C provided no clinically significant greater benefit {δ = 0.0156: 90% CI on ratio of 1600 mg C/ 800 mg C = (0.86; 1.18)} than did 800 mg C. Even though 800 mg C healed 10% more ulcers than did 400 mg C, the P-value for this comparison did not achieve statistical significance. Therefore, the mid-study analysis did not demonstrate that 800 mg C was clinically optimal as formulated in the trial objective.

3.1.5 Generalizability assessment

Table 7 provides a summary of the assessment of generalizability (poolability) of treatment effect across smoking status, baseline ulcer size and smoking status-by-baseline ulcer size.

All of the P-values are large and therefore provide no evidence of lack of generalizability of treatment effects across these subpopulations.

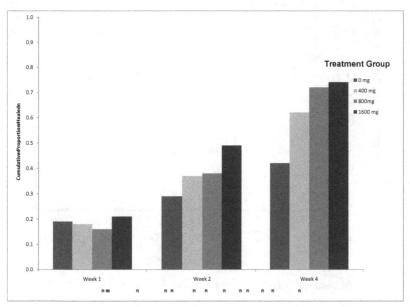

Fig. 4. Cumulative Proportion of Patients with Healed Ulcers by Week and Treatment Group

Source	F-value	P-value
Smoke x Size	1.11	0.3559
Smoke x Dose	0.40	0.7518
Size x Dose	1.12	0.3359
Smoke x Size x Dose	0.78	0.7038

Table 7. Assessment of generalizability: Smoking Status by Ulcer Size Subpopulations, Mid Study Analysis

3.1.6 Complete UGI pain relief and ulcer healing

To illustrate changes in duodenal ulcer healing and complete relief of UGI pain jointly, bivariate plots (Figure 5 and Figure 6) were generated. To develop these plots, the means (proportions) of each endpoint were computed by treatment or dose group and each endoscopy evaluation. The means, corresponding to each endoscopy evaluation and dose group identification, along with the ranges (0; 1) of each endpoint, were output to a data file. The data file was accessed by a graphical software package and a plot generated of the mean pairs by dose group. In generating the plots, the horizontal axis reflects the range of one endpoint and the vertical axis reflects the range of the other endpoint. In plotting the pairs of means for each dose group, the endoscopy evaluation corresponding to each pair appears as a floating index on the graph of each dose group.

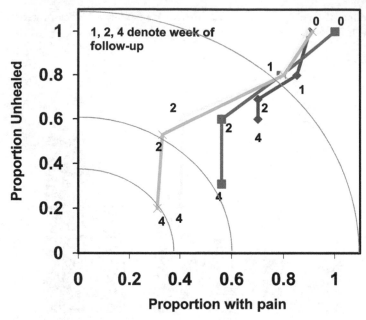

Fig. 5. Proportions of patients with Daytime Pain and Unhealed Ulcers, by Treatment Group (Mid-Study Analysis)

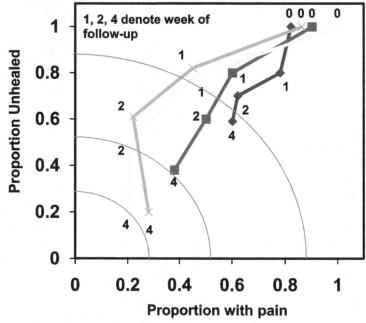

Fig. 6. Proportions of Patients with and Unhealed Nighttime Pain Ulcers, by Treatment Group (Mid-Study Analysis)

In Figures 5 and 6, the horizontal axis reflects the proportion of patients with UGI pain, and the vertical axis reflects the proportion of patients with unhealed ulcers; rather than proportions of patients without UGI pain and with healed ulcers. The (1,1) point therefore reflects where the patients are at baseline, and the (0,0) point reflects the ideal therapeutic goal of a treatment or dose by the final visit. For a broader discussion of bivariate plots, references [Peace & Tsai, 2009and Peace & Chen, 2010] may be seen.

Figure 5 is the bivariate plot of daytime UGI pain and lack of ulcer healing. Figure 6 is the bivariate plot of nighttime UGI pain and lack of ulcer healing. The fact that all dose groups do not begin at the (1,1) point is due to the fact that some patients had daytime UGI pain but not nighttime UGI pain and vice versa. Focusing on week 4 results, Figures 5 and 6 reflect a beautiful picture of dose response, both univariately and bivariately.

3.2 Final study analysis results
At the final study analysis, 168, 182, 165 and 188 patients [Young et al, 1989] were efficacy evaluatable, in the Placebo, 400 mg C, 800 mg C and 1600 mg C groups, respectively. The cumulative duodenal ulcer healing rates are summarized in Figure 7 by week of endoscopy and treatment group. The healing rates were: 17%, 16%, 15% and 21% at week 1; 30%, 40%, 42% and 48% at week 2; and 41%, 62%, 73% and 77%; for the Placebo, 400 mg C, 800 mg C and 1600 mg C groups respectively. At week 4: 800 mg C was effective ($P < 10^{-8}$) as compared to Placebo; 800 mg C was superior to 400 mg C ($P = 0.023$); and 1600 mg C provided no clinically significant greater benefit {$\delta = 0.04$: 90% CI on ratio of 1600 mg C/ 800 mg C = (0.96; 1.17)} than did 800 mg C. Therefore, the study demonstrated that 800 mg C was clinically optimal.

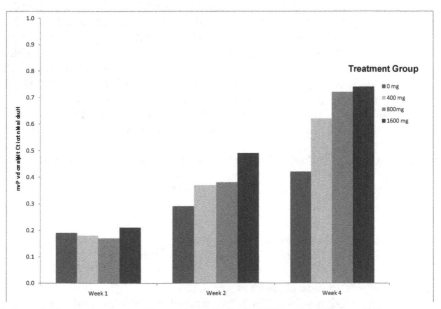

Fig. 7. Cumulative Proportion of Patients with Healed Ulcers by Week and Treatment Group (Final Study Results)

3.3 Other considerations
3.3.1 Bioequivalence trial of two-400 mg tablets and One-800 mg tablet
At the time the duodenal ulcer trial was conducted, there was no commercially available 800 mg C tablet. The commercially available 400 mg C tablet was used. Therefore a blood level trial that demonstrated bioequivalence [Randolph et al, 1986a] between a new 800 mg C tablet formulation (to be marketed) and two-400 mg C commercially available tablets had to be conducted with results available by the completion of the duodenal ulcer trial.

3.3.2 Cimetidine-by-drug interaction trials
Since C was widely prescribed (the prescription leader at the time), a change in dosage regimen, particularly a larger dose, required other trials involving the new 800 mg C regimen. We conducted specific Cimetidine-by-drug interaction trials exploring whether 800 mg C altered the circulating levels of other widely prescribed drugs. The drugs selected were Theophylline [Seaman et al, 1985; Randolph et al, 1986b; Randolph et al, 1986c] and Lidocaine [Frank et al, 1983] and Warfarin [Sax, et al, 1987].

3.3.3 Study in the elderly
At the time the duodenal ulcer trial was conducted, the FDA IND/ NDA rewrite was in progress, which among other specifics, stipulated that pharmaceutical companies should conduct studies in the elderly to explore whether doses of drugs posed a drug dose-by-age interaction. In addition, conducting clinical efficacy trials in the elderly was gaining sway. We actually developed a protocol for a small clinical trial comparing the 800 mg C to Placebo in elderly (age ≥ 65 years) patients with duodenal ulcers. The trial was to enroll 100 patients balanced across the 800 mg C and Placebo groups.

However, prior to starting the trial the author subset the final database for the trial described in this chapter and found it contained 101 elderly patients of which 19 were in the Placebo group and 23 in the 800 mg C group. Randomization in the large trial did not guarantee balance across treatment groups in this subset of elderly patients. Therefore the treatment groups were compared statistically in terms of baseline characteristics, and found to be comparable. Sixteen (16) of 23 (75.6%) elderly patients treated with 800 mg C experienced ulcer healing, as compared to 6 of 19 (32%) in the Placebo group {$\delta = 38\%$; 95% CI = (10.3%;75.6%)}. Since there was evidence in the original trial database that 800 mg C was effective in the elderly, there was no need to conduct a separate clinical efficacy trial in the elderly.

Results from the duodenal ulcer trial, the bioequivalence trial and the Cimetidine-by-drug interaction trials provided the primary data to support filing a supplemental new drug application (SNDA) to the FDA for the approval of C as a single 800 mg tablet taken at bedtime for the treatment of duodenal ulcers.

3.4 Innovative aspects of the clinical trial program
There are several aspects of this program that were rather innovative.

3.4.1 Interim analyses to drop placebo arms
Interim analyses plans that would allow dropping of the placebo arm after establishing efficacy of the doses, while allowing the dose arms to run to completion for dose discrimination, were developed.

3.4.2 Third party blinding during interim analyses

Interim analysis plans that safeguarded company personnel from knowing the identity of investigators, of patients and treatment groups were developed. These included: a. using an outside data management group who generated an analysis data set in which dummy treatment group labels, investigator id and patient id, while preserving the original randomization appeared; and b. having the outside data management group provide the blinded data set to the company statistician and to the FDA plus the file containing the IDs directly to the FDA.

3.4.3 Trial objectives as only three of six pairwise comparisons

The study objective was formulated as only 3 of six pairwise comparisons among the four dose groups while preserving the overall experiment wise Type I error across these three comparisons. The other 3 comparisons could be investigated, preferably using confidence intervals, but they should not invoke a Type I error penalty on the study objective.

3.4.4 Giving up information on center differences

Instead of using centers as a blocking factor in the primary analyses, the 12 classifications of smoking status-by-baseline ulcer size was used as the blocking factor due to small numbers of patients per treatment group per center and due to the prognostic importance of smoking status and baseline ulcer size.

3.4.5 Assessment of type of monitoring by treatment group

An assessment of differences in treatment effect between sites monitored by in-house personnel and those monitored by the CRO was conducted. There was no treatment-by-type of monitoring interaction, although the healing rates were generally lower among CRO monitored sites.

3.4.6 Association between ulcer healing and smoking status and ulcer size

The duodenal ulcer trial definitively established for the first time negative correlations between ulcer healing and smoking and ulcer healing and baseline ulcer size. Effectiveness estimates of ulcer healing were adjusted for smoking status and baseline ulcer size.

3.4.7 Utilization of bivariate graphical methods

The duodenal ulcer trial was the first to utilize bivariate plots to profile ulcer healing and UGI pain relief jointly. The plots illustrated strong dose response in terms of ulcer healing and UGI pain relief separately and jointly.

3.4.8 Establishing effectiveness based on a subset analysis

Efficacy of the 800 mg C dose was established in the elderly based on a subset analysis. The trial entered a large enough elderly population to demonstrate that 800mg C was effective in elderly. That's a plus for conducting a trial larger than necessary to establish the effectiveness of each dose.

3.4.9 Maximum use of patients screened with UGI Pain

The focus of this manuscript has been to review features of the land mark, dose comparison trial of once nightly C in the treatment of duodenal ulcer. This trial was one of three clinical trials comprising a major clinical trial program. Each center conducted three protocols: the one discussed in duodenal ulcer, but also one in gastric ulcer and one in dyspepsia.

Patients were recruited on the basis of having experienced ulcer like symptoms including epigastric UGI pain. Those who satisfied general entry criteria and who gave consent were endoscoped. If duodenal ulcer (DU) was confirmed, they entered the DU trial. If gastric ulcer (GU) was confirmed, they entered a GU trial, and if there was no DU or GU, they entered a dyspepsia trial. This latter protocol provided a rather stringent definition of dyspepsia: Ulcer like symptoms including epigastric UGI pain not explained by the presence of DU or GU. This concurrent protocol method maximized the utility of the advertisement effort to get patients to the clinic who were experiencing ulcer like symptoms.

4. Conclusions

The SNDA clinical trial program that led to approval of clinically optimal dosing of the first H2-receptor antagonist: Cimetidine, in the treatment of duodenal ulcers has been reviewed in detail as a case study. The program included a landmark clinical trial that not only definitively established 800 mg C hs for 4 weeks as the clinically optimal dosing regimen, but also was the first to definitively establish negative associations between ulcer healing and smoking status and ulcer size, as well as the first trial to establish bivariate dose response in terms of ulcer healing and relief of UGI pain. Clinical optimality of 800 mg C hs was defined as 800 mg C being effective as compared to placebo; 800 mg C being more effective than 400 mg C; and 1600 mg C not being more effective than 800 mg C.

In addition, to make maximal use of patients screened, the program included clinical trials of the 800 mg C regimen in dyspepsia and in gastric ulcers. Further, the program also included drug interaction trials of the 800 mg C dose with widely used drugs and a bioequivalence trial of a new 800 mg C tablet compared to two, 400 mg tablets of the commercially available formulation. The bioequivalence trial was required as the clinical trial in DU was conducted using the commercially available 400 mg tablet at the time of study conduct.

Since the development of Cimetidine and other H2-receptor antagonists: Ranitidine (Glaxo), Famotidine (Merck) and Zinatidine (Lilly), and the proton pump inhibitors (e.g. Prilosec and Prevacid) more is known about the causes of ulcers in the duodenum and stomach. It is now widely held that duodenal and gastric ulcers are caused by chronic use of NSAIDS: non-steroidal, anti-inflammatory medications (that decrease endogenous prostaglandin production), and by interference with the protective gastric mucosal layer from *Helicobacter pylori* infection [Thompson et al, 2010]. Current treatment consists of a combination of two antibiotics (clarithromycin and either amoxicillin or a nitroimidazole), and a proton pump inhibitor with the primary aim of eradicating H. Pylori infection [Gisbert et al, 2003]. Bismuth-based regimens are also used for second-line rescue therapy.

5. References

Barakat MH, Menon KN, Badawi AR. Cigarette Smoking and Duodenal Ulcer Healing. *Digestion*; 1984: 29: 85-90.

de Craen AJ, Moerman DE, Heisterkamp SH, Tytgat GN, Tijssen JG, Kleijnen J. Placebo effect in the treatment of duodenal ulcer. *British Journal of Clinical Pharmacology*; 1999: 48(6):853-60.

Dickson, B, Dixon, W, Peace, KE, Putterman, K, Young, MD. Cimetidine Single-Dose Active Duodenal Ulcer Protocol Design. *Post Graduate Medicine*; 1985: 78(8): 23-26.

Gisbert JP, Khorrami S, Calvet X, Gabriel R, Carballo F, Pajares JM. Meta-analysis: proton pump inhibitors vs. H2-receptor antagonists--their efficacy with antibiotics in Helicobacter pylori eradication. *Aliment Pharmacol Ther*. 2003: Oct 15;18(8):757-66).

Frank WO, Seaman JJ, Peace KE, Myerson RM, Humphries TJ. Lidocaine-cimetidine Interaction; *Ann Intern Med*; 1983: 99(3): 414-5.

Korman MG, Shaw RG, Hansky J, Schmidt GT, Stern AI. Influence of Smoking on Healing Rate of Duodenal Ulcer in Response to Cimetidine or High-dose Antacid. *Gastroenterology*; 1981: 80: 1451-1453.

Korman MG, Hansky J, Eaves ER, Schmidt GT. Influence of Cigarette Smoking on Healing and Relapse in Duodenal *Ulcer Disease. Gastroenterology*; 1983: 85: 871-874.

Lam SK, Koo J. Accurate Prediction of Duodenal Ulcer Healing Rate by Discriminant Analysis. *Gastroenterology*; 1983: 85: 403-412.

Nayak PR, Ketteringham JM. Tagamet: Repairing Ulcers without Surgery (*In Breakthroughs*); Rawson Associates, New York: 1986: 102-129.

Peace, KE. Evaluable or Evaluatable? *Biometrics*; 1984: 40(4): 1180-1181

Peace, KE. Dickson, B, Dixon, W, Putterman, K, Young, MD. A Single Nocturnal Dose of Cimetidine in Active Duodenal Ulcer: Statistical Considerations in the Design, Analysis and Interpretation of a Clinical Trial. *Post Graduate Medicine*; 1985: 78(8): 27-33.

Peace, KE. TMO: The Trial Management Organization-A New System for Reducing the Time for Clinical Trials. *Drug Information Journal*; 1990: 24: 257-264.

Peace, KE. One-Sided or Two-Sided p-Values: Which Most Appropriately Address the Question of Drug Efficacy? *Journal of Biopharmaceutical Statistics*; 1991a: 1(l): 133-138.

Peace, KE. Shortening the Time for Clinical Drug Development. *Regulatory Affairs Professionals Journal*; 1991b: 3: 3-22.

Peace KE, Tsai K-T. Bivariate or Composite Plots of Endpoints. *Journal of Biopharmaceutical Statistics*; 2009: 19: 324-331.

Peace KE, DG Chen. Clinical Trial Methodology. Chapman Hall: CRC Press (Taylor Francis), Boca Raton: 2010: 249-270.

Randolph, WC, Peace, KE, Seaman, JJ, Dickson, B, Putterman, K. Bioequivalence of a new 800 mg Cimetidine Tablet with Commercially Available 400 mg Tablets. *Current Therapeutic Research*; 1986a: 39(5): 767-772.

Randolph, WC, Seaman, JJ, Dickson, B, Peace, KE, Frank, WO, Young, MD.: The Effect of Age on Theophylline Steady-State Serum levels and clearance in normal subjects. *British Journal of Clinical Pharmacology*; 1986b: 22(5): 603-60.

Randolph, WC, Peace, KE, Frank, WD, Seaman, JJ. Age-Related Differences in Theophylline Clearance at Steady State. *Journal of the American Society for Clinical Pharmacology and Therapeutics*; 1986c: 39(2): 222-223.

Sax MJ, Randolph W, Peace KE, Chretian S, Frank WO, Gray DR, McCree L, Braverman, AB, Wyle F, Jackson BJ, Beg M. Effect of Cimetidine 800 mg hs and 300 mg q.i.d. on the Pharmaceutics of Warfarin in Patients Receiving Maintenance Warfarin Therapy. *Clinical Pharmacy*; 1987: 6(6): 492-5.

Seaman, J, Randolph, W, Peace, KE, Frank, WO, Dickson, B, Putterman, K, Young, MD. Effects of Two Cimetidine Dosage Regimens on Serum Theophylline Levels. *Post Graduate Medicine*; 1985: 78(8): 47-53.

Thomson ABR, Leung YPY, Devlin SM, Meddings J. Duodenal Ulcers; *eMedicine:* emedicine.medscape.com/article/173727-overview; Accessed Oct. 31, 2010.

Valenzuela, J., Dickson, B., Putterman, K., Young, MD., Dixon, W., Peace, K. E.,. Efficacy of a Single Nocturnal Dose of Cimetidine in Active Duodenal Ulcer: Result of a United States Multicenter Trial. *Post Graduate Medicine*; 1985: 78(8): 34-41.

Young MD, Frank WO, Dickson BD, Peace K, Braverman A, Mounce W. Determining the Optimal Dosage Regimen for H_2-Receptor Antagonist Therapy -- a Dose Validation Approach. *Alimentary Pharmacology & Therapeutics*; 1989: 3(1): 47-57.

Part 2

Treatment and Prevention Strategies of Peptic Ulcer

5

Conventional and Novel Pharmaceutical Dosage Forms on Prevention of Gastric Ulcers

Işık Özgüney
Department of Pharmaceutical Technology
Faculty of Pharmacy, University of Ege
Turkey

1. Introduction

Peptic ulcer formation in either the stomach or duedonum is due to an imbalance between erosive factors such as hydrochloric acid and pepsin and the ability of the gastroduodenal mucosal to protect and heal itself (1). Unlike duedonal ulcers, in which the importance of acid secretion is indisputable, gastric ulcers can develop despite only minimal amounts of acid.

On the other hand, it has become apparent that consumption of nonsteroidal anti-inflammatory drugs (NSAIDs) and stomach colonization by Helicobacter pylori (H.pylori) are the two most common causes of peptic ulcer disease. The prevention and management of NSAID related gastrointestinal (GI) complications are well recognized and in many cases successfully treated. However, the understanding and treatment of H. pylori-induced ulcers are still in progress (2).

2. NSAIDs induced gastric ulcers

NSAIDs are mainly indicated for mild to moderate pain of somatic origin. Due to their anti-inflammatory effect, they are among the agents most frequently used against musculoskeletal and rheumatic disorders throughout the world (3). Other indications include osteoarthritis, soft-tissue injury, renal colic, postoperative pain, and dental procedures. The efficacy of NSAIDs may vary by patient and by indication. In case of inefficacy, substitution by a NSAID from a different chemical class is a reasonable therapeutic option.

In 1899, acetylsalicylic acid was released to the pharmaceutical market (4). Almost 40 years passed before it was realized that aspirin may damage the gastric mucosa (5). Later, drugs having similar effects were recognized and thus termed `aspirin-like drugs' or NSAIDs. The main therapeutic actions proved to be analgesic, antipyretic and anti-inflammatory through inhibition of the cyclooxygenase (COX) enzyme system (6,7). During the past 15 years the number of NSAIDs has doubled. Along with the discovery in 1990 of the inducible form of the cyclooxygenase system, i.e. COX-2 (8), and development of COX-2-specific inhibitors, NSAIDs may now be classified as either (i) non-selective NSAIDs, i.e. aspirin and nonaspirin NSAIDs; (ii) COX-2 preferential inhibitors; and (iii) COX-2-specific inhibitors (coxibs) or COX-1-sparing NSAIDs (9).

NSAIDs may be grouped as salicylates (with as prominent member aspirin itself), arylalkanoic acids (diclofenac, indomethacin, nabumetone, sulindac), 2-arylproprionic acids or profens (ibuprofen, flurbiprofen, ketoprofen, naproxen), N-arylanthranilic acids or fenamic acids (mefenamic acid, meclofenamic acid), pyrazolidine derivates (phenylbutazone), oxicams (piroxicam, meloxicam), sulfonanilides (nimesulide), and others (10). As a group, NSAIDs are structurally diverse and differ in pharmacokinetic and pharmacodynamic properties, but ultimately they share the same mode of action. Like aspirin, nonaspirin NSAIDs inhibit the production of prostaglandins by blocking the COX enzyme, causing analgesic, antipyretic, and anti-inflammatory benefits, but at a risk for increased gastric bleeding (11). Two COX isoforms have been identified and referred as COX-1 and COX-2. The inducible COX-2 is an important regulator to generate prostaglandins that mediate inflammation and pain, whereas the constitutive COX-1 is responsible for maintenance of the integrity of gastric mucosa and platelet aggregation (1).

However, aspirin and nonaspirin NSAIDs differ fundamentally in the way the COX enzyme is inhibited. Aspirin inhibits COX by noncompetitive and irreversible acetylation, where an acetyl group is covalently attached to a serine residue in the active site of the COX enzyme, rendering the COX enzyme permanently inaccessible for the biotransformation of arachidonic acid into PG H_2.

Conversely, nonaspirin NSAIDs competitively and reversibly inhibit the COX enzyme during only part of their dosage interval. This distinction is exemplified by their differential effects on platelet aggregation (10).

The gastroduodenal adverse effects include dyspepsia without endoscopically proven damage, asymptomatic endoscopic lesions of submucosal haemorrhage, erosions and ulcers, and-most important-ulcer complications (3). It is highly likely that the ulcerogenic effects of NSAIDs are directly related to their ability to suppress prostaglandin synthesis in the stomach. Prostaglandins play an important role in the GI tract: they mediate several components of mucosal defence (blood flow, mucus and bicarbonate secretion and mucosal immunocyte function). There is a good correlation between the ability of an NSAID to suppress gastric prostaglandin synthesis and its ulcerogenic action. NSAIDs, including acetyl salicylic acid, also have topical irritant properties that may contribute to their ability to damage the gastric mucosa. The majority of NSAIDs are weak acids with an ionisation constant in the range of 3.5. In the strongly acid environment of gastric juice, drugs are non-ionized and freely cross the cell membrane into the mucosal cells. The elevated intracellular pH promotes dissociation to its ionized form with subsequent intra-epithelial accumulation. The phenomenon of ion trapping and/or ability of these drugs to uncouple oxidative phosphorylation represent two important steps in the topical irritancy of NSAIDs. Thus, intragastric acidic pH plays an important role in the topical or systemic adverse effects of NSAIDs on the gastroduodenal mucosa (12).

Established risk factors for NSAID-associated ulcer complications include patient-specific factors such as advanced age, female gender, a history of peptic ulcer, and drug-specific factors such as the use of non-selective NSAIDs (type, dose, duration, multiple use) and concomitant anticoagulant drugs or corticosteroids. Probable risk factors comprise H.pylori infection and heavy consumption of alcohol, whereas use of selective serotonin re-uptake inhibitors, smoking and a number of other factors have also been proposed to contribute. Knowledge of absolute risk estimates is important for clinical decision making (3).

There is consistently clear evidence that advanced age is a major risk factor for complicated ulcer disease. The risk increases at least linearly with age in both NSAID-unexposed and NSAID-exposed individuals (13,14).

There is good evidence from meta-analysis that males have a two-fold higher risk of ulcer complications compared to females (15). However, among NSAID users, women have both a greater relative risk (RR) than men (RR 5.0 versus. 3.5) (15) and a higher absolute risk, with number needed to harm (NNH) among women being about 50 versus 75 in men (13).

Patients with a history of peptic ulcer have an overall almost six-fold increased risk of ulcer complications (15, 16). Even though the relative risk of NSAID use is lower in patients without a history of ulcers than in patients with a prior ulcer (odds ratio (OR) 5.0 versus 2.5), NSAIDs are still more dangerous (17) due to the higher base-line risk of ulcer complications among the latter.

Heavy alcohol use was found to be associated with an increased risk of bleeding peptic ulcer (18,19). Previous dyspepsia may be associated with an increased risk of ulcer complications (20). NSAID-related dyspepsia is often treated with a proton pump inhibitor to heal a possible underlying ulcer. Some data suggest that the use of H_2-receptor antagonists can mask dyspepsia that may herald an ulcer bleeding. In clinical practice, therefore, proton pump inhibitors are often preferred (3).

The interaction between *H. pylori* and the use of NSAIDs in the development of gastroduodenal ulcers is less clear. *H. pylori* infection and NSAID use may represent independent but synergistic risk factors (21,22). A recent meta-analysis of 21 studies that evaluated the relationship between *H. pylori* and NSAIDs in the development of gastroduodenal ulcers found that the risk for uncomplicated ulcers was 4 times as high in *H. Pylori* positive compared with *H. pylori*-negative patients, irrespective of NSAID use (OR, 4.03), and 3 times as high in NSAID users compared with nonusers, irrespective of *H. pylori* status (OR, 3.10) (22). Furthermore, the risk of uncomplicated ulcers was almost twice as high among *H. pylori*-positive compared with *H. Pylori*-negative NSAID users (OR, 1.81), and 17.5 times higher among *H. pylori*-positive NSAID users compared with *H. pylori*-negative nonusers. Possible explanations for the increased risk of ulcers in *H. pylori*-positive NSAID users are deterioration of the mucosal barrier caused by inflammation, increased acid secretion, a higher level of apoptosis in the infected mucosa, and decreased gastric adaptation to NSAIDs (23).

Patients with rheumatoid arthritis seem to be at increased risk of having ulcer complications compared with patients with osteoarthritis (24). This difference may, however, be explained at least partly by use of higher doses of NSAIDs in patients with rheumatoid arthritis. Some studies have indicated that patients with a history of heart failure are at increased risk of ulcer complications (25). Moreover, recent data suggest that diabetes mellitus may increase the risk as well (20).

Solid evidence from landmark studies (26, 14), and good meta-analyses (15, 16) indicate that the use of ibuprofen and diclofenac is associated with a lower risk of gastroduodenal adverse effects. The use of naproxen, indomethacin and aspirin constitutes an intermediate position, while the use of piroxicam and ketoprofen is associated with a higher risk. Moreover, clear evidence indicates that a high dose of an NSAID is associated with an enhanced risk of ulcer complications in a dose-dependent fashion. (13, 16, 27, 28, 29). Moreover, users of multiple NSAIDs are at the highest risk (OR 9.0; 95% confidence interval (CI), 5.9±13.6) followed by switchers (OR 6.2; 95% CI, 4.7±8.1) compared with single-NSAID users (OR 4.6; 95% CI, 3.9-5.4) (13).

Initially, it was suggested that short duration of NSAID therapy may be associated with a higher risk of ulcer complications (26,30) perhaps explained by gastric adaptation. However, recent cohort studies and meta-analyses indicate that the risk of ulcer complications remains constant during NSAID exposure (15,31,32). After discontinuation of NSAIDs the risk of ulcer complications declines rapidly, however, being increased during 2 months before returning to the base-line level.

Whether patients are exposed to NSAIDs or not, anticoagulants increase the risk of bleeding from pre-existing ulcers because of their antihaemostatic properties. NSAIDs are prescribed to anticoagulant users in about 13% of elderly subjects, and the risk of ulcer complications is heavily increased (Relative risk (RR)12.7, 95% CI, 6.-25.7; excess risk 2.4%; and NNH_{1yr}~40) (33). Anticoagulants alone also increased both the relative and the absolute risk (RR 4.3, 95% CI, 2.6-7.2; excess risk 0.68%; NNH_{1yr} ~147).

One out of seven elderly subjects may use both NSAIDs and corticosteroids (34). Other studies (13) have confirrmed the relationship and estimated that the excess relative risk due to the interaction between NSAIDs and steroids accounts for almost 60% of all cases using both NSAIDs and steroids.

The use of selective serotonin re-uptake inhibitors (SSRI) seemed to increase the risk of upper GI bleeding threefold (OR 3.0; 95% CI, 2.1-4.4) (35). Concomitant use of NSAIDs, however, increased the risk substantially, with an OR of 15.6 (95% CI, 6.6±36.6), suggesting an important interaction between NSAIDs and SSRI.

With the discovery of the 2 COX isoenzymes, COX-1and COX-2, it was hypothesized that the continuous production of local gastroprotective prostaglandins is mainly COX-1 dependent, while the inducible production of inflammatory prostaglandins is mainly COX-2 dependent. Most traditional NSAIDs were found to be nonselective inhibitors of both COX isoforms (36). An ideal NSAID would selectively inhibit the inducible COX-2 isoform, thereby reducing inflammation and pain, without acting on the constitutive COX-1 isoform, thereby minimizing toxicity. On the basis of this hypothesis, several COX-2-selective NSAIDs were developed in the 1990s. Celecoxib (Celebrex®), rofecoxib (Vioxx®), and valdecoxib (Bextra®) received FDA approval for use in rheumatoid arthritis and osteoarthritis, while celecoxib and rofecoxib were also approved for use in acute pain. Two other COX-2 selective NSAIDs, etoricoxib (Arcoxia®) and lumircoxib (Prexige®), received European approval for use in rheumatoid arthritis, osteoarthritis, and acute gout or osteoarthritis, respectively. COX-2-selective NSAIDs demonstrate comparable analgesia and anti-inflammatory effects to nonselective NSAIDs in patients with rheumatoid arthritis and osteoarthritis (36-40). At their defined therapeutic doses, COX-2-selective NSAIDs show at least a 200- to 300-fold selectivity for inhibition of COX-2 over COX-1 (36). Many studies have evaluated the efficacy of COX-2-selective NSAIDs on reducing the risk of NSAID ulcers. In 2000, 2 pivotal outcome studies, the Celecoxib Long-term Arthritis Safety Study (CLASS) and Vioxx Gastrointestinal Outcome Research study (VIGOR), demonstrated that COX-2-selective NSAIDs decrease the risk for both endoscopic NSAID ulcers and serious NSAID ulcer complications when compared with nonselective NSAIDs (41,42).

The Multinational Etoricoxib and Diclofenac Arthritis Long-term program was a pooled intent-to-treat analysis of 3 randomized comparisons of etoricoxib (60 or 90 mg daily) and diclofenac (150 mg daily) in 34,701 rheumatoid arthritis or osteoarthritis patients (43). Overall, GI events were significantly less common with etoricoxib than with diclofenac.

In the Therapeutic Arthritis Research and GI Event Trial, 18,325 osteoarthritis patients were randomized to lumiracoxib 400 mg once daily, naproxen 500 mg twice daily, or ibuprofen

800 mg 3 times daily for 52 weeks (44). In the patients not taking aspirin, the cumulative incidence of serious NSAID ulcer complications (bleeding, perforation, or obstruction) was significantly lower with lumiracoxib than with naproxen or ibuprofen (hazard ratio, 0.21; 95% CI, 0.12 to 0.37). However, there was no significant difference in the patients concurrently taking aspirin. Furthermore, there were more myocardial infarctions with lumiracoxib, especially as compared with naproxen (0.38% versus 0.21%), although the differences were not statistically significant.

Several tentative conclusions may be drawn from these and other studies. First, the use of COX-2-selective NSAIDs significantly reduces the risk of NSAID ulcers and of serious NSAID ulcer complications. However, long-term efficacy remains debatable. Second, concurrent use of low-dose aspirin for primary or secondary prevention of cardiovascular or cerebrovascular disease negates the gastroprotective effect of COX-2-selective NSAIDs. This observation may be directly related to effect of aspirin, which irreversibly blocks COX-1 in the GI tract (45). Third, the use of COX-2-selective NSAIDs increases the risk of myocardial infarction, as compared with the nonselective NSAID naproxen (10). The highly selective COX-2 inhibitors such as rofecoxib showed reduced GI side effects but their possible role in increasing cardiac adverse effects has resulted in the withdrawal of rofecoxib and valdecoxib from the market (1).

3. Strategies to enhance the safety profile of NSAIDs

Two strategies have been employed to enhance the safety profile of NSAIDs: the use of concomitant medication to protect the gastroduodenal mucosa and the development of safer anti-inflammatory drugs: COX-2 selective inhibitors, nitric oxide-donors NSAIDs, phospholipid-coupled NSAIDs, N-enatiomers of NSAIDs (12). The other way to enhance the safety profile of NSAIDs is to use rectal drug delivery systems or modified release formulations. These are less ulcerogenic included methods to reduce topical effects such as enteric coating, rectal administration, or sustained relese oral formulations. It is now well established that the point prevalence of peptic ulcer disease in patients receiving conventional NSAID therapy ranges between 10 and 30%, which is a 10- to 30-fold increase over that found in the general population (46). In a study that examined the prevention of NSAID-related ulcer complications in 8843 arthritis patients, it was reported that, over a 6-month trial period, 0.76% of patients (or 1.5% annually) experienced upper GI complications (25). The US Food and Drug Administration (FDA) similarly estimates that 2-4% of patients taking conventional NSAID for one year experience symptomatic ulcer or potentially life-threatening ulcer complications (47). The Arthritis, Rheumatism and Aging Medical Information Systems (ARAMIS) reported that the overall annual incidence of hospitalization for GI events was 1.3%, the rate was 6 times higher in patients with RA who were taking NSAID than in those who were not (24). Despite a reduction in the rate of hospitalisation (24,48), it has been established that 1 out of 175 users of conventional NSAIDs in the USA will be hospitalised each year for NSAID-induced GI damage (49). The mortality of hospitalised patients remains about 5-10%, with an expected annual death rate of 0.08% (24).

4. Suppository formulations

The advantages of suppositories as conventional formulations compared to other dosage forms are reduction of side effects, such as GI irritation and avoidance of disagreable taste, first pass effect, and undesirable effects of meals on drug absorbtion (50-54). There are indications for using this route of administration such as when the oral administration of medication is difficult due to non-compliance of patient or when GI motility is severely impaired. In addition the oral route can not be used in some patients due to oral or oesophageal injuries or ulceration and in convulsing neonates rectal administration is easier than parenteral or oral administration (55,56).

After dissolving a suppository containing NSAID in the rectal fluids and absorption by the rectal mucosa, the NSAID will be distributed to the various body compartments. The upper haemorrhoidal vein will drain the drug into portal system while the middle and lower haemorrhoidal veins drain it directly into the inferior vena cava which explains why the drug bioavailability may be modified according to the position of the suppository into the rectum. At least a part of the drug absorbed will bypass the liver and its first pass metabolism (which is of great importance for high clearance drugs but not for low clearance drugs such as most of the NSAIDs) will be decreased. It was known that, NSAIDs are variably, but usually well absorbed rectally, thereby reducing the risk of GI ulceration and NSAID suppositories are one approach, besides many others, that is proposed to limit NSAID-induced gastropathy. This proved to be true at least in one study conducted on 45 normal volunteers who received either indomethacin or placebo suppositories, or oral indomethacin. Both suppositories seemed to be better tolerated than oral formulation (57).

Ersmark H. et al. (58) have used in their study piroxicam and indomethacin suppositories for painful coxarthrosis. Six orthopaedic clinics in Sweden made a comparison of the effects and side effects of Piroxicam (20 mg) and Indomethacin (100 mg) suppositories in 261 patients with painful coxarthrosis on the waiting list for total hip replacement. The study was designed as a single blind study over 4 weeks. Amount of pain and range of motion was registered before the trial and compared with findings after 4 weeks, including reported side effects. Both drugs gave satisfactory pain relief without any appreciable variation on weightbearing or at rest. On the other hand, the trial showed a significant difference (p = 0.0033, Student's-test) between the two drugs as regards the frequency of side effects from the lower gastrointest Glinal tract, where piroxicam had a lower rate compared with indomethacin. No serious complications occurred; 16 patients dropped out, 8 in each group.

Carrabba M. et al. (59) compared the local tolerability, safety and efficacy of meloxicam 15 mg suppositories with piroxicam 20 mg suppositories over a 3-week period in a single-blind, randomized study in patients with osteoarthritis. They found that local adverse events occurred in 11.9% of patients receiving piroxicam and 6.9% of those receiving meloxicam. Overall, GI adverse events were the most frequent of all 11.9% of piroxicam-treated patients. In both groups, about 90% of global tolerability assessments were classified, by the investigator and the patient, as either very good or good. They concluded that meloxicam 15 mg suppositories showed excellent local tolerability accompanied by good safety and efficacy in osteoarthritis, which was comparable to that of an established NSAID administered by the rectal route, and to that previously observed with oral formulations of meloxicam 15 mg.

Hatori M. et. al (60) used in their study 231 patients aged 16 to 75 years with osteoarthritis of the knee joint. Each patient received 20 mg of piroxicam daily as a suppository administered before sleep; 75% of the patients were treated for 14 days or longer. Overall treatment outcome was excellent in 34% according to physicians' ratings and in 36% according to the patients' self-ratings, good in 39% and 41%, fair in 22% and 17%, and unimproved in 5% and

7%, respectively. Side effects were reported by 3% of the patients. They concluded that treatment of osteoarthritis with piroxicam suppositories is safe and effective.

Aärynen M. and Palho J. (61) studied with 15 patients having rheumatoid arthritis or osteoarthritis. They received a single dose (20 mg) piroxicam (Felden) as suppository. Serum piroxicam concentrations were assayed by fluorometry 1, 2, 4, and 8 h after the installation of the suppository, the mean values being 1.3, 1.9, 1.8, and 1.8 mg/l, respectively. Then the patients continued on oral piroxicam 20 mg daily for maximum 3 weeks, and serum piroxicam levels (mean 6.3 mg/l) were checked at the end of this period. Nine patients then continued on piroxicam suppositories 20 mg daily for one week, and serum piroxicam levels (mean 4.5 mg/l) were again assayed at the end of this maintenance. Pain at rest, pain on motion, and joint movement restriction were scored on day 1, after oral maintenance, and after rectal maintenance. Reduced scores were found with time, but the only statistically significant effect was in the overall subjective pain relief measured after oral maintenance. Rectal irritation was recorded in one patient. They concluded that a) absorption of piroxicam from suppository was adequate, b) it was possible to maintain adequate serum piroxicam levels by repeated administration of suppository for one week, and c) the GI toleration was acceptable in these patients selected for showing poor tolerance towards other nonsteroidal antiinflammatories.

In a placebo-controlled double-blind trial analgesic effectiveness and tolerability of alpha-methyl-4-(2-thienyl-carbonyl)phenylacetic acid (suprofen, Suprol) 300 mg suppositories were evaluated for 45 informed patients suffering from chronic pain due to osteoarthritis; the subjects were treated rectally, t.i.d., for 10 days. Suprofen proved to be statistically significantly superior to placebo in all the variables considered for evaluation of the analgesic effect, i.e., pain intensity and relief scores, sum of pain intensity differences, total pain relief , global assessments by investigator and patient. In particular, the efficacy of suprofen was judged by the physician good or very good in 86.3% of the patients. Similar frequencies of rectal side-effects were observed in both treatment groups, with slightly but not significantly higher incidence in the group treated with suprofen. Haematologic and clinical chemistry laboratory tests showed no statistically significant alterations due to the treatment (62).

Efficacy and toleration of piroxicam suppositories 20 mg, given once daily for 4 weeks were assessed in 96 patients suffering from degenerative joint disease and 20 patients suffering from rheumatoid arthritis. The mean scores of objective parameters measured (tenderness, swelling, limitation of movement) decreased significantly 2 and 4 weeks after initiation of therapy. Patients' self-evaluation of pain and stiffness also significantly improved during the trial. Overall evaluation of efficacy and toleration were excellent or good in more than 80% of patients. Local toleration was excellent in all but two patients (63).

In a 15 day double-blind clinical trial 39 patients affected with rheumatic disease have been enrolled to evaluate the therapeutic effect of rectal administration of Piroxicam, in comparison with Indomethacin. At the end of the study, 20 patients had been treated with Piroxicam and 19 with Indomethacin. Nine patients in the Indomethacin group and one in the Piroxicam group dropped-out. Both drugs safety resulted good in the patients who completed the study, whereas 5 out of 10 dropped-out patients stopped the trial in consequence of severe side-effects of Indomethacin. Piroxicam induced a very good improvement in 76% of the patients, moderate in 19% and no improvement in 5%; Indomethacin induced a very good improvement in 75% of the patients, moderate in 15% and no improvement in 10%. No significative modifications resulted from the control of the laboratory blood tests. Piroxicam (30 mg/die) showed a therapeutic activity similar to Indomethacin (100 mg/die). The rectal administration of Piroxicam can be then considered a very good alternative to the oral one, particularly in the patients in which oral use of NSAID is counter-indicated (64).

Ketoprofen administered via the rectal route seemed to be valuable when given at night to patients with various rheumatic syndromes and may be particularly useful for patients who show gastric intolerance of the capsules. Anal intolerance was noted in 12% of the patients (65).

The relative risks associated with anti-inflammatory drug prescription for patients with an earlier history of drug-associated gastro-intestinal disturbance have been investigated by Bunton RW. et. al (66) in a retrospective study. Under these circumstances ibuprofen was well tolerated. The risks associated with modified salicylates (principally aspirin in enteric-coated form) and indomethacin suppositories also appeared to be relatively slight.

Together with NSAIDs a lot of other drugs such as alendronate sodium (ALD) have GI side effects. ALD is a bisphosphonate medication used in the treatment and prevention of osteoporosis. Absorption of ALD as oral formulation is very poor (0.5-1%). Its bioavailability can decrease with food effect. It has some GI adverse effects such as gastritis, gastric ulcer, and esophagitis. Asikoglo et al. (67) developed in their study a rectal formulation of ALD as an alternative to oral route and investigated the absorption of it by using gamma scintigraphy. For this reason, ALD was labelled with Technetium-99m (^{99m}Tc) by direct method. They found that the rectal absorption of ^{99m}Tc-ALD from suppository formulation was possible. According to their results, this formulation of ALD can be suggested for the therapy of osteoporosis as an alternative route. Asikoglu et al. (68) developed in another study a vaginal suppository formulation of ALD and they showed that the vaginal absorption of ^{99m}Tc-ALD from suppository formulation was also possible.

It was known that sustained release (SR) suppositories together with suppositories are other important formulations to reduce the GI side effects. In the case of drugs that are rapidly eliminated from the systemic circulation, frequent administration would be needed to maintain the therapeutic plasma concentration. To reduce the frequency of dosing, several approaches have been performed to prepare SR suppositories by using various polymer such as chitosan (69), Eudragit (70-72), cellulose acetate phthalate (73), carboxyvinyl polymer (74), and various hydrogel formulation (75,76), were also investigated. Özgüney et. al. (77) prepared SR suppositories of ketoprofen (KP). Since KP produces gastro-intestinal side effects and its administration rectally is considered as a serious alternative to the oral route (75). KP is an appropriate model drug for formulation of controlled release dosage forms due to its short plasma elimination half-life and poor solubility in unionized water, which affects its bioavailability (78). They designed KP SR suppositories according to the $3^2 \times 2^1$ factorial design as three different KP:Eudragit RL 100 ratios, three particle sizes of prepared granules and two different PEG 400:PEG 6000 ratios. The conventional KP suppositories also prepared with Witepsol H 15, Massa Estarinum B, Cremao and the mixture of PEG 400:PEG 6000. The dissolution studies of suppositories prepared was carried out according to the USP XXIII basket method and it was shown that the dissolution time was sustained to 8 hours. In addition, they determined antiinflammatory activity of SR suppository as significantly extended according to the conventional suppositories.

Güneri et. al. (79) reported that formulation of sustained-release suppositories using ibuprofen-ethylcellulose microspheres was attempted. Ibuprofen was an appropriate candidate for sustained-release formulation because of its short half-life (1.8-2 hrs) and undesired GI effects when it is administrated through oral route, such as peptic ulceration and GI bleeding.

There are a lot of studies on SR suppositories prepared with NSAIDs to reduce their GI side effects (80,81).

Liquid suppository formulations are newer SR suppository formulations according to the conventional suppository formulations. Conventional suppositories are solid forms which often cause discomfort during insertion. The leakage of suppositories from the rectum also gives uncomfortable feelings to the patients. In addition, when the solid suppositories without mucoadhesivity reach the end of the colon, the drugs can undergo the first-pass effect. To solve these problems, Choi et.al. (82) developed a novel in situ-gelling and mucoadhesive acetaminophen liquid suppository with gelation temperature at 30–36°C and suitable gel strength and bioadhesive force. Poloxamer 407 (P407) or/and poloxamer 188 (P188) were used to confer the temperature-sensitive gelation property.The mixtures of P407 (15%) and P188 (15–20%) existed as a liquid at room temperature, but gelled at 30–36°C. They studied bioadhesive polymers such as polyvinylpyrrolidone, hydroxypropylmethylcellulose, hydroxypropylcellulose, carbopol and polycarbophil to modulate the gel strength and the bioadhesive force of acetaminophen liquid suppositories. Choi et. al. (83) showed in their another study that liquid suppository A [P 407:P 188:polycarbophil:acetaminophen (15:19:0.8:2.5%)], which was strongly gelled and mucoadhesive in the rectum, showed more sustained acetaminophen release profile than did other suppositories and gave the most prolonged plasma levels of acetaminophen in vivo. Liquid suppository A also showed higher bioavailibility of acetaminophen than did the conventional formulation and it did not cause any morphological damage to the rectal tissues.

Özguney et. al. (84, 85) prepared a liquid suppository formulation using P407, P188, ketoprofen and various amounts of different bioadhesive polymers (PVP, CMC, HPMC and Carbopol 934 P). Because of the gastro-intestinal side effects ketoprofen was choosen as active ingredient. They investigated the release and mechanical characteristics of the formulations . As to the obtained results of in vitro drug release studies, Carbopol has the bigest effect on release rate among the bioadhesive polymers. It was seen that the release rate decreased with increasing of Carbopol cocentration. The release rate decreased between the formulations having highest or lowest concentrations of Carbopol in percent of 20 at 8. hour.

5. Enteric-coated formulations

Enteric-coated (EC) products are designed to minimize exposure of a drug to the acidic pH in the stomach, which could result in its degradation, or to decrease gastric side effects such as ulcers, perforations and bleeding due to the local effects of the drug on the gastric mucosa. Cellulose acetate phthalate is the polymer most commonly use for enteric coating. The core in such a formulation is coated with this polymer, which does not dissolve at a gastric pH. The dissolution of coating begins at a higher intestinal pH (generally at a pH higher than 5) as the tablet transist out of stomach into the intestine. Generally, the enteric-coated products are tablets. However, small beads or spheroids can be covered with an enteric coating and than these beads can be placed in a hard gelatin capsule (86). Ethylcellulose and cellulose acetate phthalate capsules in the form of Snap-Fit type hard gelatin capsules were developed for controlled release and enteric-coated dosage forms respectively. The capsules were drilled in different diameters by using laser and filled with concentrated drug solution. In vitro and in vivo drug releases were investigated (87). In an another study, the enteric-coated capsules were prepared using hydroxypropylmethyl cellulose phthalate and examined in vitro and in vivo drug releases (88,89).

Although diclofenac sodium (DFNa), is a conventional NSAID, it could be fully utilized without harmful side effects if it was properly formulated (90). When it comes to oral administration of DFNa, at least two requirements should be considered: (a) perfect drug retention under gastric conditions, and (b) sufficient drug release during intestinal residence time. To achieve these requirements, a variety of controlled release formulations for DFNa have already been reported. In terms of pH-responsive matrices, water-soluble matrix tablets containing DFNa coated with hydroxypropyl methylcellulose phthalate (HPMCP) for delayed release of DFNa (91) and DFNa-loaded pH-sensitive microspheres comprising of poly(vinyl alcohol) and poly(acrylic acid) interpenetrating network for the delivery of DFNa to intestines were prepared and evaluated in vitro (92). Novel enteric microcapsules were reported, and in vivo evaluation of dosage forms showed successful pharmacodynamic activities (93).

Due to the necessity to pass intact through the stomach for reaching the duodenum for absorption, the pantoprazole is formulated as solution for intravenous administration (lyophilized powder for reconstitution) or as gastric-resistant tablets (oral delayed-release dosage form). In the case of oral administration, the enteric coating prevents pantoprazole from degradation in the gastric juice (at pH 1–2, pantoprazole degrades in few minutes) (94). As a general rule, the multiple-unit products show large and uniform distribution; they are less affected by pH and there is a minor risk of dose dumping (95). Besides, these new drug delivery systems, as the polymeric microparticles, are also proposed to improve absorption, distribution, and bioavailability of acid labile drugs (96,97). As they rapidly disperse in the GI tract, they can maximize drug absorption, minimize side effects, and reduce variations in gastric emptying rates and intersubject variability (98,99).

Caldwell J.R. et al. (100) compared in their study efficacy and GI tolerability of a new enteric coated formulation of naproxen (NAP-EC) with standard immediate release naproxen (NAP-STD). For this reason one hundred seventy-nine patients with osteoarthritis and one hundred seventy-six patients with rheumatoid arthritis at high risk for developing GI side effects to NSAID therapy were enrolled in a double blind, parallel, multicenter study. All patients had either discontinued as NSAID during the previous one year or required cotreatment with antiulcer drugs for control of GI complaints related to NSAID use. The treatments were evenly divided in both diagnostic cohorts. As to the obtained results of their study, except for minor differences in alcohol consumption, baseline characteristics of patients in both treatment groups were statistically similar. Both naproxen formulations were highly efficacious by all variables of disease activity when changes were measured from baseline. No statistically significant between formulation difference was found in the primary efficacy variable, overall disease activity. Overall, between formulation differences in efficacy measures were few, though most favored NAP-STD. GI complaints were reduced by 15% (51% NAP-EC vs 60% NAP-STD, p = 0.077) and GI complaints thought to be drug related were reduced by 36% (16% NAP-EC vs 25% NAP-STD, p = 0.024). Withdrawals due to GI complaints were reduced by 37% in the NAP-EC group (12% NAP-EC vs 19% NAP-STD, p = 0.054), and withdrawals due to GI complaints judged to be drug related were reduced by 55% in the NAP-EC group (6% NAP-EC vs 12% NAP-STD, p = 0.025). They concluded that enteric coated naproxen is an effective treatment for osteoarthritis and rheumatoid arthritis. All observed differences in GI tolerability favor NAP-EC over NAP-STD.

The damaging effect of enteric-coated and plain naproxen tablets on the gastric mucosa was studied in 12 healthy subjects before and after 7 days' treatment in a randomized, double-blind, double-dummy, cross-over trial. Both formulations of the drug caused mucosal lesions, but the extent of the damage was significantly decreased after enteric-coated naproxen as compared with plain tablets. The subjects' preference was significantly in favour of the enteric-coated naproxen tablets. The plasma naproxen concentration was significantly higher after treatment with enteric-coated naproxen than after treatment with plain tablets. In conclusion, the results of the study indicate that naproxen might damage the gastric mucosa by local and systemic effects and that the local effect might be prevented by enteric coating of the tablets (101).

Aabakken L. et al. (102) studied the GI side effects of three formulations of naproxen in 18 healthy male volunteers. In a Latin-square design crossover study, the subjects received 500 mg naproxen twice daily for 7 days as plain tablets, enteric-coated tablets, or enteric-coated granules in capsules. The 51Cr-EDTA absorption test was performed before and at the end of each drug period, to evaluate changes in the distal gut. The test dose was instilled distally in the duodenum to prevent lesions in the stomach from interfering with the evaluation. Upper endoscopy was performed at the same intervals, scoring changes in the middle and distal duodenum separately from findings in the stomach and duodenal bulb. The nature and severity of adverse effects were recorded for each treatment period. Non-parametric methods were used for statistical evaluation. All drugs induced a significant increase in 51Cr-EDTA absorption, but they did not detect any difference between the three formulations. All formulations were associated with a significant increase in all the endoscopic findings monitored. Enteric-coated tablets induced significantly less lesions than enteric-coated granules in the stomach and duodenal bulb, and an advantage over plain tablets was indicated. No difference was seen in the middle and distal duodenum. The proximal endoscopic scores were not correlated to those found in the middle and distal duodenum. Evaluation of the small and large bowel should probably be included in clinical studies of NSAIDs, but their findings suggest that the importance of transfer of mucosal lesions to the distal gut by enteric coating may have been overemphasized.

The effects of plain and enteric-coated fenoprofen calcium (Nalfon, Dista, Indianapolis, Ind.) on GI microbleeding were studied in 32 normal male volunteers in a randomized, open-label, parallel trial at two inpatient research facilities. A 1-week placebo (baseline) period preceded 2 weeks of fenoprofen therapy (enteric coated or plain, 600 mg q.i.d.). Fecal blood loss was measured by 51Cr-tagged erythrocyte assay and averaged over days 4 to 7 (baseline) and 11 to 14 and 18 to 21 (active therapy). At one center GI irritation was evaluated endoscopically before and after active therapy. Endoscopy showed both formulations to cause mucosal damage not evident by subject-reported symptoms. Four of the 16 subjects developed asymptomatic duodenal ulcers. Mean daily fecal blood loss was significantly lower (P = 0.03) with enteric-coated (mean +/- SD, 1.104 +/- 0.961 ml/day) than with plain fenoprofen calcium (mean +/- SD, 1.686 +/- 0.858 ml/day), suggesting that tolerance of fenoprofen can be improved with administration in an enteric-coated form (103).

When administered on a chronic high-dosage regimen, enteric-coated aspirin granules produced significantly less gastric damage than plain aspirin or aspirin-antacid combinations. Clinically meaningful damage occurred in all subjects receiving plain aspirin, 93% of those receiving aspirin-antacid combination and only 27% and 20% of those receiving enteric-coated aspirin granules qid and bid, respectively. All three aspirin formulations were taken as 1 g qid (4 g/day) and an additional group received enteric granules administered as 2 g bid (4 g/day). Gastric damage was assessed by means of endoscopy carried out after seven days of treatment. Enteric granules are equally safe when administered on a bid or qid regimen (at same total daily dosage) and, in a bid regimen, should provide a compliance advantage for patients on high-dose therapy for diseases such as rheumatoid arthritis (104).

6. Sustained and controlled release formulations

The development of oral sustained and controlled release formulations offers some benefits: controlled administration of a therapeutic dose at the desired delivery rate, constant blood levels of the drug, reduction of side effects, minimization of dosing frequency and enhancement of patient compliance (105).

The basic rationale for the development of controlled drug delivery is to modulate the magnitude and duration of drug action(s), and to dissociate it from the inherent properties of the drug molecule. To enable optimal design of controlled release systems, a thorough understanding of the pharmacokinetics and pharmacodynamics of the drug is necessary.

In many cases, the development of SR dosage forms is somewhat empirical. It is often based on the sole objective of reducing the dosing frequency or fluctuation between peak and trough plasma concentrations (C and Cmax respectively) associated with conventional tablet or capsule formulations. The development process tends to be based on an intuitive pharmacodynamic rationale assuming that the magnitude of response elicited by the drug is closely related to changes in its plasma concentration (106).

In general, almost all drugs cause side effects or have extraneous activity in addition to their primary therapeutic function. An important principle in the design of a proper delivery system for a drug is the conconsideration that each of the pharmacologic effects of the drug has its own pharmacodynamic profile. Furthermore, while a certain pharmacological effect is considered as a therapeutic response,

larger intensities of the same effect are regarded as undesired (and possibly toxic). Thus, an important advantage of SR formulations is that by narrowing the range of drug concentrations (especially, by reducing Cmax levels) the delivery system enables the minimization of the adverse effects associated with elevated drug concentrations. This pharmacodynamic principle has been widely applied as a means to improve drug therapy (107). There are numerous examples to demonstrate modulation of adverse effect of NSAIDs by SR formulations (108-115).

Lipid-based formulations have attracted increasing attention for improvement of bioavailability of hydrophobic drugs in comparison with solid dosage forms (116). In fact, lipid microspheres composed of lecithin and soybean oil were tested as carriers for hydrophobic NSAIDs (117). Unlike many of NSAIDs, DFNa is basically watersoluble at neutral pH, making it difficult to exist in an oil-based formulation. Although self-emulsifying drug delivery system (SEDDS) composed of goat fat and Tween 65 was also applied to diclofenac (90).

Twenty-five inpatients with chronic inflammatory rheumatic disease were entered into a double blind crossover trial. Consecutive treatment regimens consisted of a single daily dose of Bi-Profenid 150 mg at 8 pm for 3 days and a single placebo tablet at 8 pm for 3 days. Order of treatment regimens was randomly assigned. Bi-Profenid proved highly superior to placebo with a very significant (p less than 0.01) difference in effectiveness on nocturnal pain, morning stiffness and pain evaluated on the pain scale. During the short treatment period no significant clinical side-effects were recorded. The authors conclude that Bi-Profenid is effective at a daily dosage of 150 mg, thus enabling to adjust prescriptions to actual needs when pain is not continuous throughout the 24 hours (118).

Schumacher HR. et al. (119) described a new extended-release formulation that maintains therapeutic plasma ketoprofen concentrations for up to 24 hours. A single 200-mg capsule thus provides daytime and nighttime symptom control. Small pellets, enclosed in a gelatin capsule, are released in the stomach but release their contained ketoprofen only after reaching the nonacidic environment of the small intestine. Diurnal fluctuations in plasma concentrations of ketoprofen are reduced, and the drug does not accumulate in plasma with extended use. The half-life of the drug from this dosage form is not significantly affected by the increasing age of the patients. The efficacy of extended-release ketoprofen in British clinical trials has been comparable to that of conventional ketoprofen or naproxen. Safety profiles have been comparable to profiles of other NSAIDs; adverse effects have usually been mild and transient, although, as with other NSAIDs, ulcers and bleeding can occur. Extended-release ketoprofen appears to be a good choice for the symptomatic treatment of rheumatoid arthritis and osteoarthritis. Convenient once-daily administration may help improve patients' compliance.

An open study was carried out in 46 patients with osteoarthritis of the hip to compare the efficacy and tolerance of treatment with ketoprofen given either as 100 mg capsules twice daily or as 2 capsules of 100 mg ketoprofen in a controlled-release formulation given once daily. The results of subjective and objective assessments before and during 3-months' treatment in the 48 patients who completed the trial showed both treatments produced improvement in all parameters, except for the time taken for inactivity stiffness to develop, and there was no significant difference between treatments in terms of efficacy. The controlled-release preparation, however, was significantly better tolerated than the ordinary capsule form. Minor haematological and biochemical changes during treatment were noted but these were not of clinical importance. Six patients, 2 receiving the controlled-release and 4 receiving the ordinary formulation of ketoprofen, were withdrawn because of lack of efficacy or unacceptable side-effects (120).

A multi-centre, double-blind, crossover study was carried out in 80 patients with rheumatoid arthritis to compare the efficacy and side-effect profiles of two formulations of indomethacin. Patients were allocated at random to receive 75 mg indomethacin per day either as 1 controlled-release tablet at night or as 1 immediate-release capsule given 3-times a day for a period of 4 weeks before being crossed over to receive the alternative treatment for a further 4 weeks. Pain scores, daily symptomatology and the requirement for escape analgesia recorded by both investigator and patient indicated that controlled-release indomethacin tablets, 75 mg given at night, was as efficacous as immediate-release indomethacin capsules given 3-times daily. However, the controlled-release formulation had a superior side-effect profile with a reduced incidence of abdominal/epigastric pain compared to the immediate-release preparation (121).

Prichard PJ. et al. (122) have compared acute gastric bleeding caused by a new slow release preparation of indomethacin (indomethacin Continus) with that caused by aspirin and other indomethacin preparations. In a randomized crossover study, blood loss into timed gastric aspirates was determined in 20 healthy volunteers after receiving, over 96 h, either placebo, aspirin (600 mg four times daily; 17 doses) indomethacin BP (50 mg three times daily; 13

doses), Indocid-R (75 mg twice daily; 9 doses) or indomethacin Continus (75 mg twice daily; 9 doses). A venous blood sample was also taken during each treatment period for subsequent determination of alpha 1-glycoprotein, and for drug assay. Gastric bleeding on placebo was 1.4 (0.7-2.8) microliters 10 min-1 (mean, 95% CI). Both aspirin and the indomethacin preparations caused significantly more bleeding (P less than 0.05). Rates of bleeding after aspirin, indomethacin BP, Indocid-R, and indomethacin Continus were respectively 22.0 (10.7-47.2) microliters 10 min-1, 4.4 (2.2-9.1) microliters 10 min-1, 10.8 (5.3-22.3) microliters 10 min-1, and 5.1 (3.0-10.6) microliters 10 min-1. 4. Rates of bleeding after indomethacin BP and indomethacin Continus, but not Indocid-R, were significantly less than after aspirin (P less than 0.01). Salicylate or indomethacin was detectable in the plasma of all subjects after the active treatment periods, except for one instance involving a subject allocated indomethacin BP. Indomethacin levels were significantly higher 2 h after Indocid-R than with indomethacin BP or indomethacin Continus. 6. alpha 1-acid glycoprotein levels were not significantly affected by prior treatment with aspirin or indomethacin.

GI blood loss was measured in 30 healthy male volunteers before and during 4 weeks of oral treatment with either tiaprofenic acid tablets 300 mg twice daily, tiaprofenic acid sustained action (SA) capsules 600 mg once daily, or indomethacin SR capsules 75 mg once daily, in an open parallel-group study of 38 days' duration. Autologous erythrocytes labelled with 51Cr were given intravenously on the first study day. GI blood loss was measured by comparing faecal and red blood cell 51Cr activity during the second and fourth weeks of drug treatment. Blood loss was significantly greater during treatment with all 3 active preparations than during the pretreatment period, but this comparison is of limited value because placebo was not given in parallel and because in 4 subjects, who had to have their erythrocytes relabelled, there was no pretreatment data. The tiaprofenic acid SA group had consistently lower blood loss than the tiaprofenic acid tablet group. Both these groups also had consistently lower blood loss than the indomethacin SR group, although the difference between the treatment groups was not significant. Blood loss during the fourth week of treatment was less than during the second week of treatment for both the tiaprofenic acid SA and indomethacin SR capsule groups. With tiaprofenic acid tablets, blood loss was very similar at weeks 2 and 4 but this result should be viewed with caution because data at week 2 were missing for 3 subjects. Thus, formulation of tiaprofenic acid as a sustained action capsule does not appear to increase gastric irritancy as measured by faecal blood loss (123).

Fourty adult patients with coxarthrosis were treated for 30 days with oral diclofenac sodium at the daily dose of 150 mg: 20 of these were administered one 150 mg prolonged-release capsule per day, the other 20 received one 50 mg enteric-coated tablet every 8 hours. The presence and severity of several symptoms and signs (various pain types, cramps, morning stiffness, impaired function capacity), the intensity of pain through the Visual Analogical Scale and some laboratory tests (Erythrocyte Sedimentation Rate, C-reactive protein, Rheuma test) were controlled to monitor drug efficacy. The routine laboratory tests of blood, liver and kidney function, the GI tolerance of the two administered formulations and the appearance of any adverse event were controlled to monitor drug tolerability. Both administration schemes yielded very positive results as to treatment efficacy, although the prolonged-release capsule often induced a somewhat quicker response. At the end of the one-month treatment more than half of patients in both groups registered disappearance of several symptoms and a noticeable reduction of the remainder ones. Systemic tolerability was also good, with superimposable results in the two groups; GI tolerance on the contrary was better in the recipients of the prolonged-release capsules (2 cases of dyspepsia) with respect to those treated with the enteric-coated tablets (2 cases of gastric pyrosis and 2 cases of gastralgia). No adverse events were registered (124).

A double-blind, double-dummy, crossover study was carried out in 8 centres to compare the efficacy and tolerability of 'controlled-release' ketoprofen tablets (200 mg) with that of indomethacin suppositories (100 mg) in out-patients with definite or classical rheumatoid arthritis. Patients were allocated at random to receive a daily bedtime dose of either 1 ketoprofen tablet or 1 indomethacin suppository plus the dummy of the other formulation for a period of 3 weeks. They were then crossed over to the alternative treatment for a further 3 weeks. Daily diary records were kept by patients of the number of night-time awakenings due to pain, pain severity at awakening in the morning and the duration of early morning stiffness. Treatment efficacy was also assessed at the end of each trial period by means of an articular index and by physician's and patient's overall evaluation of response. Adverse effects spontaneously mentioned by the patients or elicited by direct questioning using a symptom check-list were recorded. Statistical analysis of the results from 83 evaluable patients showed that the 'controlled-release' tablet formulation of 200 mg ketoprofen was equally as effective as the 100 mg indomethacin suppository in the treatment of rheumatoid arthritis, especially with regard to pain at awakening and morning stiffness. Side-effects in both groups were those commonly seen with non-steroidal anti-inflammatory drugs and, as expected, GI and CNS disturbances predominated. Overall, side-effects were fewer with ketoprofen than with indomethacin (125).

There are several histological studies which showes that controlled release formulations of NSAIDs are alternatives for preventing of gastric lesions.

Nishihata T. et al. (126) showed in their study that the increased solubility of sodium diclofenac in a suppository base in the presence of lecithin resulted in a slow release of sodium diclofenac from the base. Rat rectal mucosal damage caused by sodium diclofenac was moderated by the administration of the lecithin suppository, probably due to the low concentration of sodium diclofenac in the rectal fluid due to a slow release of sodium diclofenac from the lecithin suppository.

A mefenamic acid-alginate bead formulation (127, 128) and mefenamic acid spherical agglomerates (129) prepared with various polymethacrylates were developed in different studies and evaluated histologically. Histological studies showed that the administration of mefenamic acid in alginate beads or spherical agglomerates prevented the gastric lesions. Another work reports on a new pharmaceutical formulation for oral delivery of diclofenac sodium (DFNa). Although DFNa itself is water-soluble at neutral pH, it was readily suspended in soybean oil via complex formation with an edible lipophilic surfactant and a matrix protein. The resulting solid-in-oil (S/O) suspension containing stably encapsulated DFNa in an oil phase markedly reduced the risks for GI ulcers upon oral administration even at the LD50 level in rats (ca. 50 mg/kg DFNa) (90).

7. H. pylori induced gastric ulcers

H. pylori is a gram-negative microaerophilic non-invasive spiral bacillus which has the ability to colonize the gastric mucosa (130). It causes indolent but chronic inflammation in the gastric mucosa and its clinical course is highly variable (131). It has a powerful urease enzyme which catalyses hydrolysis of urea to ammonia, enabling the bacteria to survive in the acid milieu. Although it induces a strong host local and systemic immune response (which is important in pathogenesis) it has also developed mechanisms to evade host immunity. This means that following initial infection, which usually occurs in childhood, it is able to persist lifelong in the absence of effective treatment. This persistent infection and inflammation underlies disease, which usually occurs in adults. Worldwide, H. pylori colonizes >50% of the population and is by far the most important cause of peptic ulcers and gastric adeno-carcinoma. Its prevalence varies from more than 80% in developing countries to less than 20% in some developed countries, where it is steadily falling due to improved hygiene and sanitation, and possibly increased antibiotic use.

Only about 15% of individuals infected with H. pylori develop a peptic ulcer: who develops disease depends on bacterial, host and environmental factors (130). The infection is usually limited to the antrum, resulting in hypersecretion of acid and the development of duodenal ulcers, which is basically an acid injury. However, the infection sometimes spreads proximally, causing diffuse inflammatory damage to the gastric mucosa in the body of the stomach and resulting in a gastric ulcer. The inflammation induced by H. Pylori damages the natural defence of the gastric mucosa (131).

The risk of ulceration is higher with more virulent strains. The best-described virulence determinants are expression of active forms of a vacuolating cytotoxin (VacA) (132) and possession of a protein secretory apparatus called Cag (cytoxin-associated gene products) that stimulates the host inflammatory response (133). Cag+ strains interact more closely with epithelial cells and induce release of pro-inflammatory cytokines, thereby increasing inflammation. Host genetic susceptibility and environmental factors may affect the risk; for example, smoking is strongly associated with peptic ulceration in H. pylori-infected individuals (134). H. pylori-induced duodenal ulceration arises in people with antral-predominant gastritis (135). Gastric ulceration occurs on a background of pangastritis, often arising at the highly inflamed transitional zone between antrum and pylorus, particularly on the lesser curve. Identical hormonal changes occur, but acid production from the inflamed corpus is reduced or normal.

H. pylori appears to be responsible for 95% of the cases of gastritis and 65% of gastric ulcers (136). Although most individuals with H. pylori are asymptomatic, there is now convincing evidence that this bacterium is the major etiologic factor in chronic dyspepsia, H. pylori-positive duodenal and gastric ulcers and gastric malignancy (137, 138). Consequently, H. pylori eradication is now recognized to be the correct approach along with conventional therapies in the treatment of the disease. Options that have been considered to treat peptic ulcer disease include taking drugs such as antacids, H -blockers, antimuscarinics, proton pump inhibitors and combination therapy for gastritis associated with H. pylori. The eradication of H. pylori is limited by its principle unique characteristics. Once acquired, it penetrates the gastric mucus layer and fixes itself to various phospholipids and glycolipids on the epithelial surface, including phosphatidylethanolamine (139), GM3 ganglioside (140) and Lews antigen (141). For effective H. pylori eradication, therapeutic agents have to penetrate the gastric mucus layer to disrupt and inhibit the mechanism of colonization. This requires targeted drug delivery within the stomach environment. Although most antibiotics have very low in-vitro minimum inhibitory concentrations against H. Pylori, no single antibiotics has been able to eradicate this organism effectively. Currently, a drug combination namely "triple therapy" with bismuth salt, metronidazole and either tetracycline or amoxycillin with healing rates of up to 94% has been successfully used (142-144). The principle of triple therapy is to attack H. pylori luminally as well as systemically. The current treatment is based on frequent administration (4 times daily) of individual dosage forms of bismuth, tetracycline and metronidazole (Helidac Therapy, consisting of

262.4 mg bismuth subsalicylate, 500 mg tetracycline and 250 mg metronidazole). The associated limitations are the complex dosing regimen/frequency, large amount of dosage forms and reduced patient compliance. Therefore, a successful therapy not only includes the selection of the right drugs but also the timing and frequency as well as the formulation of the delivery system (2).

8. Dosage forms with prolonged gastric residence time

More than 50% of the pharmaceutical preparations on the market are for oral administration. The advantages of this route include the ease of administration, and avoidance of the pain and discomfort associated with injections. However, for drugs whose target is the stomach, such as antibiotics against H.pylori for local treatment of gastric ulcer, the development of oral drug delivery systems meets with physiological obstacles such as limited residence time and inefficient drug uptake by the gastric mucosa (145). Long-term monotherapy of gastric ulcer patients with amoxycillin is ineffective even at high daily doses, apparently due to limited contact time with the target site when administered in a conventional oral dosage form (138, 146-148).

The degredation of antibiotics in gastric acid may be the other reason of ineffectiveness (149). Local diffusion of the drug in the mucosa appears to be essential for achieving bactericidal levels in both healthy subjects (138) and patients: for example, more complete eradication of H. pylori was achieved by applying a new method of topical therapy in which an amoxycillin solution was kept in contact with the stomach for 1 h (150). The development of oral amoxycillin dosage forms with prolonged gastric residence time is therefore an attractive goal. Several strategies have been developed in order to prolong the gastric residence time of dosage forms and target the gastric mucosa, including the use of floating, floating in situ gelling, swelling, expanding and bioadhesive forms (151-156). A new strategy is proposed for the triple drug treatment (tetracycline, metronidazole and bismuth salt) of Helicobacter pylori associated peptic ulcers. The design of the delivery system was based on the swellable asymmetric triple layer tablet approach, with floating feature in order to prolong the gastric retention time of the delivery system. Tetracycline and metronidazole were incorporated into the core layer of the triple-layer matrix for controlled delivery, while bismuth salt could be included in one of the outer layers for instant release. Results demonstrated that sustained delivery of tetracycline and metronidazole over 6-8 h can be easily achieved while the tablet remained afloat. The floating aspect was envisaged to extend the gastric retention time of the designed system to maintain effective localized concentration of tetracycline and metronidazole. The developed delivery system has potential to increase the efficacy of the therapy and improve patient compliance (2).

Floating in situ gelling system of clarithromycin (FIGC) was prepared using gellan as gelling polymer and calcium carbonate as floating agent for potentially treating gastric ulcers, associated with H.pylori. The in vivo H. pylori clearance efficacy of prepared FIGC and clarithromycin suspension following oral administration, to H. pylori infected Mongolian gerbils was examined by polymerase chain reaction (PCR) technique and by a microbial culture method. FIGC showed a significant anti-H. pylori effect than that of clarithromycin suspension. It was concluded that prolonged GI residence time and enhanced clarithromycin stability resulting from the floating in situ gel of clarithromycin might contribute better for complete clearance of H. Pylori (157). Rajinikanth P.S et al. (149) developed in their another study a intra-gastric floating in situ gelling system for controlled delivery of amoxicillin for the treatment of peptic ulcer disease caused by H.pylori. They prepared gellan based amoxicillin floating in situ gelling systems (AFIG). The in vivo H. pylori clearance efficacy of the formulation was examined by the same technique . It showed a significant anti-H. pylori effect in the in vivo gerbil model. It was noted that the required amount of amoxicillin for eradication of H. pylori was 10 times less in AFIG than from the corresponding amoxicillin suspension. The results further substantiated that the prepared AFIG has feasibility of forming rigid gels in the gastric environment and eradicated H. pylori from the GI tract more effectively than amoxicillin suspension because of the prolonged GI residence time of the formulation.

A gastroretentive drug delivery system of DA-6034, a new synthetic flavonoid derivative, for the treatment of gastritis was developed by using effervescent floating matrix system (EFMS). The therapeutic limitations ofDA-6034 caused by its low solubility in acidic conditions were overcome by using the EFMS, which was designed to cause tablets to float in gastric fluid and release the drug continuously. The release of DA-6034 from tablets in acidic media was significantly improved by using EFMS, which is attributed to the effect of the solubilizers and the alkalizing agent such as sodium bicarbonate used as gas generating agent. DA-6034 EFMS tablets showed enhanced gastroprotective effects in gastric ulcer-induced beagle dogs, indicating the therapeutic potential of EFMS tablets for the treatment of gastritis (158).

In another example, it was found that in normal volunteers ionexchange resins achieved excellent distribution in the gastric cavity and had a prolonged gastric residence time, 20-25% remaining for 5.5 h. (155). More recent results by the same group indicate that the mechanism by which resin particles adhere to the mucosa is unlikely to be chargebased, since they persist in the stomach regardless of whether they bear a non-adhesive polymer coating and regardless of whether the stomach contains food (156). Other authors have recently shown that ion-exchange resins also interact with other mucosal surfaces, such as the nasal mucosa (159). Because of this reason, microparticles consisting of amoxycillin-loaded ion-exchange resin encapsulated in mucoadhesive polymers (polycarbophil and Carbopol 934) were prepared.

As reported in this review, the drug delivery systems have an important role on prevention of NSAID related or H.pylori induced gastric ulcers.

9. References

[1] H. Lu, D. Y. Graham. New development in the mechanistic understanding of peptic ulcer diseases. Drug Discovery Today: Disease Mechanisms 2006; 3(4): 431-437.

[2] L. Yanga, J. Eshraghib, R. Fassihia. A new intragastric delivery system for the treatment of Helicobacter pylori associated gastric ulcer: in vitro evaluation. Journal of Controlled Release 1999; 57: 215–222.

[3] C. Aalykke, K. Lauritsen. Epidemiology of NSAID-related gastroduodenal mucosal injury. Best Practice & Research Clinical Gastroenterology 2001; 15(5): 705-722.

[4] H. Dreser. Pharmacologisches Uber Aspirin (Acetylsalicylsaure). Pflügers Archiv 1899; 76: 306-318.

[5] A.H. Douthwaite & SAM Lintott. Gastroscopic observations of the effect of aspirin and certain other substances on the stomach. Lancet 1938; 2: 1222-1225.

[6] J.R. Vane. Inhibition of prostaglandin synthesis as a mechanism of action for aspirin-like drugs. Nature New Biology 1971; 231: 232-235.

[7] J.R. Vane JR & R.M. Botting. Mechanism of action of nonsteroidal anti-inflammatory drugs. American Journal of Medicine 1998; 104: 2S-8S.

[8] J.Y. Fu, J.L. Masferrer, K. Seibert et al. The induction and suppression of prostaglandin H$_2$ synthase (cyclooxygenase) in human monocytes. Journal of Biological Chemistry 1990; 265: 16 737-16 740.

[9] C.J. Hawkey. COX-2 inhibitors. Lancet 1999; 353: 307-314.

[10] H.E. Vonkeman, Mart A.F.J. van de Laar. Nonsteroidal Anti-Inflammatory Drugs: Adverse Effects andTheir Prevention. Semin Arthritis Rheum. 2010; 39: 294-312.

[11] R. Flower, R. Gryglewski, K. Herbaczynska-Cedro, J.R. Vane. Effects of anti-inflammatory drugs on prostaglandin biosynthesis. Nat New Biol 1972; 238:104-106.

[12] M. Lazzaroni, G. Bianchi Porro. Prophylaxis and treatment of non-steroidal anti-inflammatory drug-induced upper gastrointestinal side effects. Digest Liver Dis 2001; 33 (Suppl 2): 544-558.

[13] S.P. Gutthann, L.A. Garcia Rodriguez & D.S. Raiford. Individual nonsteroidal antiinflammatory drugs and other risk factors for upper gastrointestinal bleeding and perforation. Epidemiology 1997; 8: 18-24.

[14] L.A. Garcia Rodriguez & H. Jick. Risk of upper gastrointestinal bleeding and perforation associated with individual non-steroidal anti-inflammatory drugs. Lancet 1994; 343: 769-772.

[15] S. Hernandez-Diaz & L.A. Rodriguez. Association between nonsteroidal anti-inflammatory drugs and upper gastrointestinal tract bleeding/perforation: an overview of epidemiology. Archives of Internal Medicine 2000; 160: 2093-2099.

[16] D. Henry, L.L. Lim, R.L. Garcia et al. Variability in risk of gastrointestinal complications with individual non-steroidal anti-inflammatory drugs: results of a collaborative meta-analysis. British Medical Journal 1996; 312: 1563-1566.

[17] M.R. Griffin. Epidemiology of nonsteroidal anti-inflammatory drug-associated gastrointestinal injury. American Journal of Medicine 1998; 104: 23S-29S.

[18] D.W. Kaufman, J.P. Kelly, B.E. Wiholm et al. The risk of acute major upper gastrointestinal bleeding among users of aspirin and ibuprofen at various levels of alcohol consumption. American Journal of Gastroenterology 1999; 94: 3189-3196.

[19] J.P. Kelly, D.W. Kaufman, R.S. Koff et al. Alcohol consumption and the risk of major upper gastrointestinal bleeding. American Journal of Gastroenterology 1995; 90: 1058-1064.

[20] J. Weil, M.J. Langman & P. Wainwright. Peptic ulcer bleeding: accessory risk factors and interactions with non-steroidal anti-inflammatory drugs. Gut 2000; 46: 27-31.

[21] J.Q. Huang, S. Sridhar, R.H. Hunt. Role of Helicobacter pylori infection and non-steroidal anti-inflammatory drugs in peptic ulcer disease: a meta-analysis. Lancet 2002;359: 14-22.

[22] G.V. Papatheodoridis, S. Sougioultzis, A.J. Archimandritis. Effects of Helicobacter pylori and nonsteroidal anti-inflammatory drugs on peptic ulcer disease: a systematic review. Clin Gastroenterol Hepatol 2006; 4: 130-142.

[23] P. Malfertheiner, J. Labenz. Does Helicobacter pylori status affect nonsteroidal anti-inflammatory drug-associated gastroduodenal pathology? Am J Med 1998; 104: 35-40S.

[24] G. Singh & G. Triadafilopoulos. Epidemiology of NSAID induced gastrointestinal complications. Journal of Rheumatology 1999; 26 (supplement 56): 18-24.

[25] F.E. Silverstein, D.Y. Graham, J.R. Senior et al. Misoprostol reduces serious gastrointestinal complications in patients with rheumatoid arthritis recieving nonsteroidal anti-inflammatory drugs. A randomized, double-blind, placebo-controlled trial. Annals of Internal Medicine 1995; 123: 241-249.

[26] M.J.S. Langman, J. Weil, P. Wainwright et al. Risks of bleeding peptic ulcer associated with individual non-steroidal anti-inflammatory drugs. Lancet 1994; 343: 1075-1078.

[27] J.L. Carson, B.L. Strom, K.A. Soper et al. The association of nonsteroidal anti-inflammatory drugs with upper gastrointestinal tract bleeding. Archives of Internal Medicine 1987; 147: 85-88.

[28] M.R. Griffin, J.M. Piper, J.R. Daugherty et al. Nonsteroidal anti-inflammatory drug use and increased risk for peptic ulcer disease in eldery persons. Annals of Internal Medicine 1991; 114: 257-263.

[29] D. Henry, A. Robson & C. Turner. Variability in the risk of major gastrointestinal complications from nonaspirin nonsteroidal anti-inflammatory drugs. Gastroenterology 1993; 105: 1078-1088.

[30] S.E. Gabriel, L. Jaakkimainen & C. Bombardier. Risk for serious gastrointestinal complications related to use of nonsteroidal anti-inflammatory drugs. A meta-analysis. Annals of Internal Medicine 1991; 115: 787-796.

[31] T.M. MacDonald, S.V. Morant, G.C. Robinson et al. Association of upper gastrointestinal toxicity of non-steroidal anti-inflammatory drugs with continued exposure: cohort study. British Medical Journal 1997; 315: 1333-1337.

[32] G. Singh. Recent considerations in nonsteroidal anti-inflammatory drug gastropathy. American Journal of Medicine 1998; 105: 31S-38S.

[33] R.I. Shorr, W.A. Ray, J.R. Daugherty & M.R. Griffin. Concurrent use of nonsteroidal anti-inflammatory drugs and oral anticoagulants places elderly persons at high risk for hemorrhagic peptic ulcer disease. Archives of Internal Medicine 1993; 153: 1665-1670.

[34] J.M. Piper, W.A. Ray, J.R. Daugherty & M.R. Griffin. Corticosteroid use and peptic ulcer disease: role of nonsteroidal anti-inflammatory drugs. Annals of Internal Medicine 1991; 114: 735-740.

[35] F.J. De Abajo, L.A. Rodriguez & D. Montero. Association between selective serotonin reuptake inhibitors and upper gastrointestinal bleeding: population based case-control study. British Medical Journal 1999; 319: 1106-1109.

[36] G.A. FitzGerald, C. Patrono. The coxibs, selective inhibitors of cyclooxygenase-2. N Engl J Med 2001; 345: 433-442.

[37] P. Emery , H. Zeidler, T.K. Kvien, M. Guslandi, R. Naudin, H. Stead, et al. Celecoxib versus diclofenac in long-term management of rheumatoid arthritis: randomised double-blind comparison. Lancet 1999; 354: 2106-2111.

[38] G.W. Cannon, J.R. Caldwell, P. Holt, B. McLean, B. Seidenberg, J. Bolognese et al. Rofecoxib, a specific inhibitor of cyclooxygenase 2, with clinical efficacy comparable with that of diclofenac sodium: results of a one-year, randomized, clinical trial in patients with osteoarthritis of the knee and hip. Rofecoxib Phase III Protocol 035 Study Group. Arthritis Rheum 2000; 43: 978-987.

[39] W. Bensen, A. Weaver, L. Espinoza, W.W. Zhao, W. Riley, B. Paperiello et al. Efficacy and safety of valdecoxib in treating the signs and symptoms of rheumatoid arthritis: a randomized, controlled comparison with placebo and naproxen. Rheumatology (Oxford) 2002;41: 1008-1016.

[40] C.W. Wiesenhutter, J.A. Boice, A. Ko, E.A. Sheldon, F.T. Murphy, B.A. Wittmer et al. Evaluation of the comparative efficacy of etoricoxib and ibuprofen for treatment of patients with osteoarthritis: a randomized, double-blind, placebo-controlled trial. Mayo Clin Proc 2005; 80: 470-479.

[41] F.E. Silverstein, G. Faich, J.L. Goldstein, L.S. Simon, T. Pincus, A. Whelton et al. Gastrointestinal toxicity with celecoxib vs nonsteroidal anti-inflammatory drugs for osteoarthritis and rheumatoid arthritis. The CLASS study: a randomized controlled trial. JAMA 2000; 284: 1247-1255.

[42] C. Bombardier, L. Laine, A. Reicin, D. Shapiro, R . Burgos-Vargas, B. Davies et al. Comparison of upper gastrointestinal toxicity of rofecoxib and naproxen in patients with rheumatoid arthritis. VIGOR Study Group. N Engl J Med 2000; 343: 1520-1528.

[43] L. Laine, S.P. Curtis, B. Cryer, A. Kaur, C.P. Cannon. Assessment of upper gastrointestinal safety of etoricoxib and diclofenac in patients with osteoarthritis and rheumatoid arthritis in the Multinational Etoricoxib and Diclofenac Arthritis Long-term (MEDAL) programme: a randomised comparison. Lancet 2007; 369: 465-473.

[44] T.J. Schnitzer, G.R. Burmester, E. Mysler, M.C. Hochberg, M. Doherty, E. Ehrsam et al. Comparison of lumiracoxib with naproxen and ibuprofen in the Therapeutic Arthritis Research and Gastrointestinal Event Trial (TARGET), reduction in ulcer complications:randomised controlled trial. Lancet 2004; 364: 665-674.

[45] B. Cryer, M. Feldman. Effect of very low dose daily, long-term aspirin therapy on gastric, duodenal, and rectal prostaglandin levels and on mucosal injury in healthy humans. Gastroenterology 1999; 117: 17-25.

[46] J. Kremer. From prostaglandin replacement to specific COX-2 inhibition. A critical appraisal. J Rheumatol 2000; 27(Suppl 60): 9-12.

[47] H.E. Paulus. FDA Arthritis Advisory Committee meeting: serious gastrointestinal toxicity of non-steroidal anti-inflammatory drugs. Arthritis Rheumatol 1988; 31: 1450-1451.

[48] M.M. Wolfe, D.R. Lichtenstein, G. Singh. Gastrointestinal toxicity of non-steroidal anti-inflammatory drugs. N Engl J Med 1999; 340: 1888-1899.

[49] J.F. Fries. NSAID gastropathy, epidemiology. J Musculoskel Med 1991; 8: 21-28.

[50] T. Umeda, A. Matsuzawa, T. Yokoyama, K. Kuroda, T. Kuroda. Studies on sustained release dosage forms. I. preparation of indomethacin suppositories. Chem. Pharm. Bull. 1983; 31: 2793-2798.

[51] T. Nakajima, Y. Takashima, K. Iida, H. Mitsuta, M. Koishi. Preparation and in vitro evaluation of sustained-release suppositories containing microencapsulated indomethacin. Chem. Pharm. Bull. 1987; 35: 1201-1206.

[52] A.G. de Boer, D.D. Breimer, H. Mattie, J. Pronk, J.M. Gubbens-Stibble. Rectal bioavailability of lidocaine in man: partial avoidance of "first-pass"metabolism. Clin. Pharmacol. Ther. 1979; 26: 701-709.

[53] A.G. de Boer, F. Moolenaar, L.G.J. de Leede, D.D. Breimer. Rectal drug administration: clinical pharmacokinetics consideration. Clin. Pharmacokin. 1982; 7: 285-311.

[54] T. Takatori, N. Shimono, K. Higaki, T. Kimura. Evaluation of sustained release suppositories prepared with fatty base including solid fats with high melting points. Int. J. Pharm. 2004; 278: 275-282.

[55] C. King. Rectal drug administration. Journal of Equine Veterinary Science 1994; 14: 521-526.

[56] S. Corveleyna, D. Henrısta, J. P. Remona, G. VAN DER Wekenb, W. Baeyensb, J. Haustraeteb, H. Y. ABOUL-Eneınc, B. Sustronckd, P. DEPREZ. Bioavailability of racemic ketoprofen in healthy horses following rectal administration. Research in veterinary science. 1999; 67 (2): 203-204.

[57] J. P. Famaey. Suppositories for Arthritis. Clinical rheumatology 1992; 11 (1): 26-27.

[58] H. Ersmark, B. Tjornstrand, G. Gudmundsson, H. Düppe, M. Fagerlund, B. Jacobsson, G. Ordeberg, L. Wallinder. Piroxicam and indometacin suppositories for painful coxarthrosis. Clinical rheumatology 1992; 11(1): 37-40.

[59] M. Carrabba, E. Paresce, M. Angelini, A. Galanti, MG. Marini, P. Cigarini. A comparison of the local tolerability, safety and efficacy of meloxicam and piroxicam suppositories in patients with osteoarthritis: a single-blind, randomized, multicentre study. Curr Med Res Opin 1995; 13(6): 343-355 Erratum in: Curr Med Res Opin 1996; 13(7): 427-428.

[60] M. Hatori, M. Sakurai , S. Kokubun, KP. Rijal. Piroxicam suppositories in the treatment of osteoarthritis of the knee joint. Clin Ther. 1990; 12(3): 227-229.

[61] M. Aärynen, J. Palho. Piroxicam capsules versus suppositories: a pharmacokinetic and clinical trial. Arzneimittelforschung 1986; 36(4): 744-747.

[62] M. Viara, V. Menicanti, M. Nebiolo, N. Michos, C. Sarchi. Double-blind placebo-controlled study of the efficacy and tolerability of suprofen suppositories in patients with osteoarthritic pain. Arzneimittelforschung 1986; 36(7): 1113-1115.

[63] G. Heynen, P. Dessain, Piroxicam suppositories for osteoarthritis and rheumatoid arthritis: an open multicentre study in 116 patients. Eur J Rheumatol Inflamm. 1983; 6(1): 134-138.

[64] F. Maccà, L. Milani, M. Dal Follo, L. Corbetta, G. Zeni, R. Zuin. Therapeutic action of Piroxicam administered rectally in rheumatic diseases. Controlled double-blind study. Minerva Med. 1984; 75(14-15): 811-819.

[65] A. Fournie, C. Ayrolles. A clinical study of ketoprofen suppositories. Rheumatol Rehabil. 1976; Suppl:59-60.

[66] R.W. Bunton, D.C. Barrett , D.G. Palmer. Reintroduction of anti-inflammatory drug therapy after drug-associated gastro-intestinal disturbances. N Z Med J. 1982; 95(714): 582-584.

[67] M. Aşıkoğlu, I. Özgüney, İ. Özcan, O. Örümlü, T. Güneri, K. Köseoğlu, H. Özkılıç. The absorption of 99mTc-alendronate given by rectal route in rabbits. Pharmaceutical Development and Technology 2008; 13(3): 213-20.

[68] M. Aşıkoğlu, D. İlem, T. Güneri, K. Köseoğlu. Intravaginal Administration of Tc[99m]-ALD sodium. 14th International Pharmaceutical Technology Symposium, 8-10 September 2008; P-60, pp: 233-236, Antalya/Turkey.

[69] D. Ermiş, N. Tarımcı. Sustained release characteristics and pharmacokinetic parameters of ketoprofen suppositories using chitosan. Int. J. Pharm. 1997; 147: 71-77.

[70] D. Ermiş, N. Tarımcı. Preparation and in vitro evaluation of sustained release suppositories of indometacine. Ankara Ecz. Fak. Derg. 1998; 27: 11-21.

[71] G.S. Arra, S.A. Biswanath, D.R. Krishna, S. Arutla, A.K. Bandyopadhyay. Development and Evalution of Micropelleted Sustained-Release Suppositories of Terbutaline Sulfate. Drug Dev. Ind. Pharm. 1997; 23: 1233-1237.

[72] N. , T. Yokoyama, Y. Kiyohara, K. Okumura, K. Kuroda. Evalution of Indomethacin Sustained-Release Suppositories Prepared with a Methacrylic Acid-Methacrylic Asid Methyl Ester Copolymer-Polyethylene Glycol 2000 Solid Matrix. Chem. Pharm. Bull. 1988; 36: 430-434.

[73] T. Umeda, T. Yokoyama, N. Ohnishi, T. Kuroda, Y. Kita, K. Kuroda, S. Asada. Studies on Sustained-Release Dosage Forms. III. Preparation of Nifedipine Suppositories and Bioavailability in Rabbits. Chem. Pharm. Bull. 1985; 33: 3953-3959.

[74] Y. Azechi, K. Ishikawa, N. Mizuno, K. Takahashi. Sustained release of diclofenac from polymer-containing suppository and the mechanism involved. Drug Dev. Ind. Pharm. 2000; 26: 1177-1183.

[75] D. Ermiş, N. Tarımcı. Ketoprofen sustained-release suppositories containing hydroxypropylmethylcellulose phthalate in polyethylene glycol bases. Int. J. Pharm. 1995; 113: 65-71.

[76] N. Ohnishi, T. Yokoyama, T. Umeda, Y. Kiyohara, T. Kuroda, Y. Kita, K. Kuroda. Preparation of sustained-release suppositories of indomethacin using a solid dispersion system and evalution of bioavailability in rabbits. Chem. Pharm. Bull. 1986; 34: 2999-3004.

[77] I.Özgüney (Sarıgüllü), İ.Özcan, G. Ertan, T. Güneri. The preparation and evaluation of ketoprofen containing Eudragit RL 100 sustained release suppositories with factorial design. Pharmaceutical Development and Technology 2007; 12: 97-107.

[78] M.L. Vueba, L.A.E. Batista de Carvalho, F. Viega, J.J. Sousa, M.E. Pina. Influence of cellulose ether polymers on ketoprofen release from hydrophilic matrix tablets. Eur. J. Pharm. Biopharm. 2004; 58: 51-59.

[79] T. Güneri, M. Arıcı, G. Ertan Preparation and diffusional evaluation of sustained-release suppositories containing ibuprofen microspheres. FABAD J. Pharm. Sci., 2004; 29: 177-184.

[80] G. Uzunkaya, N. Bergişadi. In vitro drug liberation and kinetics of sustained release indomethacin suppository. Il Farmaco 2003; 58: 509-512.

[81] T. Kuroda , T. Yokoyama, T. Umeda , A. Matsuzawa , K. Kuroda, S. Asuda. Studies on sustained-release dosage forms. II. Pharmacokinetics after rectal administration of indomethacin suppositories in rabbits. Chem. Pharm. Bull. 1982; 31: 3319-3325.

[82] H.G. Choi, J.H. Jung , J.M. Ryu, S.J. Yoon, Y.K. Oh, C.K. Kim. Development of in situ-gelling and mucoadhesive acetaminophen liquid suppository. International Journal of Pharmaceutics 1998; 165: 33–44.

[83] H.G. Choi, Y.K. Oh, C.K. Kim. In situ gelling and mucoadhesive liquid suppository containing acetaminophen: enhanced bioavailability. International Journal of Pharmaceutics 1998; 165: 23–32.

[84] I. Özgüney, A. Kardhiqi, G. Ertan, T. G.üneri. Development of in situ-gelling and thermosensitive ketoprofen liquid suppositories. Proc. 7th Central European Symposium on Pharmaceutical Technology and Biodelivery Systems, Ljubliana, Slovenia, 2008.

[85] A. Kardhiqi, I. Özgüney. Mechanical properties of in situ-gelling and thermosensitive ketoprofen liquid suppositories. Proc. 15th International Pharmaceutical Technology Symposium, Antalya, Turkey, 2010.

[86] Gibaldi's Drug Delivery Systems In Pharmaceutical Care, Edited by Archana Desai and Mary Lee. Published by American Society of Health-System Pharmacists, Bethesda, MD, 2007.

[87] L. Kırılmaz. Two new suggestions for pharmaceutical dosage forms: ethylcellulose and cellulose acetate phthalate capsules. S.T.P. Pharma Sciences 1993; 3 (5): 374-378.

[88] E. Ö. Çetin, E. Atlıhan, O. Çağlayan, M. Aşıkoğlu, L. Kırılmaz. A new alternative for enteric-coated dosage forms: hydroxypropylmethyl cellulose phthalate capsules. Proc. 11th Pharmaceutical Technology Symposium, İstanbul, Turkey, 2002.

[89] O. Örümlü, E. Ö. Çetin, E. Atlıhan, F.G. Durak, Y.K. Dağdeviren, M. Aşıkoğlu, L. Kırılmaz. A new alternative for enteric-coated dosage forms: In vivo investigation of hydroxypropylmethyl cellulose phthalate capsules. Podium Presentations, The 4 th International Postgraduate Research Symposium on Pharmaceutics, İstanbul, Turkey, Acta Pharmaceutica Turcica Vol.46 Suppl. 2004.

[90] H. Piao, N. Kamiya, J. Watanabe , H. Yokoyama, A. Hirata, T. Fujii, I. Shimizu, S. Ito, M. Goto. Oral delivery of diclofenac sodium using a novel solid-in-oil suspension. International Journal of Pharmaceutics 2006; 313: 159-162.

[91] H.I. Kim, J.H. Park, I.W. Cheong, J.H. Kim. Swelling and drug release behavior of tablets coated with aqueous Hydroxypropylmethylcellulosephthalate (HPMCP) nanoparticles. J. Control. Release 2003; 89: 225-233.

[92] M.D. Kurkuri, T.M. Aminabhavi. Poly (vinyl alcohol) and poly (acrylic acid) sequential interpenetrating network pH-sensitive microspheres for the delivery of diclofenac sodium to the intestine. J. Control. Release 2004; 96: 9-20.

[93] S.S. Biju, S. Saisivam, N.S. Maria, G. Rajan, P.R. Mishra. Dual coated erodible microcapsules for modified release of diclofenac sodium. Eur. J. Pharm. Biopharm. 2004; 58: 61-67.

[94] G.M. Ferron, S. Ku, M.Abell, M. Unruh, J. Getsy, P.R. Mayer, J. Paul. Oral bioavailability of pantoprazole suspended in sodium bicarbonate solution. Am. J. Health Syst. Pharm. 2003; 60 (13): 1324-1329.

[95] S.Y. Lin, Y.H. Kao. Tablet study of spray-dried sodium diclofenac enteric-coated microcapsules. Pharm. Res. 1991; 8 (7): 919-924.

[96] P. O'Donnell, J. McGinity. Preparation of microspheres by the solvent evaporation technique. Adv. Drug Deliv. Rev. 1997; 28: 25-42.

[97] Y. Yamagata, M. Misaki, T. Kurokawa, K. Taira, S. Takada. Preparation of a copoly(DL-lactic/glycolic acid)-zinc oxide complex and its utilization to microcapsules containing recombinant human growth hormone. Int. J. Pharm. 2003; 251: 133-141.

[98] K.A. Mehta, M.S. Kislalioglu, W. Phuapradit, A.W. Malick, N.H. Shah. Release performance of a poorly soluble drug from a novel, Eudragit®-based multi-unit erosion matrix. Int. J. Pharm. 2001; 213: 7-12.

[99] R.P. Raffin, L.M. Colome´, A.R. Pohlmann, S.S. Guterres. Preparation, characterization, and in vivo anti-ulcer evaluation of pantoprazole-loaded microparticles. European Journal of Pharmaceutics and Biopharmaceutics. 2006; 63: 198-204.

[100] J.R. Caldwell, S.H. Roth. A double blind study comparing the efficacy and safety of enteric coated naproxen to naproxen in the management of NSAID intolerant

patients with rheumatoid arthritis and osteoarthritis. Naproxen EC Study Group. J Rheumatol. 1994; 21(4): 689-95.

[101] R.I. Trondstad, E. Aadland, T. Holler, B. Olaussen. Gastroscopic findings after treatment with enteric-coated and plain naproxen tablets in healthy subjects. Scand J Gastroenterol. 1985; 20(2): 239-42.

[102] L. Aabakken, B.A Bjornbeth, B. Hofstad, B. Olaussen, S. Larsen, M. Osnes. Comparison of the gastrointestinal side effects of naproxen formulated as plain tablets, enteric-coated tablets, or enteric-coated granules in capsules. Scand J Gastroenterol Suppl. 1989; 163: 65-73.

[103] J.R. Ryan, W.A. Riley, R. Vargas, W.W Offen, C.M. Gruber. Enteric coating of fenoprofen calcium reduces gastrointestinal microbleeding. Clin Pharmacol Ther. 1987; 42(1): 28-32.

[104] F.L. Lanza, M.F. Rack, G.S. Wagner, T.K. Balm. Reduction in gastric mucosal hemorrhage and ulceration with chronic high-level dosing of enteric-coated aspirin granules two and four times a day. Dig Dis Sci. 1985; 30(6) :509-512.

[105] Y. W. Chien, Controlled- and modulated-release drug-delivery systems. in: J. Swarbrick, J. C. Boylan (Eds). Encyclopedia of Pharmaceutical Technology, Marcel Dekker, New York, 2001; 203-226.

[106] G. Castaneda-Henandez, G. Caille, P. du Souich. Influence of drug formulation on drug concentration–effect relationships. Clin. Pharmacokinet. 1994; 26: 135–143.

[107] A. Hoffman. Pharmacodynamic aspects of sustained release preparations. Advanced Drug Delivery Reviews 1998; 33: 185–199.

[108] A.T. Florence, P.U. Jani, Novel oral formulations: their potential in modulating adverse effects. Drug Safety 1994; 10: 233–266.

[109] F.P. Maesen, J.J. Smeets. Comparison of a controlled-release tablet of salbutamol given twice daily with a standard tablet given four times daily in the management of chronic obstructive lung disease. Eur. J. Clin. Pharmacol. 1986; 31: 431–436.

[110] I. Özgüney (Sarıgüllü), G. Ertan, T. Güneri. Dissolution Characteristics of Megaloporous Tablets Prepared with Two Kinds of Matrix Granules. Il Farmaco 2004; 59(7): 549-555.

[111] E. Karasulu, H. Y. Karasulu, G. Ertan, L. Kırılmaz and T. Güneri. Extended release lipophilic indomethacin microspheres: formulation factors and mathematical equations fitted drug release rates. European Journal of Pharmaceutical Sciences. 2003; 19(2-3); 99-104.

[112] L. Kırılmaz, A. Şahin, Z. Sarçin, F. Taneri. A preliminary investigation on the estimation of the sustained-release of indomethacin from agar beads. Part I., Acta Pharm. Turcica. 1997; XXXIX, (3): 119-132.

[113] L. Yang, R. Fasihsi. Modulation of diclofenac release from a totally soluble controlled release drug delivery system. Journal of Controlled Release 1997: 44 (2-3); 135-140.

[114] J. A. Herrera, A. Millán, R. Ramos, P. Fuentes, M. González. Evaluation of the effectiveness and tolerability of controlled-release diclofenac-potassium versus immediate-release diclofenac-potassium in the treatment of knee osteoarthritis. Current Therapeutic Research 2007; 68(2): 82-93.

[115] M. Halsas, J. Hietala, P. Veski, H. Jürjenson, M. Marvola. Morning versus evening dosing of ibuprofen using conventional and time-controlled release formulations. International Journal of Pharmaceutics. 1999; 189(2,5): 179-185.

[116] C.W. Pouton. Lipid formulations for oral administration of drugs: nonemulsifying, self-emulsifying and 'self-microemulsifying' drug delivery systems. Eur. J. Pharm. Sci. 2000; 11: 93–98.

[117] O. Ohmukai. Lipo-NSAID preparation. Adv. Drug Deliv. Rev. 1996; 20: 203–207.

[118] J.M. Harrewyn, B. Amor. Double-blind comparative study of slow-release ketoprofen and a placebo in chronic inflammatory rheumatism. Sem Hop. 1983; 59(46): 3225-3228.

[119] H.R. Schumacher. Ketoprofen extended-release capsules: a new formulation for the treatment of osteoarthritis and rheumatoid arthritis. Jr Clin Ther. 1994; 16(2): 145-159.

[120] K.D. Morley, R.M. Bernstein, G.R. Hughes, C.M. Black, C.N. Rajapakse, L.A. Wilson. Comparative trial of a controlled-release formulation of ketoprofen ('Oruvail') and a conventional capsule formulation of ketoprofen ('Orudis') in patients with osteoarthritis of the hip. Curr Med Res Opin. 1984; 9(1): 28-34.

[121] P. Bacon, R.A. Luqmani, C. Barry, D. Foley-Nolan, R. Grahame, J. West, B.L. Hazleman, A.O. Adebajo, G.R. Hughes, M. Abdullah et al. A comparison of two formulations of indomethacin ('Flexin Continus' tablets and 'Indocid' capsules) in the treatment of rheumatoid arthritis. Curr Med Res Opin. 1990; 12(2): 121-127. Erratum in: Curr Med Res Opin 1990; 12(3): 142.

[122] P.J. Prichard, T.J. Poniatowska, J.E. Willars, A.T. Ravenscroft, C.J. Hawkey. Effect in man of aspirin, standard indomethacin, and sustained release indomethacin preparations on gastric bleeding. Br J Clin Pharmacol. 1988; 26(2): 167-72.

[123] S.J. Warrington, J. Dana-Haeri, M.A. Horton, E.J. Thornton. Drugs Comparison of gastrointestinal blood loss in healthy male volunteers during repeated administration of standard and sustained action tiaprofenic acid and sustained release indomethacin. Drugs 1988; 35 Suppl 1: 90-94.

[124] C. Varese, A. Palazzini. Open study of a diclofenac sodium prolonged-release in patients suffering from coxarthrosis. Eur Rev Med Pharmacol Sci. 1997; 1(1-3): 57-62.

[125] P. Uddenfeldt, I. Leden, B. Rubin. A double-blind comparison of oral ketoprofen 'controlled release' and indomethacin suppository in the treatment of rheumatoid arthritis with special regard to morning stiffness and pain on awakening. Curr Med Res Opin. 1993; 13(3): 127-32.

[126] T. Nishihata, H. Wada, A. Kamada. Sustained-release of sodium diclofenac from suppository. International Journal of Pharmaceutics 1985: 27 (2-3): 245-253.

[127] F. Sevgi, B. Kaynarsoy, G. Ertan. An anti-inflammatory drug (mefenamic acid) incorporated in biodegradable alginate beads: development and optimization of the process using factorial design. Pharm Dev Technol. 2008; 13(1): 5-13.

[128] F. Sevgi, B. Kaynarsoy, M. Özyazıcı, C. Pekçetin and D. Özyurt. A Comparative Histological Study of Alginate Beads as a Promising Controlled Release Delivery for Mefenamic Acid. Pharmaceutical Development and Technology 2008; 13: 387-392.

[129] M. Özyazıcı, F. Sevgi, C. Pekçetin, B. Sarpaş and Ş. Sayın. Sustained release spherical agglomerates of polymethacrylates containing mefenamic acid: in vitro release, micromeritic properties and histological studies. Pharmaceutical Development and Technology (In Press). (doi: 10.3109/10837450.2010.550621).

[130] D. Majumdar, J. Bebb, J. Atherton. Helicobacter pylori infection and peptic ulcers. Medicine. 2007; 35 (4): 204-209.

[131] L. H. Lai, J. J.Y. Sung. Helicobacter pylori and benign upper digestive disease. Best Practice & Research Clinical Gastroenterology. 2007; 21 (2): 261-279.

[132] J.C. Atherton, P. Cao, R.M. Peek, M.K.R. Tummuru, M.J. Blaser, T.L. Cover. Mosaicism in vacuolating cytotoxin alleles of Helicobacter-Pylori association of specific vaca types with cytotoxin production andpeptic-ulceration. J Biol Chemil 1995; 270: 17771-17777.

[133] J. Viala, C. Chaput, I.G. Boneca. et al. Nod1 responds to peptidoglycan delivered by the Helicobacter pylori cag pathogenicity island. Nat Immun 2004; 5: 1166-1174.

[134] T.S. Chen , Y.C. Lee, F.Y. Li, F.Y. Chang. Smoking and hyperpepsinogenemia are associated with increased risk for duodenal ulcer in Helicobacter pylori-infected patients. J Clin Gastroenterol 2005; 39: 699-703.

[135] S.F. Moss, S. Legon, A.E. Bishop, J.M. Polak, J. Calam. Effect of Helicobacter-pylori on gastric somatostatin in duodenal-ulcer disease. Lancet 1992; 340: 930-932.

[136] A. Lee. The nature of Helicobacter pylori. Scand. J. Gastroenterol. 1996; 31(Suppl. 214): 5-8.

[137] G.N. Tytgat. Current indications for Helicobacter pylori eradication therapy. Scand. J. Gastroenterol. 1996; 31(Suppl. 215): 70-73.

[138] M.P. Cooreman, P. Krausgrill, K.J. Hengels. Local gastric and serum amoxicillin concentrations after different oral application forms. Antimicrob. Agents Chemother. 1993; 37: 1506-1509.

[139] B.D. Gold, M. Huesca, P.M. Sherman, et al. Helicobacter mustelae and Helicobacter pylori bind to common lipid receptors in vitro. Infect. Immun. 1993; 61: 2632-2638.

[140] B.L. Slomiany, J. Piotrowski, A. Samanta et al. Campylobacter pylori colonization factors shows specificity for lactosylceramide sulfate and GM3 ganglioside. Biochem. Internat. 1989; 19: 929-936.

[141] T. Bore´n, P. Falk, K.A. Roth, et al., Attachment of Helicobacter pylori to human gastric epithelium mediated by blood group antigens. Science 1993; 262: 1892-1895.

[142] A.L. Blum, Helicobacter pylori and peptic ulcer disease. Scand. J. Gastroenterol. 1996; 31(Suppl. 214): 24-27.

[143] R.V. Heatley. The treatment of Helicobacter pylori infection. Aliment. Pharmacol. Ther. 1992; 6: 291-303.

[144] A.T.R. Axon. Helicobacter pylori therapy: effect on peptic ulcer disease. J. Gastroenterol. Hepatol. 1991; 6: 131-137.

[145] M. Cuna, M.J. Alonso, D. Torres. Preparation and in vivo evaluation of mucoadhesive microparticles containing amoxicillin-resin complexes for drug delivery to the gastric mucosa. European Journal of Pharmaceutics and Biopharmaceutics 2001; 51: 199-205.

[146] D.Y. Graham, G.M.A. Borsch. The who's and when's of therapy for Helicobacter pylori. Am. J. Gastroenterol. 1990; 85: 1552-1555.

[147] A. Ateshkadi, N.P. Lam, C.A. Johnson. Helicobacter pylori and peptic ulcer disease. Clin. Pharm. 1993; 12: 34-48.

[148] J.C. Atherton, A. Cockayne, M. Balsitis, G.E. Kirk, C.J. Hawkey, R.C. Spiller. Detection of the intragastric sites at which Helicobacter pylori evades treatment with amoxycillin and cimetidine. Gut 1995; 36: 670-674.

[149] P.S. Rajinikanth, J. Balasubramaniam, B. Mishra. Development and evaluation of a novel floating in situ gelling system of amoxicillin for eradication of Helicobacter pylori. International Journal of Pharmaceutics 2007; 335: 114–122.

[150] K. Kimura, K. Ido, K. Saifuku, Y. Taniguchi, K. Kihira, K. Satoh, T. Takimoto, Y. Yoshida. A 1-h topical therapy for the treatment of Helicobacter pylori infection. Am. J. Gastroenterol. 1995; 90: 60-63.

[151] N. Nagahara, Y. Akiyama, M. Nakao, M. Tada, M. Kitano, Y. Ogawa. Mucoadhesive microspheres containing amoxicillin for clearance of Helicobacter pylori. Antimicrob. Agents Chemother. 1998; 38: 2492-2494.

[152] A.K. Hilton, P.B. Deasy. In vitro and in vivo evaluation of an oral sustained-release floating dosage form of amoxycillin trihydrate. Int. J. Pharm. 1992; 86: 79-88.

[153] V.R. Patel, M.M. Amiji. Preparation and characterization of freezedried chitosan-poly(ethylene oxide) hydrogels for site-specific antibiotic delivery in the stomach. Pharm. Res. 1996; 13: 588-593.

[154] S. Shah, R. Qaqish, V. Patel, M. Amiji. Evaluation of the factors influencing stomach-specific delivery of antibacterial agents for Helicobacter pylori infection. J. Pharm. Pharmacol. 1999; 51: 667-672.

[155] S. Burton, N. Washington, R.J.C. Steele, R. Musson, L. Feely. Intragastric distribution of ion-exchange resins: a drug delivery system for the topical treatment of the gastric mucosa. J. Pharm. Pharmacol. 1995; 47: 901-906.

[156] S. Thairs, S. Ruck, S.J. Jackson, R.J.C. Steele, L.C. Freely, C. Washington, N. Washington. Effect of dose size, food and surface coating on the gastric residence and distribution of an ion Exchange resin. Int. J. Pharm. 1998; 176: 47-53.

[157] P.S. Rajinikanth, B. Mishra. Floating in situ gelling system for stomach site-specific delivery of clarithromycin to eradicate H. Pylori. Journal of Controlled Release 2008; 125: 33–41.

[158] S.W. Jang, J.W. Lee, S.H. Park, J. H. Kima, M. Yoo, D.H. Na, K.C. Lee. Gastroretentive drug delivery system of DA-6034, a new flavonoid derivative, for the treatment of gastritis. International Journal of Pharmaceutics. 2008; 356: 88–94.

[159] M. Takenaga, Y. Serizawa, Y. Azechi, A. Ochiai, Y. Kosaka, R. Igarashi, Y. Mizushima. Microparticle resins as a potential nasal drug delivery system for insulin. J. Control. Release 1998; 52: 81-87.

6

Ethnopharmacology as Current Strategy in the Search of Novel Anti-Ulcerogenic Drugs: Case of a Brazilian Medicinal Plant (*Maytenus ilicifolia* Mart. ex. Reissek)

Rômulo Dias Novaes and João Paulo Viana Leite
Federal University of Viçosa
Brazil

1. Introduction

Several medical products of natural origin were conceived in traditional systems of knowledge and practice that has been transmitted over centuries and which continuously change. In actual scenario, researchers of many countries involved in the modern drug discovery processes are becoming increasingly aware of the value of their traditional knowledge, while global pharmaceutical industry is looking for alternative solutions to reduce the crescent innovation deficit and enhance the development of new products.

Has been systematically showed that aleatory screening of plants used traditionally by pharmaceutical industries in the search for new leads or drugs is vastly expensive and requires much time. On the other hand, ethnodirected approach to traditional knowledge has been extremely useful in screening and identification of plants with bioactive compounds with potential application in drug development. This approach consists in selecting species according to the indication of specific population groups in certain contexts of use. The ethnodirected approach has significantly increased the chances of discovery of new biomolecules with potential therapeutic application while reduce the cost and time involved in this process. Beyond this approach provide a shortcut to the discovery of active compounds that could serve as a basis for rational drug development, it also provides a mechanism for pre-screening on the therapeutic properties of the species collected. Most of these compounds are part of routinely used traditional medicines and hence their tolerance and safety are relatively better known than any other chemical entities that are new for human use. Thus, traditional medicine based on ethnodirected bioprospecting offers an unmatched structural variety as promising new leads.

In the context of ethnodirected studies, the ethnopharmacological research has shown a great contribution in selecting plants and discovery of compounds with pharmacological potential. Ethnopharmacology is a strategy used in the investigation of plants with medicinal properties, combining information acquired from users of medicinal plants (traditional communities and experts), with chemical and pharmacological studies. While in the past the typical industrial drug discovery process made the use of aleatory selection and systematic bioassays to find promising compounds for a particular target, ethnopharmacology goes the opposite way, tries to understand the pharmacological basis of culturally important medicinal plants, testing their efficacy in the laboratory.

Currently, research centers and pharmaceutical industries have driven the search for new drugs of plant origin with effective activity to fight several diseases that today present a limited treatment, including gastrointestinal ailments. In the case of gastric ulcers, several plants extracts described in the specific cultural context are being investigated in the search for sources of effective biomolecules in reducing the damage to gastric mucosa.

Gastric hyperacidity and ulceration of the stomach mucosa due to various factors are serious health problems of global concern. Peptic ulcer disease (encompassing gastric ulcer and duodenal ulcer) affect a large portion of the world population and are triggered by several factors, including stress, smoking, nutritional deficiencies, and ingestion of non-steroidal anti inflammatory drugs. Today, there are two main approaches for treating peptic ulcer. The first deals with reducing the production of gastric acid and the second with re-enforcing gastric mucosal protection. Although a number of anti-ulcer drugs such as H_2 receptor antagonists, proton pump inhibitors and cytoprotective agents are available, all these modern pharmacological approach have side effects and limitations. Moreover, development of drug tolerance and incidence of recurrences make the efficacy of allopathic drugs arguable. Therefore, there is urgent need to find alternatives that have antiulcerogenic properties. This has been the basis for the development of new anti-ulcer agents, which include herbal substances that could serve as leads for the development of new drugs.

In view of the importance of finding new plant compounds for the management of gastric ulcers in the context of current health, this chapter aims to show plant species and crud drug preparations with antiulcer activity identified within the ethnopharmacological approach. Furthermore, will be described the main phytochemicals responsible for the antiulcer therapeutic properties of plant extracts. Finally, by analyzing the case of *Maytenus ilicifolia*, will address aspects from preliminary phytochemical analysis and experimental tests with different preparations of this plant, and the process of isolation of fractions of the ethanol extract of *Maytenus ilicifolia* for identification of bioactive constituents related to its gastroprotective action.

2. Contribution of ethnopharmacology in the selection of natural products with potential application in health care

Chemical substances derived from plants have been used to treat human diseases since the dawn of medicine. Currently, the health care based in natural products is still the mainstay of about 75 - 80% of the whole world population, and the major part of traditional therapy involves the use of plant extracts (Gilani & Atta-ur-Rahman, 2005). Recognizably, natural products remain an important source for the discovery of new drugs and is estimated that about 13000 plant species worldwide are known to have been used in drugs formulation. About 60% of anticancer and 75% of anti-infective drugs approved from 1981-2002 could be traced to natural origins (Patwardhan & Vaidyab, 2010). Studies on sources of new drugs from 1981 to 2007 reveal that almost half of the drugs approved since 1994 are based on natural products (Harvey, 2008). Currently, it is estimated that about 80% of molecules used in drugs sold worldwide are derived from natural products and that over hundred new natural product-based leads are in clinical development (Butler, 2008; Bhutani & Gohil, 2010). Moreover, despite the tremendous development of chemical synthesis today, 25% of prescribed drugs in the world are of vegetable origin (Balunas & Kinghorn, 2005; Bhutani &

Gohil, 2010). Aspirin, atropine, artimesinin, colchicine, digoxin, ephedrine, morphine, physostigmine, pilocarpine, quinine, quinidine, reserpine, taxol, tubocurarine, vincristine and vinblastine are a few important examples of what medicinal plants have given us in the past. Most of these plant-derived drugs were originally discovered through the study of traditional cures and folk knowledge of indigenous people and some of these could not be substituted despite the enormous advancement in synthetic chemistry (Sekar et al., 2010).

Due to growing drug discovery from natural products, researchers and pharmaceutical industries has been increasing interest in traditional health practices used around the world (Patwardhan, 2005). This interest has been renovated for decades due to systematic demonstrations that plants are the richest resource of drugs of traditional systems of medicine, modern medicines, nutraceuticals, food supplements, folk medicines, pharmaceutical intermediates and chemical entities for synthetic drugs (Hammer et al., 1999). Since the reported data so far available on plants are comparatively meager before the number of plant population, ethnopharmacologists, botanists, microbiologists and natural-product chemists world over today, is constantly still in search of medicinal efficacy of plants and their phytochemicals. Furthermore, the wide spectrum of therapeutic activity makes the natural products attractive candidates for further research (Vlietinck & Van Den Berghe, 1991). In this context, a new recognition has been given to ethnopharmacology, traditional, complementary and alternative medicines, which re-emerging as new strategic options in health attention, has provided valuable clues of plants with bioactive compounds potentially usable in the production of new drugs (Harvey et al., 2010; Patwardhan & Vaidyab, 2010). The World Health Organization's Commission on Intellectual Property and Innovation in Public Health also has duly recognized the promise and role of traditional medicine in developing affordable drugs for the treatment of health problems (Patwardhan, 2005a; Patwardhan & Vaidyab, 2010).

The ethnopharmacological approach is currently employed to study numerous medicinal plants and vegetable preparations from traditional ethnic groups (Elisabetsky & Nunes, 1990). Although the clinical efficacy of these preparations is reported by traditional practices, they have not been scientifically validated. Thus, ethnopharmacologists typically develop working hypotheses derived from field observations having as one of its main goals to enhance the knowledge of local communities incorporating scientific findings to traditional accounts. In this context, the central questions that direct the ethnopharmacological research is if a specific plant extract used in the cultural context to cure some diseases present a pharmacological basis that explains the effects traditionally indicated. In this process, ethnopharmacological discoveries started with field observations and ended in new pharmacological insights (Gertsch, 2009). Therefore, ethnopharmacology research is transdisciplinary, touching on areas like anthropology, ethnobiology, and as the name implies, pharmacology (Raza, 2006; Gertsch, 2009).

The systematic screening ethnopharmacology-based of plant species with the purpose of discovering new potential bioactive compounds is a routine activity in many laboratories (Elisabetsky, 2002). Traditionally, the etnopharmacological research on the medicinal plants should be extended with the identification and isolation of specific phytochemicals. After these processes, only from the careful scientific examination of these isolated compounds could lead to standardization and quality control of the products to ensure their safety. It is after such evaluation that vegetable derivatives can be approved for the development of new products used in health care (Vlietinck & Van Den Berghe, 1991, Elisabetsky, 2002; Patwardhan, 2005b).

Several advantages can be achieved with the adoption of ethnodirected method for screening bioactive components. Due to traditional use of vegetable products in specific communities for the prevention or treatment of various health conditions, it is possible to meet preliminary criteria for safety for human consumption and any adverse effects of such use (Elisabetsky & Nunes, 1990; Vlietinck & Van Den Berghe, 1991). Coupled with better cultural acceptability of natural products and reduced cost is encouraging for both the consuming public and national health care institutions to consider plant medicines as a complementary practice to synthetic drugs (Elisabetsky & Nunes, 1990; Elisabetsky, 2002; Patwardhan, 2005a).

3. Peptic ulcers and herbal medicine

Peptic ulcer disease (PUD) is one of the most common, chronic gastrointestinal disorder in modern era. Now it has become a common global health problem affecting a large number of people worldwide and also still a major cause of morbidity and mortality (Sen et al., 2009). An estimated 15,000 deaths occur each year as a consequence of PUD (Dharmani & Palit, 2006).

Ulcer is an open sore that develops on the inside lining of the stomach (a gastric ulcer) or the small intestine (a duodenal ulcer). Both types of ulcers are also referred to as PUD and can be characterized by inflamed lesions or excavations of the mucosa and tissue that protect the gastrointestinal tract. The most common symptom of a peptic ulcer is a burning or gnawing pain in the center of the abdomen (stomach) (Tarnawski, 2005, Vyawahare et al., 2009).

In the past, it was mistakenly thought that the main causes of peptic ulcers were lifestyle factors, such as diet, smoking, alcohol and stress. While these factors may play a limited role, it is known that the leading cause of peptic ulcers is a type of bacteria called *Helicobacter pylori* (*H. pylori*) can infect the stomach and small intestine; and in some people, the bacteria can irritate the inner layer of the stomach and small intestine, leading to the formation of an ulcer (Dulcie et al., 1997). Peptic ulcer occurs due to an imbalance between the aggressive (acid, pepsin and *H. pylori*) and the defensive (gastric mucus, bicarbonate secretion, prostaglandins, nitric oxide, growth factors and innate resistance of the mucosal cells) factors (Falcão et al., 2008b). Painkillers known as nonsteroidal anti-inflammatory drugs (NSAIDs), which include aspirin and ibuprofen, are the second most common cause of peptic ulcers that can irritate the lining of the stomach and small intestine in some people, particularly if they are taken on a long-term basis (Tarnawski, 2005; Vyawahare et al., 2009).

Traditionally, there are two main approaches for treating peptic ulcer. The first deals with reducing the production of gastric acid and the second with re-enforcing gastric mucosal protection (Sen et al., 2009). According to the old hypothesis, acid secretion was thought to be the sole cause of ulcer formation and reduction in acid secretion was thought to be the major approach towards therapy. However, in the light of recent evidences this concept has changed. The modern approach for the ulcer treatment mainly targets the potentiation of the gastrointestinal defensive system preventing ulceration by inhibiting acid secretion, increase gastroprotection, increase epithelial cell proliferation and stop apoptosis for effective ulcer healing process (Bandhopadhyay et al., 2002).

Recently, there has been a rapid progress in the understanding of the pathogenesis of peptic ulcer. Most of the studies focus on newer and better drug therapy for the prevention and treatment of peptic ulcer. These have been made possible largely by the availability of the proton pump inhibitors, histamine receptor antagonists, drugs affecting the mucosal barrier and prostaglandin analogues (primarily misoprostol) (Hoogerwerf & Pasricha, 2006). However, the clinical evaluation of these drugs showed development of tolerance and incidence of relapses and side effects that make their efficacy arguable. Furthermore, most of these drugs produce several serious adverse reactions including toxicities, arrhythmias, impotence, gynaecomastia, arthralgia, hypergastrinemia, haemopoeitic changes and even may alter biochemical mechanisms of the body upon chronic usage (Vyawahare et al., 2009). This has been the rationale for the development of alternative approach in recent days for the research of new antiulcer drugs medicaments from traditional medicinal system, which includes herbal drugs.

For many years, herbal medicines were generally indicated only as coadjutant gastrointestinal therapy to conventional drugs and when these drugs presented adverse effects and are used during a long-term. Due to several plants encountered in many countries have been reported to poses marked antiulcerogenic activity, the role of natural medicine in management of gastrointestinal diseases has been rethought (Schmeda-Hirschmann & Yesilada, 2005). Thus, the investigation of traditional knowledge, popular medicine and the development of new medicaments based in natural products for the treatment of diseases like peptic ulcer have been indicated as a absolute requirement of our time (Sen et al., 2009).

Medicinal plants and their derivatives have been an invaluable source of therapeutic agents to treat various disorders including PUD (Borrelli & Izzo, 2000). The use of vegetable extracts used in popular medicine and their phyto-constituents as drug therapy to treat major ailments has proved to be clinically effective for the treatment of PUD (Dharmani and Palit, 2006). Furthermore, the use of plants and their phytoconstituents in the treatment of gastrointestinal diseases is promising due to the broad spectrum of action on various defensive mechanisms like antioxidant, antinflamatory, imunomodulatory, cytoprotective and antisecretory (Newall et al., 1996).

Although several plants have showed beneficial gastroprotective effects, earlier publications, and researchers from around the world, have pointed out that relatively little of the world's plant biodiversity has been extensively screened for bioactivity (Harvey et al., 2010), and this scenario extends to most plants that have traditional indication for the management of gastric ulcers.

4. Ethnopharmacological discovery of antiulcer crude drugs

Treatment of gastrointestinal ailments with natural products is quite common in traditional medicine worldwide. The importance of ethnopharmacological studies in the search for plants with gastroprotective activity is emphasized by the observation that the first drug effective against gastric ulcer was carbenoxolone, discovered as a result of research on a commonly used indigenous plant, *Glycyrrhiza glabra*. Also, studies on cabbage, previously employed as an anti-ulcer agent in folk medicine, has led to the development of gefarnate, a drug used for the treatment of gastric ulcers (Akhtar & Munir, 1989). Thus, a search among medicinal plants is still important, despite the progress in conventional chemistry and pharmacology in producing effective drugs (Harvey et al., 2010).

Currently, new therapeutic approaches with medicinal plants based in traditional knowledge and in ethnopharmacological screening have received particular attention in the prevention and/or treatment of gastric diseases such as PUD. In this context, there are reports of a large variety of plants species with antiulcerogenic potential in several countries. Examples of plants and their phytochemicals with antiulcer activity investigated in ethnopharmacological studies are sowed in table 1.

Botanical name	Parts used*	Actives phytochemicals	Ulcer model
Aclepiadaceae			
Hemidesmus indicus	root	alkaloids, tannins, phenols, saponins	aspirin, pylorus ligation, cyteamine
Anacardiaceae			
Anacardium occidentale	leaves	glycosylated quercetin, glycosylated myricitin, catechin, proanthocyanidin, biflavonoid amentoflavone	ethanol + HCl
Asteraceae			
Centaurea solstitialis	spiny flowers	sesquiterpene lactones, chlorojanerin 13-acetylsolstitialin A, solstitialin A	ethanol, HCl, indometacin cold stress, serotonin
Clusiaceae			
Calophyllum brasiliense	stem bark	flavones, flavonols, triterpenoids, xanthones, steroids	ethanol, indomethacin, cold stress, pyloric ligation
Combretaceae			
Anogeissus latifolia	bark	glycosides, leucocyanidin, ellagic and flavellagic acid, galic acid	ethanol, aspirin, cold stress, pylorus ligation
Euphorbiaceae			
Alchornea castanaefolia	leaves, bark	quercetin-3-O-β-D-galactopyranoside, quercetin-3-O-α-L-arabinopyranoside, myrecetin-3-O-α-L-arabinopyranoside, quercetin, galic acid, amentoflavone, glycolipids, free sugars	ethanol + HCl, acetic acid cold stress, pylorus ligation, indomethacin
Emblica officinalis	fruits	flavonoids, phenols, curcuminoides, phyllembelic acid, tannins,	ethanol, aspirin, cold stress, pylorus ligation,

Fabaceae

Desmodium gangeticum	root	alkaloids, steroids, pterocarpanoids flavone, isoflavonoid glycosides, N-oxides, b-amyrone, tryptamines,	ethanol, aspirin, cold stress, pylorus ligation
		phospholipids	
Spartium junceum	flowers	alkaloids, saponins, spartitrioside	ethanol, pylorus ligation, cold stress

Labiatae

Ocimum sanctum	leaves	eugenol, carvacrol, caryophyllene,	ethanol, acetic acid,
		apigenin, luteolin, orientin,	aspirin, reserpine,
		molludistin, ursolic acid	pylorus ligation

Liliaceae

Aloe vera	leaves	alkaloids, sterols, gelonins, saponins, fatty acid, glycoproteins	HCl, pylorus ligation
Asparagus racemosus	root	alkaloids, steroids, saponins, flavonoids, phenols, tannins, terpenes	ethanol, aspirin, cold stress, pylorus ligation,

Malphiaceae

Byrsonima crassa	leaves	quercetin-3-o-b-D-galactopyranoside quercetin-3-o-a-L-arabinopyranoside amentoflavone, catechin, epicatechin	ethanol + HCl

Meliaceae

Azadirachta indica	bark	phenols, phenolic diterpenoids, glycosides, isoprenoids, essential oils	ethanol, aspirin, indomethacin, histamin
		flavonoids, tannins	

Oleaceae

Jasminum grandiflorum	leaves	alkaloids, saponins, phenois flavonoids, carotenoids, glycosides	pylorus ligation + aspirin ethanol, acetic acid

Sapindaceae			
Allophylus serratus	leaves	ß-sitosterol, phenacetamide, flavonoids, glycosides	ethanol, aspirin, acetic acid, cold stress
Rhizophoraceae			
Rhizophora mangle	bark	polyphenols, catechin, epicatechin, chlorogenic, gallic and ellagic acids, gallotannins, elagitannins	diclofenac
Rubiaceae			
Rubia cordifolia	root	anthraquinones, iridoid glycoside, bicyclic hexapeptides, triterpenes	pylorus ligation
Scrophulariaceae			
Scoparia dulcis	aerial parts	cirsitakaoside and quercetin	pylorus ligation, histamine, bethanechol
Simaroubaceae			
Quassia amara	bark	alkaloids, b-carbonile, cantin-6, steroids, quassinoids, terpenes	ethanol, HCl
Solanaceae			
Solanum nigrum	Fruits	tannins, alkaloids, carbohydrates, anthocyanins	ethanol, indomethacin, pylorus ligation, cold stress
Utleria salicifolia	rhizome	steroids, alkaloids, terpenoids, saponins, tannins	ethanol, acetic acid cold stress, pylorus ligation
Zingiberaceae			
Zingiber officinalis	Root	alkaloids, flavonoids, phenols, monoterpenoids, sesquiterpenoids	methanol, acetone, HCl
Amomum subulatum	fruits	anthocyanins, aurone, flavone, essestial oils	ethanol, aspirin, pylorus ligation

Table 1. Plants with antiulcerogenic activity from ethnopharmacological studies.
*Gastroprotective effects were obtained using crude preparations of all the plants described

Important questions related with crude drugs are the necessary amount of plant part to provide a healing response, traditional way of preparation (infusion, decoction and maceration), concentration (plant/solvent ratio), frequency and duration of treatment. Unfortunately, this basic information is not always present in ethnopharmacological studies and this fact is surprising as there should be a realistic approach to the doses to confirm the reputed effectiveness of the crude drugs. Extraction yields and doses recommended in traditional medicine were not taken into account in most cases. This fact clearly suggested the need for guidelines when looking for gastroprotective crude drugs or gastroprotective compounds from medicinal plants (Schmeda-Hirschmann & Yesilada, 2005).

In anthropological and ethnobiological investigations of popular herbal therapies practices has been indicated that as a common way of preparation, plants are used in traditional medicine as infusions or decoctions, but in some localities also as macerates, either in water or in alcoholic beverages (Schmeda-Hirschmann & Rojas de Arias, 1990). In particular cases, the treatment may also be applied by direct ingestion of the material.

As a common popular practice, the plant material (in the range of 5–50 g of dry plant material per liter) is placed in a pot of solvent (most commonly hot or coldwater), while resinous materials which would not dissolve in polar solvents are directly swallowed. As the percent (w/w) extraction yields of plant material presents a great variability depending on the extraction solvent, processing temperature and time, doses corresponding to 5–50 g of dry plant material are about 0.5–10 g extract for an adult user (60–70 kg) corresponding to ca. 100–150 mg of crude extract per kg of body weight. In the current scenario, it has been observed that most studies have investigated the antiulcerogenic properties using different animal models at doses of plant extracts ranging from 5 to about 2000 mg/kg. However, the doses between 25 and 800 mg/kg have indicated great gastroprotective effect of crude plant extracts, range that is more realistic considering the tolerable human consumption. Higher doses may not be realistic since they will not be used or recommended in traditional medicine (Schmeda-Hirschmann & Yesilada, 2005).

Although crude drugs obtained through the use of herbal preparations with fresh or dried plants and concentrated plant extracts have broad applicability in folk medicine, the viability of this practice in the pharmaceutical industry is arguable. Is widely recognized that crude drugs exhibit a wide spectrum of phytochemicals with different biological activities. However, few of these compounds have pharmacological activities of interest for the treatment of specific health conditions, and although these compounds are present in crude drugs, can also be phytochemicals with antagonistic activity or even harmful to human health. Furthermore, another important aspect is the difficulty of standardization in the phytochemical composition of these crude drugs since there is a wide variation in levels of the chemical components related to where the raw material was obtained (Leite, 2009).

In this context, following the identification of the efficacy of crude herbal preparations in different health conditions, the method ethnopharmacological predicts the development of several research stages aiming to identify, concentrate and isolate phytochemical components to test the biological activities of each compound identified in the crude drug. In this process, it is possible to focus the investigations on the phytochemicals responsible for the desired biological effects (Fabricant & Farnsworth, 2001; Bhutani & Gohil, 2010). Thus, through this approach it is possible to achieve the level of control required in pharmacological studies in order to determine the therapeutic dose, toxicity and mode of use of specific phytochemicals, criteria that must be strictly defined where the intention is to discover and develop new pharmaceuticals derived from plants for commercial purposes

(Koehn & Carter, 2005). A basic scheme of the ethnopharmacological method is represented in the figure 1. Based in this method several phytochemicals with antiulcer activity were discovered, and was clearly demonstrated that the main benefits of these crude drugs are linked to alkaloids, flavonoids, saponins and tannins.

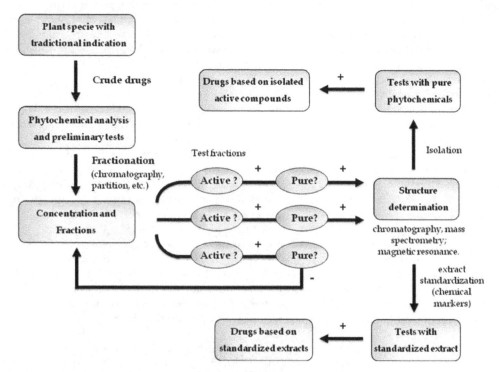

Fig. 1. Generic representation of ethnopharmacological method in a bioassay-guided fractionation for the investigation of phytochemicals with therapeutic properties used in drugs development (adapted from Koehn and Carter, 2005).

5. Antiulcer properties of specific phytochemicals

5.1 Alkaloids

The alkaloids are a diverse group of low molecular weight nitrogen-containing compounds derived mostly from amino acids. These secondary metabolites are found in about 20 % of plant species (Ziegler & Facchini, 2008). Plants containing alkaloids with antiulcer properties are showed in table 2. Furthermore, these phytochemicals represent a group of natural products that has had a recognized impact in medicine and are being used in management of gastrointestinal ailments. Clinically, alkaloids they are used to block the muscarinic activity of acetylcholine showing antispasmodic and antisecretory effects in the treatment of spastic colitis, gastroenteritis and peptic ulcer. In a previous literature review were identified fifty-five naturally derived alkaloids with antiulcer activity such as imidazole, indole, isoquinoline, non-nitrogen heterocycle alkaloid, phenylalkylamide, piperidine, pyrazine, pyridine, pyrrolidine, pyrrolizidine, quinolizidine and tropane alkaloids (Falcão et al., 2008a).

Botanical name	Parts used	Ulcer model
Apocynaceae *Himatanthus lancifolius*	bark	ethanol, pylorus ligation
Annonaceae *Enantia chlorantha*	bark	ethanol, HCl pylorus ligation
Apocynaceae *Voacanga africana*	fruits	ethanol, HCl, pylorus ligation, indomethacin
Asteraceae *Mikania cordata*	leaves	diclofenac
Senecio brasiliensis	flowers	ethanol, HCl, pylorus ligation, indomethacin
Buxaceae *Pachysandra terminalis*	leaves	cols stress
Flabaceae *Sophora flavescens*	leaves	acetic acid, cold stress
Ranunculaceae *Coptis chinensis*	rhizoma	ethanol, acetic acid pylorus ligation
Coptis japonica	rhizoma	ethanol
Rubiaceae *Pausinystalia yohimbe*	bark	cold stress
Rutaceae *Galipea longiflora*	bark	ethanol, HCl, bethanecol

Table 2. Plants containing alkaloids with anti-ulcer activity.

Among the different alkaloids showing potent pharmacological properties are the narcotic analgesic morphine, the antimicrobial berberine and the sympathomimetic ephedrine. These isoquinoline alkaloids occur mainly in plants belonging to families Papaveraceae, Berberidaceae and Ephedraceae (Ziegler & Facchini, 2008). In murine model of gastric damage induced by reserpine, aspirin or indomethacin, morphine and ephedrine presented significant antiulcer activity (Al-Shabanah et al., 1993; Sandor & Cuparencu, 1977). In addition, the alkaloid 7,8-dihydro-8-hydroxypalmatine obtained from the bark of *Enantia chlorantha* was effective to increase gastric mucus and accelerated ulcer-healing production after gastric lesions caused by acetic acid. Positive effect was also evidenced when ulceration of gastric mucosa was induced using HCl/ethanol and pylorus ligature (Tan et al., 2000). Other alkaloids isolated from *Coptidis* rhizome, coptisine and 8-oxocoptisine, showed protection of gastric mucosa similar to that offered by gastroprotective conventional drugs such as cimetidine and sucralfate (Hirano et al., 2000, 2001).

Alkaloids derived from *Voacanga africana* was assayed for cytoprotective, anti-secretory and ulcer healing actions. Through enteral administration, alkaloid fraction inhibited ulcer formation in a dose-dependent way in several models of gastric damage (HCl/ethanol, absolute ethanol, HCl/ethanol/ indomethacin, pylorus ligation, cold restraint stress, and histamine). These alkaloids have gastric anti-secretory effects similar to histamine receptor blockers and decreased the gastric acid secretion. Moreover, its cytoprotective and ulcer healing effects are associated to its property to strengthen gastric mucosal defenses by stimulating mucus synthesis (Tan & Nyasse, 2000). When combined with ranitidine, a synergistic anti-secretory effect was observed (Tan et al., 2002). In addition, alkaloids such as matrine, 13-alpha-hydroxymatrine and oxy-matrine isolated from *Sophora flavescens* were able to decrease the acid secretion and inhibited the gastric motility in experimental model of gastric ulcers induced by pylorus ligature (Zhu et al., 1993; Yamazaki, 2000).

The pyrrolizidine alkaloids integerrimine, retrorsine, senecionine, usaramine and seneciphylline were extracted from *Senecio brasiliensis*. These alkaloids demonstrate significant activity in acute and chronic gastric ulcers. In this investigation, gastroprotective effects of alkaloids were associated to the stimulation prostaglandin synthesis in gastric mucosal and free mucus, reduction of exfoliation of superficial cells, hemorrhages and blood cell infiltration, events that can be mediated by increased expression of epidermal growth factors (Toma et al., 2004).

5.2 Flavonoids

Flavonoids are important constituents in human diet that are also found in several medicinal plants used in popular medicine around the world (Di Carlo et al., 1999). These molecules represent a highly diverse class of secondary metabolites derived from vegetable material comprising about 9,000 structures with a wide range of biological effects, including antiulcer activity (Mota et al., 2009).

There are several studies with flavonoids naturally derived were found to be able to protect the gastric mucosa reducing the number and intensity of the lesions induced by a variety of ulcerogenic agents such as ethanol, HCl, acetic acid, aspirin, diclofenac, indomethacin, reserpine, cold stress and pylorus ligation (Borrelli & Izzo, 2000). Currently, the flavonoids catechin, flavanone, flavone, kaempferol, naringin, naringenin, quercetin, and rutin have been most commonly cited as having important gastroprotective effect in experimental models of duodenal and gastric ulcers.

Several mechanisms have been proposed to explain the gastroprotective effects of flavonoids; these include increase of mucosal prostaglandin content, decrease of histamine secretion from mast cells and inhibition of *H. pylori* growth (Beil et al., 1995). Furthemore, flavonoids have been found to be free radical scavengers with an important role in protection against ulcerative and erosive lesions of the gastrointestinal tract. Due to low toxicity, flavonoids could have a therapeutic potential ideal for treatment of gastrointestinal diseases associated with *H. pylori* infection, i.e. type B gastritis and duodenal ulcer (Di Carlo et al., 1999, Martín et al., 2000). Common flavonoids with antiulcer activity are shown in Figure 2.

In experiments with murine model of ethanol-induced gastric ulcers, the flavonoids naringin and quercetin displayed marked antiulcerogenic effects. In particular, naringin at a dose of 400 mg/kg had a significant gastroprotective effect, reducing the number and severity of ulcerative lesions. It is suggested that the gastroprotective property of naringin occurs through a complex non-prostaglandin dependent mechanism that involved an increase in the mucus synthesis and their viscosity. Free-radical scavenging also seems to be implicated in this protective activity (Martín et al., 2000).

Butein

citoprotection, antioxidant, increase mucus production, ulcer healing

Catechin

antioxidant, increases mucus synthesis, hormone inhibition, ulcer healing

Dihydroxychalcone

citoprotection, reduce intestinal transit, acid inhibition

Flavanone

cyclooxygenase and lypoxigenase inhibition, proton pump and H. pylori inhibition

Kaempferol

antioxidant, proton pump inhibition mucus synthesis, leucotriene inhibition

Luteolin

antioxidant, lipoxygenase and acid inhibition

Myricetin

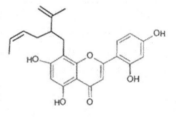

antioxidant,
antinflamatory,
lipoxygenase and
coxigenase inhibition,
motility stimulation

Naringenin

antioxidant,
lipoxygenase, proton
pump inhibition, mucus
and prostaglandin
synthesis

Naringin

antioxidant,
lipoxygenase and acid
inhibition, mucus
synthesis

Quercetin

antinflamatory,
histamine, lipoxygenase,
proton pump and H.
pylori inhibition, mucus
synthesis

Rutin

antinflamatory,
antioxidant,
lipoxygenase
inhibition, mucus
synthesis

Vexibinol

acid inhibition,
antioxidant, mucus and
prostaglandin synthesis

Fig. 2. Flavonoids with antiulcerogenic properties and their mechanisms of action.

Administration of Quercetin at a dose of 200 mg/kg also showed beneficial effects by reducing the occurrence of ulcers and increased the amount of glycoprotein content of gastric mucus. A proposed mechanism of action for the effects of Quercetin is a cytoprotective effect mediated by antioxidant properties, stimulation of prostaglandin and inhibition of leukotriene production, events that reinforce the defensive compounds of the gastrointestinal wall (Alarcon de la Lastra et al., 1994; Di Carlo et al., 1999). In a rat model of gastric damage induced by acidified ethanol, the antiulcer effects of flavone, quercetin, naringin, rutin and kaempferol were previously related to the synthesis of platelet activating factor (PAF), a recognized ulcerogenic agent (Izzo, 1996). In this study, intraperitoneal administration of quercetin, rutin and kaempferol reduced tissue erosion in a dose-dependent manner (25-50 mg/kg), while naringin reduced gastric damage only at high dose levels (200-400 mg/kg) and flavone was inactive. Gastric mucosa of rats exposed to acidified ethanol presented large amounts of PAF and the treatment with flavonoids proved to have protective effects against the gastric damage when the doses utilized were able to reduce PAF synthesis. Although other protective mechanisms cannot be excluded, evidences indicate that the degree of PAF inhibition produced by flavonoids was an important factor associated with the reduction of gastric injuries (Izzo et al., 1994; Di Carlo et al., 1999).

The influence of flavonoids on gastric acid secretion, mucosal prostaglandin production and *H. pylori* growth were also previously investigated (Beil et al., 1995). In this study, the flavonoids Flavone, Flavanone and Quercetin reduced *H. pylori* growth and the acid production in response to histamine and dibutyryl cyclic AMP stimulation. All flavonoids tested also inhibited the gastric proton pump (H^+/K^+), however, no inhibitory action was observed on the formation of prostaglandin E. In this context, flavone and flavanone increased PGE release, and quercetin was inactive in this process. Thus, was possible concluded that due to low toxicity of flavonoids and the effective gastroprotective properties described (antisecretory action, stimulation of prostaglandins, inhibition of *H. pylori*), these compounds presented a promissory therapeutic potential for the direct treatment of ulcerative diseases or for the development of drugs with this purpose (Di Carlo et al., 1999).

5.3 Saponins

Saponins are largely distributed in plants and are characterized as a specific kind of glycosides. They exhibit haemolytic properties and are highly toxic in direct contact with the blood stream. According to the structure of the aglycone or sapogenin two forms of saponin are recognized, the steroidal and triterpenoid type, the latter form being found in high concentrations in many plant species (Samuelsson, 1992; Borrelli & Izzo, 2000).

Antiulcer activity of several plant species containing high amounts of Saponins has been continuously indicated in different experimental ulcer models. The main species investigated in ethnopharmacological studies are shown in Table 3. Was previously demonstrated that liquorice root contains about 2%-12% of glycyrrhizic acid and the seeds of the horse-chestnut up to 13% of aescin (Newall et al., 1996; Borrelli & Izzo, 2000). Among these, saponins isolated from the rhizome of *Panax japonicus* and the fruit of *Kochia scoparia* (with about 20% of saponins) showed significant gastro-protective properties by inhibiting the amount and severity of ulcerative lesions (Matsuda et al., 1998). Furthemore, oleanolic acid oligoglycosides extracted from the same plants showed antiulcer effects on ethanol- and indomethacin-induced gastric damage. In another study, methanol extract of *Panax japonicus* rhizome also was able to protect gastric mucosa against stress- or HCl-induced ulcers (Yamahara et al., 1987; Borrelli & Izzo, 2000).

Aescin, a mixture of saponins encoutered in the seeds of *Aesculus hippocastanum*, has been shown to possess a marked antiulcer property (Marhuenda et al., 1993). For this compound, the gastroprotective effect has been associated with an inhibition of gastric acid and pepsinogen secretion. However, in a model of gastric ulceration ethanol-inducedm aescin was also effective in preventing gastric lesions (Marhuenda et al., 1994; Borrelli & Izzo, 2000). As in this model acid and pepsin do not play a significant role, the evidences indicates that other protective mechanisms are involved in the antiulcer action of aescin Furthermore,

Botanical name	Parts used	Materials tested	Ulcer model
Araliaceae			
Polyscias balfouriana	leaves, roots	ethanolic extract	aspirin
Asteraceae			
Aster squamatus	aerial parts	hydroalcoholic extract	ethanol, pylorus ligation
Chenopodiaceae			
Kochia scoparia	fruits	isolated saponin	ethanol, indomethacin
Combretaceae			
Pteleopsis suberosa	bark	aqueous extract	indomethacin
Compositae			
Calendula officinalis	rhizome	isolated saponin	arsenic, butadione, pylorus ligattion
Dilleniaceae			
Davilla rugosa	stem	hydroalcoholic extract	acetic acid, ethanol, HCl, cold stress
Fabaceae			
Spartium junceum	Flowers	ethanolic extract	ethanol
Icacinaceae			
Pyrenacantha staudtii	Leaves	aqueous extract	indomethacin, serotonin, cold stress
Menispermaceae			
Rhigiocarya racemifera	Leaves	aqueous extract	indomethacin, serotonin, reserpine
Mimosaceae			
Calliandra portoticensis	Leaves	ethanolic, aqueous extract	cold stress, pylorus ligation
Sapindaceae			
Aesculus hippocastanum	seed	mix of saponins	ethanol, pylorus ligation cold stress
Sapindus saponaria	fruits, leaves	hydroalcoholic extract	cold stress
Sapotaceae			
Mimusops elengi	bark	hydroalcoholic extract	ethanol, pylorus ligation

Ethnopharmacology as Current Strategy in the Search of Novel Anti-Ulcerogenic Drugs: Case of a Brazilian
Medicinal Plant (Maytenus ilicifolia Mart. ex. Reissek)

115

Scarabaeoidea

Panax binnatifidus   rhizome   isolated saponin   psychological stress

Theaceae

Camellia sinensis   seed   methanolic extract   ethanol

Table 3. Plants containing saponins with anti-ulcer activity.

mucus synthesis mediated by prostaglandin seems not to be an able mechanism to explain the role of aescin-induced gastro-protection due to inability of saponin to stimulate the prostaglandin production in model of ethanol-induced gastric ulceration (Marhuenda et al., 1994; Borrelli & Izzo, 2000).

In a general context, the current information indicate that the antiulcer protective activities of the saponins are not due to inhibition of gastric acid secretion but probably due to activation of mucous membrane protective factors (Borrelli & Izzo, 2000).

5.4 Tannins

Plants produce tannins as protective substances, found in the outer and inner tissues. Tannins are by definition phenol compound with sufficiently high molecular weight and different chemical structures occurring in medicinal and food plants that are utilized world-wide. This phytochemical presents several remarkable biological and pharmacological activities and an important meaning for human health. Tannins are used in medicine primarily because of their astringent properties, which are due to the fact that they react with the proteins of the layers of tissue with which they come into contact (Samuelsson, 1992; Borrelli & Izzo, 2000). Moreover, the used of tannins against peptic ulcer, diarrhea and as an antidote in poisoning by heavy metals are described in medical literature.

Several plants with anti-ulcer activity containing high levels of tannins are showed in Table 4. In a previous investigation, a crude extract of *Linderae umbellatae* exhibited a marked anti-peptic and antiulcerogenic activity (Ezaki et al., 1985; Borrelli & Izzo, 2000). In this study, condensed tannins such as (+)-catechin, (-)-epicatechin, proanthocyanidin, cinnamtannin B1 and D1 (monomers, dimers, trimers and tetramers) have been isolated and their anti-peptic and anti-ulcer activity confirmed in experimental models of gastric lesions induced by pylorus-ligation in rats and stress in mice. Significant biological differences were observed between the chemicals structures of tannins. Monomers and dimers, did not presented inhibitory activity on peptic activity in vitro, while trimers exhibited higher inhibition of peptic activity compared to tetramers. In mice with pylorus ligation, trimers and tetramers markedly reduced the peptic activity of gastric juice. Furthermore, monomers and dimers slightly suppressed the peptic activity in this experimental model (Ezaki et al., 1985; Borrelli & Izzo, 2000). As monomers and dimers proved to be inactive in vitro, it is possible that their activity is not related to the direct inhibition of pepsin in vivo, but mainly related to influence on the secretion mechanism of pepsin.

Additional mechanisms have been related to the antiulcer action of tannins. This phytochemicals are known to coat the outermost layer of the mucosa and to render it less permeable and more resistant to chemical and mechanical injury or irritation (Asuzu & Onu, 1990; Borrelli & Izzo, 2000). When a low concentration of tannins is applied to the mucosa,

Botanical name	Parts used	Extract	Ulcer model
Anacardiaceae			
Myracrodruon urundeuva	bark	ethyl-acetate tannin fraction	ethanol, indomethacin
Schinus terebinthifolius	bark	aqueous	cold stress
Celastraceae			
Maytenus ilicifolia	leaves	aqueous	indomethacin
Combretaceae			
Combretum dolichopetalum	roots	ethanolic	indomethacin, cold
Pteleopsis suberosa	bark	chloroform, aqueous	Indomethacin, cold stress
Euphorbiaceae			
Excoecaria agallocha	bark	aqueous	diclofenac
Fabaceae			
Sesbania grandiflora	bark	ethanolic	indomethacin
Fagaceae			
Quercus suber *Quercus coccifera*	leaves	isolated tannins	ethanol
Lauraceae			
Linderae umbellatae	steam	isolated tannins	cold stress
Meliaceae			
Entandrophragma utile	bark	aqueous	ethanol
Menispermaceae			
Rhigiocarya racemifera	leaves	aqueous	reserpine, serotonin,
Myrtaceae			
Syzygium cumini	bark	isolated tannin	ethanol + HCl
Scrophulariaceae			
Veronica officinalis	aerial parts	hydroalcoholic	indomethacin, reserpine

Table 4. Plants containing tannins with anti-ulcer activity.

only the outermost layer is tanned, becoming less permeable and affording an increased protection to the subjacent layers against the action of bacteria, chemical irritation, and, to a certain extent, against mechanical irritation. In another hand, high concentrations of tannins often cause coagulation of the proteins of the deeper layer of the mucosa, resulting in inflammation, diarrhea and vomiting. The discovery of the inhibitory effects of tannins on lipid peroxidation in rat liver mitochondria and microsomes was followed by the uncovering of several effects related to improving the several gastrointestinal symptoms, activity that may be related to inhibition of lipoxygenase products related to metabolism of arachidonic acid (Okuda, 2005; Borrelli & Izzo, 2000). In addition, gastroprotective protective effects are related to antioxidant, vasoconstricting and antihemorrhagic properties of tannins (Borrelli & Izzo, 2000), which has also been linked to inhibition of *H. pylori* growth by several hydrolysable tannins (Funatogawa et al., 2004).

6. Screening of the constituents from *Maytenus ilicifolia* with anti-ulcerogenic activity

The beneficial medicinal effects of plant materials typically result from the secondary products present in the plant, and usually are not attributed to a single compound but a combination of the metabolites. In an extensive literature review, was identified, in quantitative terms, that the gastroprotective properties of crude drugs plant-based are attributed mainly to the presence of flavonoids, being found about 53 flavonoid compounds with antiulcer activity (Mota et al., 2009). However, currently there are sufficient evidence that in crude vegetables preparations the gastroprotective effects are also deeply influenced by other phytochemicals such as alkaloids, saponins and tannins. Therefore, efforts should be directed towards isolation and characterization of the active principles and elucidation of the relationship between structure and activity, followed by attempts for modulation of its activity potential by chemical modification. Furthermore, detailed analysis of the active constituents of natural drugs should be directed towards clinical relevance and to maintain indispensable reproducible quality in biological evaluation.

The ethnopharmacology constitutes an important and reliable method in bioprospecting of phytochemicals with anti-ulcer activity. The case of the discovery of the gastroprotective activity of *Maytenus ilicifolia* constitutes an appropriate example that clearly demonstrates the important role of ethnopharmacology in elucidating the pharmacological basis that is associated with a large part of traditional knowledge about medicinal plants and that waiting to be discovered.

Maytenus ilicifolia Mart. ex. Reissek belongs to the Celastraceae, a pantropical family native to southern Brazil, Paraguay, Uruguay, and northern Argentina. The plant is a small medicinal evergreen shrub that grows to a height of five meters bearing leaves and berries that resemble holly and is popularly known as "espinheira santa" (holy spine), "cancerosa", "cangorosa", "maiteno" and "espinheira divina" (divine spine) (Cordeiro et al., 2006). *Maytenus ilicifolia* is widely used as a traditional medicine in many countries of South America and its leaves are traditionally used as a remedy for gastrointestinal diseases, including dyspepsia and gastric ulcers (Leite et al., 2001, 2010). They are found in the local commerce as capsules, powders, dried leaves, or as aqueous or aqueous-alcoholic preparations.

The antiulcerogenic activity of *Maytenus ilicifolia* leaves is well documented. Has been showed that its aqueous extract causes significant reduction in the number of gastric ulcers induced by both indomethacin and cold-restraint stress in rats. This protection was similar to that observed with cimetidine, a well known histamine H2 receptor antagonist. Chemical constituents obtained from this plant extracts with solvents of different polarities are terpenoids, flavonoids, tannins and polysaccharides (Leite et al., 2001).

Souza-Formigoni et al., (1991) used boiling water extract of *Maytenus ilicifolia* leaves against ulcer lesions induced by indomethacin and cold-restraint stress in rats and found that both the oral and intraperitoneal administration of the extract had a potent antiulcerogenic effect against both types of ulcers. In this study, several phytochemicals were identified in crud extract of *Maytenus ilicifolia* and apparently polyphenols and flavonoids were the main compounds linked to gastroprotective effects evidenced. However, in a study conducted by Martins et al., (2003), antiulcer effects of *Maytenus ilicifolia* spray-dried powders obtained of an ethanol extract was mainly related to the tannins content in the crude extract. Thus, results of these studies suggested that a number of active constituents might be present in crude extract to control ulcerative lesions. However, of the major bioactive component of *Maytenus ilicifolia* that offers antiulcer effects remained still not well understood.

In a previous study, Baggio and collaborators reported the potent *in vivo* gastroprotective properties of a flavonoid-rich fraction separated from the leaves of *Maytenus ilicifolia*, *Maytenus ilicifolia*, containing epicatechin (3.1%) and catechin (2%) as major constituents, which was correlated with the in vitro inhibition of rabbit gastric H+,K+-ATPase activity (Baggio et al., 2007). Aiming to further the investigation on the bioactive constituents from *Maytenus ilicifolia* leaves, Leite et al., (2010) carried out a phytochemical investigation of an ethanol extract of *Maytenus ilicifolia* leaves for the isolation of compounds which were further used as chemical markers to monitorize an activity-guided fractionation of a lyophilized aqueous extract of *Maytenus ilicifolia* leaves. Finally, high performance liquid chromatography analyses of aqueous extract and its chromatographic fractions were carried out, aiming at establishing a correlation between gastroprotective effect and chemical composition. In this study, fractionation of aqueous extract led to 5 fractions containing different flavonoids such as the tri-flavonoid glycosides mauritianin, trifolin, hyperin, epicatechin, a tetra-glycoside kaempferol derivate and the monosaccharide galactitol. Chemical structures of the phytochemicals identified are showed in Figure 3. These fractions were evaluated in rats for their effects on gastric secretion volume and pH in a model of pylorus ligation. Considering the results of the study it was possible to conclude that only fractions containing mauritianin and tetra-glycoside kaempferol derivate caused significant increase of gastric volume and pH, thus indicating that these glycosides play an important role on the gastroprotective effect of *Maytenus ilicifolia* leaves. Compounds identified in the other fractions had a less important contribution to gastroprotective effect since they have not disclosed significant activity on gastric volume and pH of rats. Gastric mucus is believed to play an important role in the defensive mechanism against gastric ulceration. The protective effect of mucus as an active barrier may be attributed to the glycoproteins, which have the property of holding water in the interstices, thus obstructing the diffusion of hydrogen ions. Stress has been shown to decrease the amount of mucus adhering to the gastric mucosa (Jorge et al., 2004). Hence, increase in synthesis of mucus, according to results obtained in this study with *Maytenus ilicifolia*, is consistent to those found by some authors (Bravo et al., 1990; Sairam et al., 2002), suggesting that such increase is an important factor for antiulcer protection.

Because of mucosa protection, extracts of *Maytenus ilicifolia* may represent an important clinical alternative in antiulcerogenic therapeutic, though, further studies are needed to evaluate the real usefulness of this extract in the prevention and treatment of peptic ulcers. Thus, the screening of the constituents from *Maytenus ilicifolia* with antiulcer activity used in this study, clearly illustrate as a phytochemical investigation directed by an ethnopharmacologycal approach can be of great value in the search for compounds with potential use for the development of new and more efficient drugs used in management of ulcerative diseases and others health disorders. The occurrence of tetra-glycosylated flavonoids in this specie afford a valuable chemical marker for the quality control of the Brazilian *Maytenus* marketed as phytomedicines.

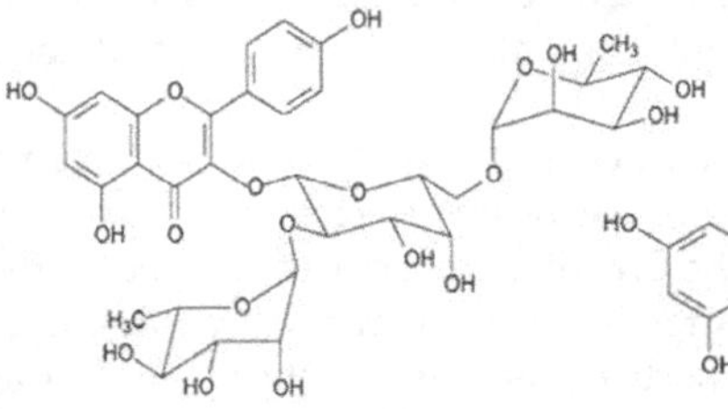

1. mauritianin

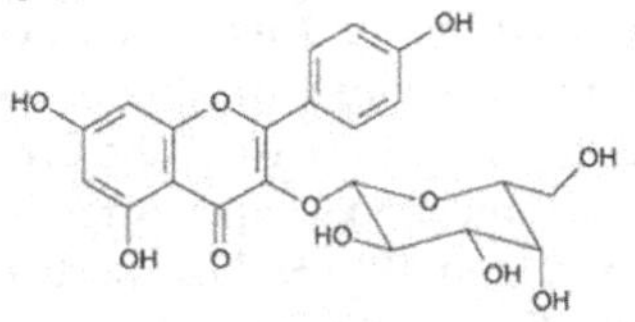

2. trifolin

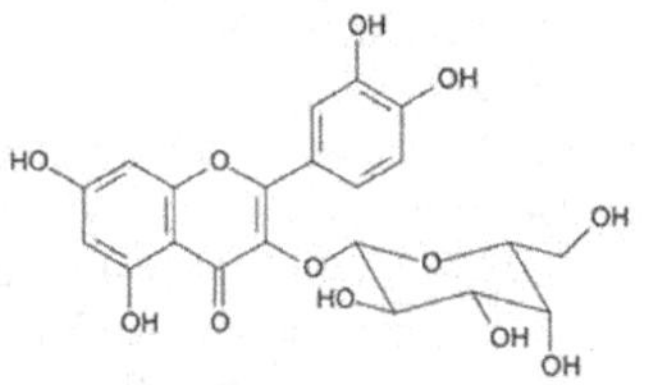

3. hyperin

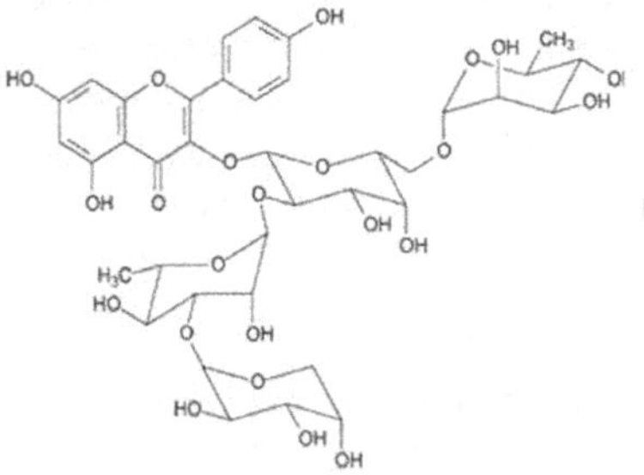

4. tetra-glycoside kaempferol derivative

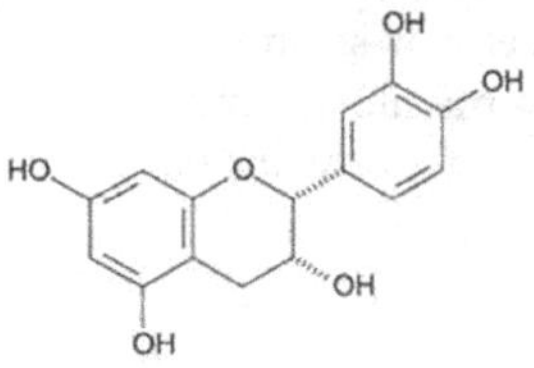

5. epi-catechin

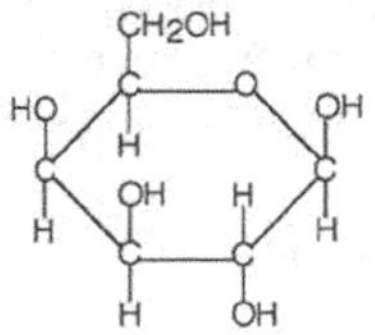

6. galactiol

Fig. 3. Phytochemicals identified in a lyophilized aqueous extract of *Maytenus ilicifolia* leaves.

7. Conclusion

Currently, there is a positive trend in favor of traditional, complementar and integrative therapies both in scientific research and health care. Furthermore, in recent decades has been observed strengthening of approaches related to health care such as ethnopharmacology, reverse pharmacology, phytotherapy, systems biology and personalized medicine. Ethnopharmacology has already played recognized importance in the discovery of plants with medicinal potential and in the development of natural health care practices, and is likely to play more significant role in the years to come. It would not be surprising to see that the use of herbal medicines will be gradually accepted in the main stream of conventional medicine. Due to acceptance that the diversity of chemical substances found in vegetable materials may have different biological effects of interest with potential applications in many different health conditions, it is believe that there will be a growing trend in the use of novel natural products and development of chemical libraries based on these products in drug discovery campaigns.

Plant resources have proved to be an important source for the discovery of new substances with antiulcer potential. Researches in this area have been targeted for both the isolation of active principles, such as to obtain standardized extracts. Polyphenolic compounds, including flavonoids, have been the subject of increasing interest since *in vitro* and *in vivo* biological assays indicated that flavonoids can mediate a range of mechanisms related to anticancer, antitumor, and anti-oxidant activities, among other. The contribution of the flavonoids to the dietary intake of polyphenolics compounds is considerable. In fact, cereals, legume seeds, fruits, wine, and tea contain significant amounts of flavonoids and their derivatives.

In Brazil, studies of the species *Maytenus ilicifolia* have advanced considerably, reinforcing the use in folk medicine, where preparations from the leaves of this species are used as an antiulcer treatment. This species is part of the cast of the Brazilian Pharmacopoeia, being the phenolic constituents used as chemical markers. After several chemical investigations, preclinical and clinical (Phase I, II and III) studies, herbal preparations that include this species obtained registration with the Health Surveillance Agency (ANVISA), the Brazilian agency that regulates the registration of these products. The species is also included in the list of herbal medicines that the Brazilian government provides in the pharmaceutical assistance of the Unified Health System (SUS), and their herbal medicine, therefore, proven by the government as to its effectiveness and safety. In *Maytenus ilicifolia* the 3-O-glycosides of quercetin and kaempferol are the most common group of flavonoids. It is known that the sugar moiety is an important factor for the bioavailability of the flavonoid derivatives.

8. References

Alarcon de la Lastra, C.; Martin M.J. & Motilva, V. (1994). Antiulcer and gastroprotective effects of quercetin: a gross and histologic study. *Pharmacology*, Vol. 48, No. 1, pp. 56-62, ISSN 0031-7012

Akhtar, M.S. & Munir, M. (1989). Evaluation of the gastric antiulcerogenic effects of solanum nigrum, brassica oleracea and ocimum basilicum in rats. *Journal of Ethnophannacology*, Vol. 27, No. 1-2, pp. 163-176 ISSN 0378-8741

Al-Shabanah, O.A.; Islam, M.W.; Al-Gharably, N.M. & Al-Harbi, M.M. (1993). Effect of khatamines and their enantiomers on aspirin, indomethacin, phenylbutazone and reserpine induced gastric ulcers in rats. *Research Communications in Substance of Abuse*, Vol. 14, No. 1, pp. 81-94, ISSN 0193 -0818

Asuzu, I.U. & Onu, O.U. (1990). Anti-Ulcer activity of the ethanolic extract of *Combretum dolichopetalum* Root. *Pharmaceutical Biology*, Vol. 28, No. 1 , pp. 27-32, ISSN 1388-0209

Baggio, C.H.; Freitas, C.S.; Otofuji, G.M.; Cipriani, T.R.; Souza, L.M.; Sassaki, G.L.; Iacomini, M.; Marques, M.C.A. & Mesia-Vela, S. (2007). Flavonoid-rich fraction of *Maytenus ilicifolia* Mart. ex. Reiss protects the gastric mucosa of rodents through inhibition of both H+, K+-ATPase activity and formation of nitric oxide. *Journal of Ethnopharmacology*, Vol. 113, No. 3, pp. 433-440, ISSN 0378-8741

Balunas, M.J. & Kinghorn, A.D. (2005). Drug Discovery from Medicinal Plants. *Life Sciences*, Vol. 78, No. 5, pp. 431-441, ISSN 0024-3205

Bandhopadhyay, U.; Biswas, K.; Chatterjee, R.; Bandyopadhyay, D.; Chattopadhyay, I.; Ganguly, C.K.; Chakraborty, T.; Bhattacharya, K. & Banerjee, R.K. (2002). Gastroprotective effect of Neem (*Azadiracta indica*) bark extract: possible involvement of H + K + ATPase inhibition and scavenging of hydroxyl radical. *Life Sciences*, Vol. 71, No. 24, pp. 2845-865, ISSN 0024-3205

Beil, W.; Birkholz, C. & Sewing, K.F. (1995). Effects of flavonoids on parietal cell acid secretion, gastric mucosal prostaglandin production and Helicobacter pylori growth. *Arzneimittel-Forschung,*Vol. 45, No. 6, pp. 697-700, ISSN 0004-4172

Bhutani, K.K. & Gohil, V.M. (2010). Natural products drug discovery research in India: Status and appraisal . *Indian Journal of Experimental Biology*, Vol. 48, No. 3, pp. 199-207, ISSN 0975-1009

Borrelli, F. & Izzo, A.A. (2000). The plant kingdom as a source of anti-ulcer remedies. *Phytotherapy Research*, Vol. 14, No. 8, pp. 581–591, ISSN 0951-418X

Bravo, L.; Escolar, G.; Navarro, C.; Fontarnau, R. & Bulbena, O. (1990). Effect of zinc acexamate on gastric lesions induced by aspirin: a morphological study. *European Journal of Pharmacology*, Vol. 190, No. 1-2, pp. 59-65, ISSN 0014-2999

Butler, M.S. (2008). Natural products to drugs: natural product-derived compounds in clinical trials. *Natural Product Reports*, Vol. 28, No. 3, pp. 475-516, ISSN 0265-0568

Cordeiro, D.S.; Raghavan, G.S.V. & Oliveira, W.P. (2006). Equilibrium moisture content models for *Maytenus ilicifolia* leaves. *Biosystems Engineering*, Vol. 94, No. 2, pp. 221-228, ISSN 1537-5129

Dharmani, P. & Palit, G. (2006). Exploring Indian medicinal plants for antiulcer activity. *Indian Journal of Pharmacology*, Vol. 38, No. 2, pp. 95-92, ISSN 0253-7613

Di Carlo, G.; Mascolo, N.; Izzo, A.A. & Capasso, F. (1999). Flavonoids: old and new aspects of a class of natural therapeutic drugs. *Life Sciences*, Vol. 65, No. 4, pp. 337-353, ISSN 0024-3205

Dulcie, A.M.; Vikash, S.; Roy, O.; Karl, H.P. & Joseph, D.C. (1997). Cucurbitane triterpenoids from the leaves of *Momordica foetida*. *Phytochemistry*, vol. 45, No. 2, pp. 391-395, ISSN 0031-9422

Elisabetsky, E. (2002). Traditional medicines and the new paradigm of psychotropic drug action, In: *Ethnomedicine and drug development, advances phytomedicine*, Iwu MM and Wootton J Editors, pp. 133-144, Elsevier, ISBN 044450852X, Oxford

Elisabetsky, E.& Nunes, D.S. (1990). Ethnopharmacology and its role in developing countries. *AMBIO: A Journal of the Human Environment* vol. 19, No. 8, pp. 419-421. ISSN 1654-7209

Ezaki, N.; Kato, M.; Takizawa, N.; Morimoyo, S.; Nonaka, G.; Nishioca, I. (1985). Pharmacological studies *on Linderae umbellata* Ramus. IV. Effects of condensed tannin related compounds on pepitic acitivity and stressinduced gastric lesions in mice. *Planta Medica*, , v. 52, No.1, p. 34-38, ISSN 0032-0943

Falcão, H.S.; Leite, J.A.; Barbosa-Filho, J.M.; Athayde-Filho, P.F.; Chaves, M.C.O.; Moura, M.D.; Ferreira, A.L.; Almeida, A.B.A.; Souza-Brito, A.R.M.; Diniz, M.F.F.M. & Batista, LM. (2008a). Gastric and Duodenal Antiulcer Activity of Alkaloids: a review. *Molecules*, Vol. 13, No. 12, pp. 3198-3223, ISSN 1420-3049.

Falcão, H.S.; Mariath, I.R.; Diniz, M.F.F.M.; Batista, L.M. & Barbosa-Filho, J.M. (2008b). Plants of the American continent with antiulcer activity. *Phytomedicine*, Vol. 15, No. 1-2, pp. 132-146, ISSN 0944-7113

Fabricant, D.S. & Farnsworth, N.R. (2001). The Value of Plants Used in Traditional Medicine for Drug Discovery. *Environmental Health Perspectives*, Vol. 109, Suppl. 1, ISSN 0091-6765

Funatogawa, K.; Hayashi, S.; Shimomura, H.; Yoshida, T.; Hatano, T.; Ito, H. & Hirai, Y. (2004). Antibacterial activity of hydrolysable tannins derived from medicinal plants against *Helicobacter pylori. Microbiology and Immunology*. Vol. 48, No. 4, pp. 251–261, ISSN 1348-0421

Gertsch, J. (2009). How scientific is the science in ethnopharmacology? Historical perspectives and epistemological problems. *Journal of Ethnopharmacology*, Vol. 122, No. 2, pp. 177-183, ISSN 0378-8741

Gilani, A.H. & Atta-ur-Rahman. (2005). Trends in ethnopharmacology. *Journal of Ethnopharmacology*, Vol. 100, No. 1-2, pp. 43-49, ISSN 0378-8741

Hammer, K.A.; Carson, C.F. & Riley, T.V. (1999). Antimicrobial activity of essential oils and other plant extracts. *Journal of Applied Microbiology*, Vol. 86, No. 6, p. 985, ISSN 1364-5072

Harvey, A.L. (2008). Natural products in drug discovery. *Drug Discovery Today*. Vol. 13, No. 19-20, pp. 894-901, ISSN 1359-6446

Harvey, A.L, Clark, R.L.; Mackay, S.P. & Johnston, B.F. (2010). Current strategies for drug discovery through natural products. *Expert Opinion on Drug Discovery*, Vol. 5, No. 6, pp. 559-568, ISSN 1746-0441

Hirano, H.; Tokuhira, T.; Yoshioka, Y.; Yokoi, T. & Shingu, T. (2000). Analysis of gastric mucosus membrane-protective compounds in *Coptidis* rhizoma. *Natural Medicine*. Vol. 54, No. 5, pp.209-212, ISSN 1340-3443

Hirano, H.; Osawa, E.; Yamaoka, Y. & Yokoi, T. (2001). Gastric-mucous membrane protection activity of coptisine derivatives. *Biological and Pharmaceutical Bulletin*, Vol. 24, No. 11, pp. 1277-1281, ISSN 1347-5215

Hoogerwerf, W.A. & Pasricha, P.J. (2006). Pharmacotherapy of gastric acidity, peptic ulcers, and gastroesophageal reflux disease. In: *Goodman & Gilman's the pharmacological basis of therapeutics*, Brunton LL, Lazo JS and Parker KL Editors, pp. 1005-1020, McGraw-Hill Medical Publishing Division, ISBN 0071354697, NewYork

Izzo, A.A.; Di Carlo, G.; Mascolg, N.; Autgre, G. & Capasso, F. (1994). *Phytotherapy Research*, Vol. 8, No. 3, pp. 179-181, ISSN 0951-418X

Izzo, A.A. (1996). PAF and the digestive tract. A review. *Journal of Pharmacy and Pharmacology*, Vol. 48, No. 11, pp. 1103-1111, ISSN 0022-3573

Jorge, R.M.; Leite, J.P.; Oliveira, A.B. & Tagliati, C.A. (2004). Evaluation of antinociceptive, anti-inflammatory and antiulcerogenic activities of *Maytenus ilicifolia. Journal of Ethnophamacology*, Vol. 94, No. 1, pp. 93-100, ISSN ISSN 0378-8741

Koehn, F.E. & Carter, G.T. (2005). The evolving role of natural products in drug discovery. *Nature Reviews Drug Discovery*, Vol. 4, No. 3, pp. 206-220, ISSN 1474-1776

Leite, J.P.V.; Rastrelli, L.; Romussi, G.; Oliveira, A.B.; Vilegas, J.H.Y.; Vilegas, W. & Pizza, C. (2001). Isolation and HPLC quantitative analysis of flavonoid glycosides from brazilian beverages (*Maytenus ilicifolia* and *M. aquifolium*). *Journal of Agricultural and Food Chemistry*, Vol. 49, No. 8, pp. 3796–3801, ISSN 1520-5118

Leite, J.P.V. (2009). *Fitoterapia, bases científicas e tecnológicas*. Atheneu (1ª edição), ISBN 978-85-7379-237-9, São Paulo

Leite, J.P.V.; Braga, F.C.; Romussi, G.; Persoli, R.M.; Tabach, R.; Carlinid, E.A. & Oliveira, A.B. (2010). Constituents from *Maytenus ilicifolia* leaves and bioguided fractionation for gastroprotective activity. *Journal of Brazilian Chemical Society*, Vol. 21, No. 2, pp. 248-254, ISSN 0103-5053

Marhuenda, E.; Martin, M.J. & Alarcon de la Lastra, C. (1993). Antiulcerogenic activity of aescine in different experimental models. *Phytotherapy Research*, Vol. 7, No. 1, pp. 13-16. ISSN 0951-418X

Marhuenda, E.; Alarcón de la Lastra, C. & Martín, M.J. (1994). Antisecretory and gastroprotective effects of aescine in rats. *General Pharmacology*. Vol. 25, No. 6, pp. 1213-1239, ISSN 0306-3623

Martín, M.J.; Alarcón De La Lastra, C.; Motilva, V. & La Casa, C. (2000). Antiulcer and gastroprotective activity of flavonic compounds: mechanisms involved, In: *Studies in natural products chemistry, bioactive natural products*, Atta-ur-Rahman Editor, pp. 419-456, Elsevier, ISBN 0444518789, Oxford

Martins, A.G.; Guterres, S.S. & González-Ortega, G. (2003). Anti-ulcer Activity of Spray-dried Powders prepared from Leaf Extracts of *Maytenus ilicifolia* Martius ex Reiss. *Acta Farmacéutica Bonaerense*, Vol. 22, No. 1, pp. 39-44, ISSN 0326-2383

Matsuda, H.; Li, Y.; Murakami, T.; Yamahara, J. & Yoshikawa M. (1998). Protective effects of oleanolic acid oligoglycosides on ethanol- or indomethacin-induced gastric mucosal lesions in rats. *Life Sciences*, Vol. 63, No. 17, pp. 245-250, ISSN 0024-3205

Mota, K.S.L.; Dias, G.E.N.; Pinto, M.E.F.; Luiz-Ferreira, A.; Souza-Brito, A.R.M.; Hiruma-Lima, C.A.; Barbosa-Filho, J.M. & Batista, LM. (2009). Flavonoids with gastroprotective activity. Molecules, Vol. 14, No. 3, pp. 979-1012, ISSN 1420-3049

Newall, C.A.; Anderson, L.A. & Phillipson, J.D. (1996). *Herbal medicines: a guide for health care professionals*, The Pharmaceutical Press (1ª edition), ISBN 0853692890, London.

Okuda, T. (2005). Systematics and health effects of chemically distinct tannins in medicinal plants. *Phytochemistry*, Vol. 66, No. 17, pp. 2012–2031, ISSN 0031-9422

Patwardhan, B. (2005a). Traditional Medicine: Modern approach for affordable   global health. In: Commission on Intellectual Property Rights IaPHC, [World Health Organization (WHO). Geneva: WHO].

Patwardhan, B. (2005b) Ethnopharmacology and drug discovery. *Journal of Ethnopharmacology*, Vol. 100, No. 1-2, pp. 50-52, ISSN 0378-8741

Patwardhan, B. & Vaidyab, A.D.B. (2010). Natural products drug discovery: Accelerating the clinical candidate development using reverse pharmacology approaches. Indian Journal of Experimental Biology, Vol. 48, No. 3, pp. 220-227, ISSN 0975-1009

Raza, M. (2006). A role for physicians in ethnopharmacology and drug discovery. *Journal of Ethnopharmacology*, Vol. 104, No. 3, pp. 297-301, ISSN 0378-8741

Sairam, K.; Rao, Ch.V.; Babu, M,D.; Kumar, K.V.; Agrawal, V.K. & Goel, R.K. (2002). Antiulcerogenic effect of methanolic extract of *Emblica officinalis*: an experimental study. *Journal of Ethnopharmacology*, Vol. 82, No. 1, pp. 1-9, ISSN 0378-8741

Samuelsson, G. (1992). *Drugs of natural origin, a textbook of pharmacognosy* , Swedish Pharmaceutical Press (6ª edition), ISBN 1439838577, Stockhlm

Sekar, T.; Ayyanar, M. & Gopalakrishnan, M. (2010). Medicinal plants and herbal drugs. *Current Science*, Vol. 98, No. 12, pp. 1558-1559, ISSN 0011- 3891

Sandor, V. & Cuparencu, B. (1977). Analysis of the mechanism of the protective activity of some sympathomimetic amines in experimental ulcers. *Pharmacology*, Vol. 15, No. 3, pp. 208-217, ISSN 0031-7012

Sen, S.; Chakraborty, R.; De, B. & Mazumder, J. (2009). Plants and phytochemicals for peptic ulcer: An overview. *Pharmacognosy Review*, Vol. 3, No. 6, pp. 270-279, ISSN 0976-2787

Schmeda-Hirschmann, G. & Rojas de Arias, A. (1990). A survey of medicinal plants of Minas Gerais, Brazil. *Journal of Ethnopharmacology*, Vol. 29, No. 2, pp. 159-172, ISSN 0378-8741

Schmeda-Hirschmann, G. & Yesilada, E. (2005). Traditional medicine and gastroprotective crude drugs. *Journal of Ethnopharmacology*, Vol. 100, No. 1-2, pp. 61-66, ISSN 0378-8741

Souza-Formigoni, M.L.; Oliveira, M.G.; Monteiro, M.G.; da Silveira-Filho, N.G.; Braz, S. & Carlini, E.A. (1991). Antiulcerogenic effects of two Maytenus species in laboratory animals. *Journal of Ethnopharmacology*, Vol. 34, No. 1, pp. 21-27, ISSN 0378-8741

Tan, P.V. & Nyasse, B. (2000). Anti-ulcer compound from *Voacanga africana* with possible histamine H_2 receptor blocking activity. *Phytomedicine*, Vol. 7, No. 6, pp. 509-515, ISSN 0944-7113

Tan, P.V.; Nyasse, B.; Enow-Orock, G.E.; Wafo, P. & Forcha, E.A. (2000). Prophylactic and healing properties of a new anti-ulcer compound from *Enantia chlorantha* in rats. *Phytomedicine*, Vol. 7, No. 4, pp. 291-296, ISSN 0944-7113

Tan, P.V.; Nyasse, B.; Dimo, T.; Wafo, P. & Akahkuh, B.T. (2002). Synergistic and potentiating effects of ranitidine and two new anti-ulcer compounds from Enantia chlorantha and Voacanga africana in experimental animal models. *Die Pharmazie*. Vol. 57, No. 6, pp. 409-412, ISSN 0031-7144

Tarnawski, A.S. (2005). Cellular and molecular mechanisms of gastrointestinal ulcer healing. *Digestive Diseases and Sciences*, Vol. 50, Suppl. 1, pp. 24-33, ISSN 0163-2116

Toma, W.; Trigo, J.R.; Bensuaski de Paula, A.C. & Souza Brito, A.R.M. (2004). Preventive activity of pyrrolizidine alkaloids from *Senecio brasiliensis* (Asteraceae) on gastric and duodenal induced ulcer on mice and rats. *Journal of Ethnopharmacology*, Vol. 95, No. 2-3, pp. 345-351, ISSN 0378-8741

Vlietinck, A.J. & Van Den Berghe, D.A.J. (1991). Can ethnopharmacology contribute to the development of antiviral drugs? *Journal of Ethnopharmacology*, Vol. 32, No. 1-3, pp. 141-153, ISSN 0378-8741

Vyawahare, N.S.; Deshmukh, V.V.; Gadkari, M.R. & Kagathara, VG. (2009). Plants with Antiulcer Activity. *Pharmacognosy Reviews*, Vol. 3, No. 5, pp. 118-125, ISSN 0973-7847

Yamahara, J.; Kubomura, Y.; Miki, K. & Fujimura, H. 1987. Antiulcer action of *Panax japonicus* rhizome. *Journal of Ethnopharmacology*, Vol. 19, No. 1, pp. 95-101, ISSN 0378-8741

Yamazaki, M. (2000). The pharmacological studies on matrine and oxymatrine. *Yakugaku Zasshi*, Vol. 120, No. 10, pp. 1025-1033, ISSN 0031-6903

Ziegler, J. & Facchini, P.J. (2008). Alkaloid biosynthesis: metabolism and trafficking. *Annual Review of Plant Biology*, Vol. 59, pp. 735-769, ISSN 1543-5008

Zhu, Z.P.; Zhang, M.F. & Shen, Y.Q. (1993). Antiulcer components of *Sophora viciifolia* alkaloids. *Tianran Chanwu Yanjiu Yu Kaifa*, Vol. 5, pp. 26-29, ISSN 1001-6880

7

Spices as Alternative Agents for Gastric Ulcer Prevention and Treatment

Ibrahim Abdulkarim Al Mofleh
College of Medicine, King Saud University
Kingdom of Saudi Arabia

1. Introduction

1.1 Important aspects on ulcer pathogenesis

World-wide, peptic Ulcer disease (PUD) is considered as a common gastrointestinal disorder. It develops as a result of altered balance between offensive and defensive factors. Offensive (aggressive) factors disrupt normal mucosal integrity and allow H+ back diffusion with a subsequent cellular injury. Helicobacter pylori (H. pylori) and nonsteroidal anti-inflammatory drugs (NSAID) represent the major aggressive factors associated with PUD. Experimentally induced gastric ulcer has expanded our knowledge on ulcer pathogenesis. Indomethacine, 80% ethanol and pyloric ligation are the methods commonly applied in experimental ulcer models. Other universally accepted experimental ulcer models include 0.2 mol/L NaOH, 25% NaCl, stress induced by swimming (1), acetylsalicylic acid (2), cold-restraint (3) and hypothermic restraint (4).

A major event in the pathogenesis of NSAID induced gastric ulcer is represented by inhibition of prostaglandin (PG) synthesis, enhancement of gastric acid secretion, suppression of bicarbonate secretion, glutathione (GSH) levels, mucosal circulation, cell proliferation and growth as well as alteration of gastric mucosal barrier integrity. Inhibition of PG biosynthesis enhances generation of leukotrienes and other products of the 5-lipoxygenase pathway (5). These products disrupt the mucosal barrier with subsequent enhancement of gastric mucosal permeability for H + ions and Na+ ions and reduction of transmucosal potential difference (6, 7). Furthermore, NSAID uncouple mitochondrial oxidative phosphorylation, affect mitochondrial morphology, reduce the intracellular ATP levels and alter the normal regulatory cellular function (8). These processes promote erosions and ulcer formation. In addition, generation of reactive oxygen species (ROS) is also considered as a major factor contributing to ulcer pathogenesis. Another, prostaglandin-independent pathway of gastric ulcer pathogenesis is induced by enhanced endothelial adhesion, activation of polymorphonuclear cells (PMN) with subsequent release of oxidative byproducts (9, 10). PMN activation induces depletion of GSH and sulfhydryl compounds (SH) in tissue with enhanced mucosal myeloperoxidase (MPO) and malondialdehyde (MDA) concentration (11). Myeloperoxidase is considered as a marker of oxidative process induced by PMN tissue infiltration.

Similarly, in ethanol-induced gastric mucosal injury there is enough evidence to suggest the role of oxidative burst. Ethanol-induced oxidative damage is commonly associated with generation of ROS, leading to oxidative stress. Acute ethanol treatment induced oxidative damage is associated with a decreased GSH content in gastric tissue along with an increased MDA and xanthine oxidase activity (12). The oxygen free radicals-induced lipid peroxidation affects mitochondrial energy metabolism and plays a critical role in the pathogenesis of acute ethanol-induced gastric mucosal injuries (13). On the mitochondrial level, ethanol-induced intracellular oxidative stress causes also mitochondrial permeability transition with mitochondrial depolarization that precedes gastric mucosal cells necrosis. This process can be prevented by intracellular antioxidants, such as GSH (14). Acute ethanol administration is also associated with inhibition of catalase and, glutathione peroxidase (GPx) activities with significant increase of MDA contents, MPO activity, and cellular apoptosis (15). Furthermore, ethanol induces inhibition of SH with enhancement of superoxide dismutase (SOD) and glutathione reductase (GR) activities (16). The extent of oxidative damage in stomach as indicated by the ulcer index, gastric mucosal MDA content and alteration of mitochondrial ultrastructure is correlated with ethanol exposure and concentration (13).

2. Introduction in spices

Spices are used in several parts in the world as food additives and carminatives. Since ancient times they are also applied in the traditional management of a variety of disorders. Currently their therapeutic value has gained a considerable interest and several investigators have reported their effects in laboratory animals and in man. It has been experimentally demonstrated that spices, herbs, and their extracts possess antibacterial (17) antifungal (18,19), vermicidal, nematocidal, molluscicidal properties (20-22), anti-inflammatory and antirheumatic activity (23-25), hepatoprotective (26,27), nephro-protective (28), antimutagenic, anticancer potentials (28-30) and antihypercholesterimc potentials (31-34).

A tremendous number of studies have evaluated the antiulcer effect of spices. Although some investigators have reported deleterious effect of certain spices such as red and black pepper, the majority have demonstrated rather a cytoprotective activity in animal (35-37) as well as in human (38).

3. Factors involved in ulcer healing

In the presence of mucosal barrier disruption, several factors including acid, bile acids, NSAID and ethanol promote H+ back diffusion and enhance the susceptibility to develop ulcer. On the other hand, optimal mucosal microcirculation and bicarbonate secretion with formation of an alkaline buffer layer at the epithelial surface is considered as a first line of mucosal defense and gastroprotection. Other factors including prostaglandins (PG), growth factors (GF), nitric oxide (NO) or calcitonin gene-related peptide (CGRP), as well as some gut hormones such as gastrin, cholecystokinin (CCK), leptin, ghrelin, gastrin-releasing peptide (GRP) and melatonin are involved in mucosal defense system and the ulcer healing process. The protective action of gut hormones is attributed to the release of cyclooxygenase-2 (COX-2) and PGE2 at the ulcer margins (39, 40) or activation of sensory nerves (41). In addition, Tumor necrosis factor – α (TNF-α), released during gastric mucosal injury, activates PG pathway and promotes epithelial cell repair and healing (42). EGF and other growth factors are also pivotal for the process of mucosal healing. Furthermore, in response to gastric injury and inflammation, gastrin and parietal cells contribute to the regulation of mucosal proliferation (43).

4. Why spices, herbs and plant extracts are considered as an alternative ulcer therapy?

Ulcer healing and prevention of recurrence represent the central goals of treatment. The treatment is targeted at either counteracting aggressive factors like acid, pepsin, active oxidants, platelet aggravating factor (PAF), leukotrienes, endothelins, bile or exogenous factors including (NSAID) or enhancing mucosal defense such as mucus, bicarbonate, blood flow, PG and NO (44). Antiscretory drugs including H_2-receptor antagonists (H_2-RA) and proton pump inhibitors (PPI) alone or combined with antibiotics in the presence of H. pylori infection are currently considered as the most acceptable drugs for ulcer treatment. The main action of antisecretory drugs is acid suppression. These agents lack effect on other factors involved in ulcer pathogenesis and therefore, do not meet all treatment goals. In addition, acid suppressors are expensive and associated with adverse effects and ulcer recurrence. Hence, efforts are on to search for suitable alternative treatment from medicinal plants resources. Already a large percentage of world population relies on medicinal plants to treat a variety of disorders including PUD. In addition to their ability to act on various pathogenetic factors, they are cheap and easily accessible. Furthermore, a large number of spices and plant extracts evaluated by various researchers for their anti-ulcer effects have a favorable outcome. (29, 45-48)

The antiulcer effect of spices/herbs is based on the activities of their chemical constituents, which attenuate the gastric secretion, enhance mucosal integrity, interfere with oxidative burst, NO, SH compounds and inhibit H. pylori growth. Due to their variable phytochemical constituens they may exhibit antisecretory, cytoprotective, antoxidant or combined activities.

5. Herbs and gastric secretion

A variety of spices and their extracts possess a potent antiscretory activity. Pylorus-ligation in rats represents the model of antisecretory studies. A number of spices, herbs and plants methanolic or aqueous extracts possess an antisecrertoy activity. For instance, Cissus quadrangularis , Maytenus ilicifolia, phytosphingosine, Cecropia glaziovii Sneth (Cecropiaceae), alkaloid extract and 2-phenylquinoline obtained from the bark of Galipea longiflora (Rutaceae) and Landolphia owariensis induce significant inhibition of acidity, pepsin content and ulcer index (49-54), respectively. This potent antisecretory action of spices and plant extracts is likely related to their flavonoid content. Maytenus ilcifolia is considered among flavenoid-rich plant extracts (55).

In rats with pylorus ligation, antisecretory effect of methanolic extract of Momordica charantia L. is demonstrated by decrease in acidity, pepsin content and ulcer index with an increase in gastric mucosal content (56).

Likewise, the protective effect of Cissus quadrangularis extract is mediated by inhibition of gastric secretion with decrease in ulcer index as well as enhancement of mucosal defense (49).

6. Herbs and cytoprotection

Several spices and plants extracts promotes ulcer healing via enhancing gastric mucosal content beside their antisecretory activity in pylorus-ligated rats. Ginger rhizome extract-induced cytoprotective activity is based on its antioxidative and gastric mucosal protective activities (1). Total carotenoid and astaxanthin esters protect mucin, enhance antioxidants enzymes level and H+, K+-ATPase inhibitory activity (57). Furthermore, boswellic acid-induced gastroprotection depends on generation of cytoprotective PG, enhanced gastric mucosal resistance, and inhibition of leukotriene synthesis (3). Similarly, Galipea longiflora (Rutaceae) protect gastric mucosa by enhancement of mucus content and antisecretory activity (53). In addition to its antioxidant activity, Cissus sicyoides , induce increase of NO and SH compounds and enhances defense mechanism (58). In pylorus-ligated rats, beside its antiscretory action, Momordica charantia L. extract also significantly increases gastric mucosal content (56). Increase in Glycoprotein level, gastric mucin content and SH concentration are essential for the gastroprotection. Their levels are raised by treatment with Cissus quadrangularis extract (49)

7. Herbs and antioxidants

Recently, oxidants are found to play a critical role in PUD pathogenesis. Experimental NSAID and ethanol induced microvascular and gastric mucosal injuries are at least partially caused by ORS release (59). Therefore, implementations of agents with antioxidative properties are useful for the prevention of injuries and promotion of gastric ulcer healing. Many spices have phytochemicals with antioxidative activities. For instance, Coriander contains many antioxidant constituents including d-linalool, borneol, geraniol, geranyl acetate, camphor, carvone, which are responsible for its antioxidative property (60). Black cumin (Nigella sativa), peperine and thymoquinone, the active constituents of pepper and Nigella sativa, respectively have also the ability to inhibit ROS in experimentally induced gastric lesions in rats (29, 60, 61).

Many other spices/herbs and plant extracts protect against experimentally-induced gastric mucosal injuries through their potential antioxidative effect. These include ginger rhizome, carotenoid and astaxanthin esters, Cissus sicyoides extract, isopulegol and the herb collection Korniozil (1, 57, 58, 62, 63), respectively. Through the interaction with endogenous PG and antioxidative properties, isopulegol, monoterpene a constituent of essential oils of several aromatic plants, induce significant gastroprotection. Total carotenoid and astaxanthin esters increase the levels of the antioxidant enzymes catalase, SOD, and GPx in gastric homogenate and protect gastric mucin (57). Korniozil also protects against experimentally induced stress ulcers, with restoration of lipid peroxidation and antioxidative system function along with enhancement of gastric mucous coat regeneration (63). Ginger rhizome extract gastroprotective activity is also based on restoration of antioxidant enzymes and gastric mucin generation in addition to inhibitory effect on H. pylori growth (1). Due to its antioxidative properties, Cissus sicyoides oral extract increase also NO and SH and induces also protection [58]

The alkaloid indigo, obtained from the leaves of Indigofera truxillensis Kunth (Fabaceae), prevents ethanol induced depletion of SH and GPx activity, inhibits GR and MPO activities and partially inhibits gastric mucosa DNA damage caused by ethanol (64).

8. Herbs combined activities

Due the presence of several active constituents, some spices/herbs and plant extracts protect the gastric mucosa via different mechanisms. For instance, Weikang decoction acts as antisecretory, cytoprotective and antioxidative agent. It enhances mucosal thickness, NO in gastric tissue, PGE2 in plasma, (EGF) content in gastric juice and SOD in plasma. In addition it inhibits also MDA and endothelin in plasma (65). Many other spices like Rocket Eruca sativa, black cumin, black pepper, clove, cardamom, caraway , peppermint, saffron, coriander and anise possess also antisecretory, cytoprotctive and antioxidative activities (4, 29, 66-73). They also replenish gastric wall mucus concentration and SH levels and significantly reduce MDA level.

Besides its H. pylori bactericidal effect, Davilla elliptica also enhances NO, H_2O_2, TNF - α production and GSH bioavailability. These activities are related to its phytochemical constituents acylglycoflavonoids, phenolic acid derivatives and tannins (74). Also Brazilian medicinal plant methanolic extracts have an anti-H. pylori effect and protect the gastric mucosa by increasing PGE2, antisecretory and gastroprotective properties (75) The gastroprotection of Vochysia tucanorum Mart. methanolic extract and buthanolic fraction provided by the antioxidant activity and maintenance of gastric mucosa NO levels is interrelated to its phytochemical constituent Triterpenoid (76)

9. Herbs- PG interaction

Gastric protection is maintained in a state of equilibrium between aggressive and protective factors. In experimental ulcer model, indomethacin increases acid secretion, activates oxidative stress and inhibits the release of cyclooxygenase-1 (COX-1), PGE2, bicarbonate, and mucus (77). Similar to conventional NSAID, COX-2 inhibitors also delay the healing of chronic gastric ulcer and suppress the epithelial cell proliferation, angiogenesis and maturation of the granulation tissue in experimental animals. COX-2 is important for gastric mucosal defense (78). Indomethacin- induced gastric damage is associated with an increase of acid and oxidative parameters and inhibition of protective factors such as COX- 1, PGE2, bicarbonate, and mucus release (77).

Generally, PG are products of arachidonic acid and their biosynthesis is influenced by local, hormonal and neural factors. They stimulate gastric and duodenal bicarbonate secretion and the production of mucus glycoproteins. PG are also able to protect the gastric mucosa against experimentally induced gastric injuries in an acid independent manner known as "cytoprotection" (79). PG play a pivotal role in the gastric mucosal defensive system and contribute to the overall protective process against gastric mucosal injuries. They exhibit a variety of defensive mechanisms including mucus-alkaline secretion, mucosal hydrophobicity, mucosal microcirculation, tissue lysosomes stabilization, SH preservation, rapid proliferation and mucosal cells renewal. Mucosal integrity protection can also be accomplished even by small quantities of PG. Gastroprotection is attained by stimulation of mucosal protective PG biosynthesis or by the inhibition of preulcerogenic arachidonic acid metabolites (80). In addition, PG antiulcer activity is determined mainly by their antioxidant property with inhibition of lipid peroxidation as well as SOD and catalase activities (81).

Other mediators involved in gastric mucosal protection besides PG include growth factors, NO, CGRP and some gut hormones such as gastrin and CCK. In addition, leptin, ghrelin and gastrin-releasing peptide (GRP) have also the ability to protect gastric mucosa against corrosive agents-induced mucosal damage. Gut hormones protective activity is attributed to PG release (41). Ulcer healing is controlled by contribution of growth factors and gut hormones, increase of COX-2 induction and local PGE release in the ulcer area. Endogenous PG generated at ulcer margin play a key role in ulcer cure (82)

In acute injury, in the presence of PG-mediated paracellular space closure, mucosal permeability, PG helps the mucosal permeability to recover with epithelial restitution (83,

84). The ulcer healing by endogenous PG is mediated by PGEP4 receptors, as well as involvement of COX-2 in the early stage and COX-1 in the late stage of healing. Bacterial lipopolysaccharide contributes also through COX and endogenous PG genes activation to gastric mucosal protection in rats (85).

Mainly through their effect on PG, several plant extracts promote ulcer healing. For instance, Hyptis spicigera essential oil major constituents, monoterpenes, enhances PGE2-induced gastric mucus and reduces ulcer size in addition to increasing COX-2 and EGF expression in gastric mucosa and acceleration of ulcer healing (86).

Other spices and plant extracts involved in activation of PG synthesis and healing of gastric mucosal injuries include Boswellic acid, isopulegol, Teucrium polium (3, 62, 87). Endogenous PG and PGEP1 receptors play a key role in the adaptive protection (88). Chilli is believed to be detrimental to the gastric mucosa, however, its active ingredient capsaicin, decreases acid secretion and activates the defensive system by enhancing mucus, alkali secretions as well as mucosal microcirculation and hence, it prevents ulcer formation. Furthermore, capsaicin stimulates afferent neurons in the stomach and transmits signals to the central nervous system, which trigger an anti-inflammatory response and gastroprotection (89). Furthermore, Citrus lemon, Alchornea triplinervia and Myristica malabarica have demonstrated gastroprotective effect. Citrus lemon belongs to Rutaceae family and contains two main components, limonene and β-pinene. In ethanol and indomethacin gastric ulcer models, while Citrus lemon and limonene induce complete gastroprotection, β-pinene is not effective. Citrus lemon and limonene protective effect is linked with PGE2 and mediated by enhancing mucus secretion, HSP-70 and VIP (90). The antiulcer effect of ethyl acetate fraction of Alchornea triplinervia, a medicinal plant used in Brazil to treat gastrointestinal ulcers, is mainly related to its flavonoids content and mediated by increasing gastric mucosal prostaglandin PGE2 levels (75).

While PGE2, and vascular endothelial Growth Factor (VEGF) levels decrease, EGF and endostatin levels increase in indomethacin- induced ulceration in mice. Through modulation of PG synthesis and angiogenesis, Myristica malabarica plant extract restores these parameters. In comparison omeprazole, which offered similar healing, did not alter these parameters (91).

Coenzymes Q10, an essential cofactor in the mitochondrial electron transport pathway possess a potent antioxidant action. Pretreatment of indomethacin induced gastropathy with CoQ10 prevents ROS generation, mitochondrial dysfunction, vascular permeability erosions, ulcers and helps to restore PGE_2, NO and GSH levels (92).

10. Herbs and EGF

Growth factors and their receptors are also important for maintaining physiological function of gastric mucosa. They maintain and enhance defensive and inhibit aggressive factors. Following acute mucosal injury and during the initial stages of experimental gastric ulcer healing, R-associated tyrosine kinase is essential for regulation of cell proliferation, EGFR gene activation, EGFR phosphorylation, and increased mitogen-activated protein (MAP) kinase activity. H. pylori is a major cause of PUD and contributes also to inhibition of healing. In experimental gastric ulcer model, H. pylori vacuolating cytotoxin interfers with ulcer healing and inhibits cell proliferation, binding of EGF to its receptor, EGF-induced EGFR phosphorylation, and MAP and extracellular signal-related kinase (ERK-2) activation (93,94).. Growth factors and their receptors are pivotal for the process of gastroprotection and ulcer healing. EGF and transforming growth factor (TGF)-α and their common receptor (EGFR) inhibit gastric secretion, boost overexpression of growth factors, blood flow at ulcer margin and promote cell proliferation with ulcer healing (95). The process of gastric mucosal tissue repair and healing is controlled by EGFR activation (96). EGF-induced gastric epithelial cells proliferation is likely intervened by ERK /COX-2 pathway (97). Various GF exhibit different functions of the mucosal repair. They are implicated in the process of tissue healing with cell migration, proliferation, differentiation, secretion, and degradation of extracellular matrix. While EGF , TGF- α , and trefoil factors (TFFs), usually present in the gastric juice or mucosa, as well as hepatocyte growth factor (HGF) are responsible for epithelial structure reconstitution, basic fibroblast growth factor (bFGF), (VEGF), transforming growth factor-β (TGF-β) and platelet derived growth factor (PDGF), are essential for connective tissue reconstitution(98,99).

In gastric mucosal injury, EGF released from salivary glands and TGF-α from gastric mucosa are of particular value in mucosal integrity maintenance and repair. EGF and TGF-α have similar spectra of biological activity in the repair mechanism. Accumulation of EGF and EGFR overexpression in the ulcer area contributes together to repair process. During the ulcer healing process they activate cells migration from the ulcer margin and cell proliferation along with formation of granulation tissue and microvessels, angiogenesis (100). During initial stage of experimental ulcer healing, EGFR-associated tyrosine kinase plays an essential role in the regulation of cell proliferation by activation of the EGFR gene, EGFR phosphorylation, and enhancement of MAP kinase activitay. The presence of H. pylori vacuolating cytotoxin counteracts this process (93).

Numerous growth factors accelerate gastric epithelial and mesenchymal injury healing in vitro with acceleration of cell migration and proliferation. Gastric epithelial healing is mainly accelerated by a group of growth factors including EGF, TGF-α and HGF, while mesenchymal healing is predominantly accelerated by TGF-β and bFGF. Both, gastric epithelial and mesenchymal injury healing are significantly accelerated by PDGF, factor-betabeta and insulin-like growth factor-1 (IGF-1). During the healing process, IGF-1 regulates the gastric epithelial-mesenchymal interaction (96,101).

In injured gastric mucosa, growth factors TGF-α, HGF and IGF accelerate epithelial restitution and variably regulate the regeneration of human gastric epithelial cells through modulation of cell shape adaptation, migration and proliferation (102). Growth factors endorse EGFR-dependent PI3K activation, which promotes cell migration and restitution in injured human gastric epithelial monolayers (103).

Smoking is known as a risk factor for PUD. The detrimental effect of smoking is exhibited by inhibition of cell proliferation, mucus secretion and angiogenesis due to deficiency in EGF biosynthesis and its mRNA expression. The shortage of these factors is responsible for the delay in ulcer healing (104).

Several spices and plant extracts such as Mexican tea herb and pilular adina herb, Chuanxiong spices, Capsaicin, Kuiyangping, Weitongning and Angelica sinensis interact with EGF synthesis and hence contribute to the gastroprotection. For instance, Mexican tea herb and pilular adina herb stimulate NO, EGF secretion and EGFR expression and herewith protect the gastric mucosa integrity (105). Capsaicin-sensitive nerves induced ulcer healing is mediated by stimulation of EGF expression in salivary glands, serum and gastric mucosa (106). Also Kuiyangping, promotes ulcer healing in rats and decreases recurrence via increased expression of EGF and EGFR mRNA (107). Furthermore, Weitongning herb increases EGF and NO content in ulcer scars, and hence improves ulcer healing and reduces recurrence (108). In experimental myocardial infarction, Angelica and Chuanxiong spices promote endothelial cell proliferation and VEGF expression(109) and likewise may also promote angiogenesis and tissue repair in experimental ulcer. In indomethacin-induced gastric mucosal injury, crude extract from Angelica sinensis promotes EGF-mediated gastric mucosal healing via DNA synthesis, stimulation and augmentation of EGF mRNA expression (110). Picrorhiza kurroa (Scrofulariaceae) rhizomes possess an antioxidative property indicated by reduction of thiobarbituric acid reactive substances (TBARS) and protein carbonyl in addition to enhancing expression of EGF, VEGF, COX-1 and 2 enzymes associated with an increase of mucin and mucosal PGE2, which explain its ability to heal indomethacin-induced acute gastric injury in mice (111). Similarly, Myristica malabarica spice constituting two major antioxidants, malabaricone B and malabaricone C suppressed thiobarbituric acid reactive substances and protein carbonyls levels. Malabaricone C is more potent in modulating expression of EGF receptor and COX isoforms, mucin secretion, PGE2 synthesis and in controlling all these factors (112). Furthermore, ulcer cure by malabaricone B and malabaricone C is related to their ability to modulate angionetic factors. They significantly increase the mucosal EGF level serum VEGF level and microvessels formation. In contrary, the healing effect of misopristol and omeprazole is not correlated with angiogenesis enhancement (113).

11. Herbs and nitric oxide

In combination with other factors, NO significantly add to mucosal protection. The inflammatory process is mediated by inducible nitric oxide synthase (iNOS) and interleukin-8 (IL-8). Nitric oxide donors (SIN-1 and NOC-18) augment IL-8 and nitrite in mRNA, expression of IL-8. Production of large amounts of NO by iNOS may activate NF-kappaB and AP-1 and the expression of IL-8 in gastric epithelial cells (114). While iNOS is found in inflammatory cells in ulcer bed, NOS is located at the vascular endothelium and mucosal cells in normal and ulcerated gastric tissues. Endothelial NOS and NO significantly contribute to ulcer healing (106,115). Maintenance of NO synthesis is essential for an adequate mucosal defense. Conversely, Inhibition of NO synthesis in mucosal injury models is associated with an increase in ulcer index and asymmetric dimethylarginine (ADMA) levels along with a significantly decreased dimethylarginine dimethylaminohydrolase (DDAH) activity. ADMA Administration is associated with an inflammatory process with inhibition of NO synthesis and elevation of TNF-α levels and indicates the importance of ADMA in precipitating gastric mucosal injury (116). Such a process can be prevented by the use of extracts obtained from herbs and plants rich in phenolic compounds. Methanolic extract and buthanolic fraction of Vochysia tucanorum Mart., possess an antioxidant activity and protect NO levels in gastric mucosa. This protective effect is probably mediated by its phenolic compounds containing various active phytochemical constituents, triterpenoids (76). Triterpenoids are also active constituents of Croton reflexifolius and may explain its gastroprotective effect. Pretreatment with NOS inhibitor attenuates the gastroprotective effect induced by polyalthic acid (117). Furthermore, plant-extract-induced gastroprotective activity is likely related to the enhancing effect on release of NO in addition to NOS inhibitor expression and gastric microcirculation (118).

12. Herbs and SH compounds

The pathogenesis of gastric ulcer is complex. Several endogenous substances including SH compounds are important for the cytoprotection. They are involved in motivation of PG synthesis, protection of gastric mucosal integrity as well as in the antioxidative process. SH mucosal concentration is suppressed, especially in ethanol-induced gastric mucosal injuries. Preservation of mucosal microcirculation for rapid restitution and cell proliferation is considered as a key target of gastroprotection by either PG or SH compounds (119).

Several spices and plant extracts have protective effect against ethanol-induced SH depletion. Among these spices, Black seed, coriander, peppermint, black pepper, clove, anise aqueous suspension, and rocket replenishe ethanol-induced gastric wall mucus and SH depletion in experimental studies (4,66,67,71-73). Similarly, Ginkgo biloba extract preserves mucosal function via inhibition of ethanol-induced SH and gastric wall mucus depletion and lipid peroxidation (120). Methanolic extracts of C. sicyoides and Commiphora opobalsamum (L.) Engl. (Balessan) also enhances the defense system in rodents and inhibits gastric injuries through SH and NO involvement (58).

13. Herbs and cytokines

Altered immune system function significantly contributes to the pathogenesis of ulcer disease, particularly T-helper lymphocytes and released cytokines. The gastroprotection induced by Phyllanthus emblica L. also upregulates anti-inflammatory cytokine IL-10 concentration through its antioxidative activity, modulates anti-inflammatory cytokines and inhibits pro-inflammatory cytokines TNF-α and IL-1β (121).

The process of ulcer formation is considerably induced and regulated by IL-1β, TNF-α, IL-4, -6, -8, -12 cytokines. Cytokines, IL-1β and IL-1RN genes modulate the inflammatory response and therefore play an important role in the course of the disease (122).

In many gastric injuries, TNF-α is involved in the induction of chemokine expression. It increases the number of macrophages and monocyte chemotactic protein-1 (MCP-1) mRNA expression in mucosal scar. Increased MCP-1 may play a key role in regulating leukocyte recruitment and chemokine expression in gastric ulcer. TNF-α increases also macrophage inflammatory protein (MIP)-2 and cytokine-induced neutrophil chemoattractant (CINC-2α) mRNA expression and MPO activity (123). Cytokine gene polymorphisms influence mucosal cytokine expression and the degree of inflammation in H. pylori infection (124).

Furthermore, IL-1β enhances adhesion molecules expression, intercellular adhesion molecule 1 and leucocytic β2 integrins as well as the concentrations of TNF-α in ulcer scar and contributes to the recurrence of gastric ulcers in rats. The presence of gastric acid is important for the recurrence process of IL-1β-induced gastric ulcer. Gastric acid activates the inflammatory process in scarred mucosa during ulcer recurrence (125).

The outcome of H. pylori infection is influenced by the host response, which in susceptible individuals determines the development of ulcer. In H. pylori infected antral mucosa response is associated with an increase of proinflammatory IL-1β , IL-6, TNF α cytokines, and IL-8; the immunoregulatory gamma interferon (IFN-γ); and the anti-inflammatory TGF-β (126). A correlation between genetic polymorphisms and H. pylori-related diseases is well-established. While IFN-γ +874 AA genotype is associated with cagA positive infections, IL-10 −819 TT and TNF-A −857 TT are associated with intestinal metaplasia and duodenal ulcer, respectively (127).

Among various gastropathies gastritis is the only gastric disorder associated with significant oxidative stress marker expression of TNF-α, IL-8 and H. pylori cagA+/vacAs1 genotype. These probably represent the main oxidative markers responsible for ROS level increase with a decrease of the expression of the Manganese superoxide dismutase (MnSOD) and GPx (128).

In Western countries, polymorphism of pro-inflammatory cytokine genes is associated with the development of duodenal ulcer and gastric cancer. Similarly, polymorphisms in TNF-α rather than IL-1β are associated with an increased risk for gastric ulcers and gastric cancer in Japan. Increased risk of gastric ulcer development is associated with carriage of the alleles TNF-α-857 T, TNF-α-863 A and TNF-α-1031 C. Simultaneous carriage of more than one high-producer allele of TNF-α further increase the risks for gastric ulcer and cancer (129). In chronic H. pylori infection Pro-inflammatory cytokines are produced in the gastric mucosa by inflammatory cells. In contrast to Asians, in western population the inflammatory cytokine gene polymorphisms IL-4-590, IL-6-572 and IL-8-251 are more associated with development of PUD. Polymorphisms of these and other cytokines such as IL-1β, IL-1RN and TNF-α, may help to predict those at higher risk to develop peptic ulcer and those , who require H. pylori eradication(130).

Spices and other plant extracts may interfere with cytokines function, regulate the inflammatory process and help in ulcer healing. In gastric ulcer model, both curcumin and bisdemethoxycurcumin, a yellow pigment in rhizomes of Curcuma longa, promote gastric ulcer healing. While curcumin suppress iNOS and TNF-α protein production, bisdemethoxycurcumin lowers the increased iNOS protein expression level without any effect on TNF-α. The gastroprotective property of bisdemethoxycurcumin is related to its capability to decrease gastric acid secretion and suppress iNOS-mediated inflammation (131). Medicinal plants may also modulate lipopolysaccharide-induced proinflammatory cytokine production in murine macrophage cells and in mice treated with the stimulant lipopolysaccaharide. This has been demonstrated by the use of three herbal constituents, apigenin (chamomile), ginsenoside Rb1 (ginseng) and parthenolide (feverfew). All of these herbal constituents have inhibited lipopolysaccaharide-induced IL-6 and/or TNF-α production in culture(132).

14. Herbs and H. pylori

H, pylori represents the main cause for PUD and its eradication is imperative for ulcer healing and reduction of ulcer recurrence rate. The current eradication rate is below 90% and the resistance rate is growing up. Therefore, the search for potent H. pylori bactericidal agents from plants resources is emerging. Several spices and plant extracts possess H. pylori growth inhibitory activities. Curcumin (133), black cumin (134), eugenol, cinemaldeyde (135), turmeric, cumin, ginger, chilli, borage, black caraway, oregano and parsley (136) have an anti-H. pylori activity. Oil extract of Chamomilla recutita affects H. pylori morphological and fermentative properties and inhibits urease production (137). H. pylori adhesion to the gastric mucosa, an important stage of infection is inhibited by extracts of turmeric, borage and parsley (136), curcumin and its methanolic extract restrain the growth of all strains of H. pylori in vitro (133)]. Moreover, eugenol and cinnamaldehyde have prevented growth of H. pylori obtained from human gastric tissue, and inhibited the growth of all 30 tested H. pylori strains, with a lack of resistance (135). Besides, phenolic compounds of Oregano (Origanum vulgare L.), a Mediterranean herb, possess an inhibitory effect on H. pylori growth (138).

Also, aqueous-ethanol extracts of over 25 of Pakistani medicinal plants including Mal. philippines (Lam) Muell. Mallotus philippines (Lam) Muell., Curcuma amada Roxb., Myrisctica fragrans Houtt., and Psoralea corylifolia L have potent anti-H. pylori activity (139). In addition, methanolic extract of 25 0f 50 Taiwanese folk medicinal plants have also demonstrated compelling anti-H. pylori action (140). Furthermore, of 53 Mexican traditional medicinal plants especially extracts of Artemisia ludoviciana subsp. mexicana, Cuphea aequipetala, Ludwigia repens,and Mentha x piperita and methanolic extracts of Persea americana, Annona cherimola, Guaiacum coulteri, and Moussonia deppeana have verified a persuasive H. pylori inhibitory effect (141).

At last, the anti- H. pylori effect of 70 Greek plant extracts and a variety of commercially available herbs used in traditional medicine such as extracts of Chamomilla recutita, Conyza albida, Origanum vulgare Anthemis melanolepis, Cerastium candidissimum, Dittrichia viscosa, and Stachys alopecuros have inhibited a standard strain and 15 H. pylori clinical isolates (142).

15. Adverse events

Spices, herbs and other plant extracts have been used in traditional medicine for thousands of years. Recently, in several parts of the world there is a growing acceptance for using these agents to treat various conditions including PUD. Most of these extracts have been effective; however their safety and toxicity have not been well-evaluated. The increasing use of herbal medicine is expected to be more frequently associated with adverse reactions. Clinical evaluation of these adverse effects is not easy due lack of standardization, randomization, adequate number of patients and difficulty in using an appropriate placebo. Herbs are believed to be safe and have no adverse effect. However similar to other drugs they may induce intrinsic or extrinsic adverse effects. Some of their multiple constituents, such as anti-cancer plant-derived drugs, digitalis and the pyrrolizidine alkaloids are cytotoxic. Nevertheless, their adverse effects are less frequent than those of synthetic drugs (143).

Hepatotoxicity induced by curcumin and its derivatives (144) as well as by turmeric and its ethanolic extract in vulnerable mice has been reported (145). Also animals treated with Cinnamon zeylanicum, Piper longum and R. chalepensis have developed abnormalities in liver, spleen, lung or reproductive organs, in addition to an increase in count and motility of sperm and decrease in hemoglobin level (146,147). Kava (Piper methysticum), used as anxiolytic herb in Western countries has been potentially found to be hepatotoxic. Its hepatotoxicity is correlated with overdose, prolonged treatment, concurrent medication, and the quality of raw material (148). Suspected herb-induced liver injury (HILI) is evaluated by the causality score using this multidisciplinary approach and Roussel Uclaf Causality Assessment Method (RUCAM) (149).

In addition to hepatic toxicity, alteration of body weight has been described in rodents treated with Foeniculum vulgare ethanolic extracts and Ruta chalepensis (150). Furthermore, in experimental model, piperine has decreased mating performance and fertility and intrauterine injection has caused loss of implants without histological abnormalities (151). Herbal-induced toxicity is influenced by herbs related factors (quality, dose and nature of constituents) and individual risk factors (genetics, age, concomitant drugs, and concomitant diseases) (152). Therefore, simultaneous administration of herbs with conventional medications should generally be discouraged (153).

Herbal medicine-associated adverse reactions are expected to occur more frequently as a result of the fast mounting use of these agents in treatment. Some commonly used herbs like St John's wort (Hypericum perforatum), a popular herbal anti-depressant, lead to a decrease of the activity of immunosuppressive agents i.e.cyclosporine and subsequent tissue rejection in transplanted patients. Like other medicinal plants it also interferes with cytochrome P450 activity and metabolism of other drugs (154).

Examples of Drugs known to interact with St John's wort include besides cyclosporine tacrolimus as well as HIV non-nucleoside and protease inhibitors (155). Other drugs interfering with St. John's wort CYP 3A4 induction include , oral contraceptives.and indinavir(156).

Literature review of 128 case reports or case series, and 80 clinical trials have revealed that St John's wort-induced cytochrome P450 and P-glycoprotein induction, decreases plasma levels of a large variety and frequently used medications. Clearance of caffeine and midazolam may be influenced by Echinacea (157).

Herbal agents such as St. John's wort, interact differently with various drugs. It may increase the clearance of some medications via cytochrome P-450 mixed-function oxidase or through P-glycoprotein efflux pump modulation. On the other hand, it may decrease digoxin, theophylline, warfarin, protease inhibitors, cyclosporine, tacrolimus, and tricyclic antidepressants concentration with subsequent reduction of their therapeutic effect. A third category of drugs such as procainamide carbamazepine and mycophenolic acid are not affected by St. John's wort. herb (158).

Therapeutic drug monitoring is usually estimated by immunoassay technique. The potential interference St. John's wort, with commonly by this method monitored drugs has been evaluated. A significant interference with digoxin, quinidine, procainamide, N-acetyl procainamide theophylline, tricyclic antidepressants, phenytoin, carbamazepine, valproic acid and phenobarbital serum levels is lacking (159). Due to unwanted effects, ginseng and ginkgo should not be combined with anticoagulants and valerian with barbiturates (160). Elderly patients are more likely to develop diseases and ingest more medications. They are also prone to develop suppression of cytochrome P450 (CYP) activity. Taking herbal agents make them more vulnerable to herb-drug interactions (161). Herbal toxicity may also affect other central organs like the kidney. Case reports of interstitial fibrosis progressing to chronic renal failure and termed as aristolochic acid nephropathy may complicate treatment with slimming herbs belonging to Aristolochia family (162). Despite all of these reports of adverse events, spices are generally safe when used in standared doses. Popular traditional Chinese medicine has relatively less adverse effects and appears safer than other drugs (163).

The safety of herbal agents during pregnancy has been evaluated in 392 pregnant women 8% have reported taking chamomile, licorice, fennel, aloe, valerian, Echinacea oil 27, propolis and cranberry. Only four out 109 have reported insignificant adverse events in form of constipation after tisane, rash and itching after local application of aloe or almond oil. A higher incidence of threatening miscarriage and preterm labors was observed among regular users of chamomile and licorice (164).

In disparity, many spices and plant extracts, in commonly used dose, up to 500mg/kg body weight have not exhibited adverse effect. These include cardamom (62, 68), black pepper (66), clove (67), caraway (69), saffron (70),coriander(71), peppermint (72), anise (73), davilla elliptica and nitida (74) ,Brazilian medical plants (75) and Alchornea triplinervia (76) and Hyptis spicigera Lam (86). Even in pregnancy, ginger, peppermint, and Cannabis have been used to treat nausea were effective and lack clinical evidence of harm (165). Clinically, spices like turmeric and curcumin have been well-tolerated even with high doses and lack any toxicity (166).

16. References

[1] Nanjundaiah SM, Annaiah HN, M Dharmesh S. Gastroprotective Effect of Ginger Rhizome (Zingiber officinale) Extract: Role of Gallic Acid and Cinnamic Acid in

H+, K+-ATPase/H. pylori Inhibition and Anti-oxidative Mechanism. Evid Based Complement Alternat Med. 2009: 1-13.

[2] Choi SM, Shin JH, Kang KK, Ahn BO, Yoo M. Gastroprotective effects of DA-6034, a new flavonoid derivative, in various gastric mucosal damage models. Dig Dis Sci 2007;52: 3075–3080. [PubMed]

[3] Singh S, Khajuria A, Taneja SC, Khajuria RK, Singh J, Johri RK, Qazi GN. The gastric ulcer protective effect of boswellic acids, a leukotriene inhibitor from Boswellia serrata, in rats. Phytomedicine 2008; 15:408–415. [PubMed]

[4] Alqasoumi S, Al-Sohaibani M, Al-Howiriny T, Al-Yahya M, Rafatullah S. Rocket "Eruca sativa": a salad herb with potential gastric anti-ulcer activity. World J Gastroenterol 2009;15:1958–1965. [PubMed]

[5] Chernomorets NN, Seleznev AV, Revutskiĭ BI, Alifanova RE, Kravchenko ZV, Cherkasskaia EP. [The differentiated phytotherapy of patients with duodenal peptic ulcer] Lik Sprava 1992:112–115. [PubMed]

[6] Chakŭrski I, Matev M, Stefanov G, Koĭchev A, Angelova I. [Treanntment of duodenal ulcers and gastroduodenitis with a herbal combination of Symphitum officinalis and Calendula officinalis with and without antacids] Vutr Boles 1981;20:44–47.

[7] Al-Howiriny T, Al-Sohaibani M, Al-Said M, Al-Yahya M, El-Tahir K, Rafatullah S. Effect of Commiphora opobalsamum (L.) Engl. (Balessan) on experimental gastric ulcers and secretion in rats. J Ethnopharmacol 2005;98:287–294. [PubMed]

[8] Schiestl RH, Chan WS, Gietz RD, Mehta RD, Hastings PJ. Safrole, eugenol and methyleugenol induce intrachromosomal recombination in yeast. Mutat Res 1989;224:427–436. [PubMed]

[9] Lo YC, Yang YC, Wu IC, Kuo FC, Liu CM, Wang HW, Kuo CH, Wu JY, Wu DC. Capsaicin-induced cell death in a human gastric adenocarcinoma cell line. World J Gastroenterol 2005;11:6254–6257. [PubMed]

[10] Mothana RA, Gruenert R, Bednarski PJ, Lindequist U. Evaluation of the in vitro anticancer, antimicrobial and antioxidant activities of some Yemeni plants used in folk medicine. Pharmazie 2009;64:260–268. [PubMed]

[11] Lichtenberger LM, Romero JJ, Carryl OR, Illich PA, Walters ET. Effect of pepper and bismuth subsalicylate on gastric pain and surface hydrophobicity in the rat. Aliment Pharmacol Ther 1998;12:483–490. [PubMed]

[12] Al Mofleh IA, Alhaider AA, Mossa JS, Al-Sohaibani MO, Al-Yahya MA, Rafatullah S, Shaik SA. Gastroprotective effect of an aqueous suspension of black cumin Nigella sativa on necrotizing agents-induced gastric injury in experimental animals. Saudi J Gastroenterol 2008;14:128–134. [PubMed]

[13] Pan JS, He SZ, Xu HZ, Zhan XJ, Yang XN, Xiao HM, Shi HX, Ren JL. Oxidative stress disturbs energy metabolism of mitochondria in ethanol-induced gastric mucosa injury. World J Gastroenterol 2008 ; 14;14 :5857-5867.

[14] Hirokawa M, Miura S, Yoshida H, Kurose I, Shigematsu T, Hokari R, Higuchi H, Watanabe N, Yokoyama Y, Kimura H, Kato S, Ishii H. Oxidative stress and mitochondrial damage precedes gastric mucosal cell death induced by ethanol administration. Alcohol Clin Exp Res 1998 ;22(3 Suppl):111S-114S.

[15] Li NS, Luo XJ, Zhang YS, He L, Liu YZ, Peng J. Phloroglucinol protects gastric mucosa against ethanol-induced injury through regulating myeloperoxidase and catalase activities. Fundam Clin Pharmacol. 2010. [Epub ahead of print] PMID: 20880383)

[16] Farias-Silva E, Cola M, Calvo TR, Barbastefano V, Ferreira AL, De Paula Michelatto D, Alves de Almeida AC, Hiruma-Lima CA, Vilegas W, Brito AR. Antioxidant activity of indigo and its preventive effect against ethanol-induced DNA damage in rat gastric mucosa. Planta Med 2007 ;73 :1241-1246.

[17] Liu CS, Cham TM, Yang CH, Chang HW, Chen CH, Chuang LY. Antibacterial properties of Chinese herbal medicines against nosocomial antibiotic resistant strains of Pseudomonas aeruginosa in Taiwan. Am J Chin Med 2007;35:1047-1060. [PubMed]

[18] Seneviratne CJ, Wong RW, Samaranayake LP. Potent anti-microbial activity of traditional Chinese medicine herbs against Candida species. Mycoses 2008;51:30-34. [PubMed]

[19] Hitokoto H, Morozumi S, Wauke T, Sakai S, Kurata H. Inhibitory effects of spices on growth and toxin production of toxigenic fungi. Appl Environ Microbiol 1980;39:818-822. [PubMed]

[20] Karapinar M. Inhibitory effects of anethole and eugenol on the growth and toxin production of Aspergillus parasiticus. Int J Food Microbiol 1990;10:193-199. [PubMed]

[21] El Garhy MF, Mahmoud LH. Anthelminthic efficacy of traditional herbs on Ascaris lumbricoides. J Egypt Soc Parasitol 2002;32:893-900. [PubMed]

[22] Kiuchi F, Goto Y, Sugimoto N, Akao N, Kondo K, Tsuda Y. Nematocidal activity of turmeric: synergistic action of curcuminoids. Chem Pharm Bull (Tokyo) 1993;41:1640-1643. [PubMed]

[23] Sharma JN, Srivastava KC, Gan EK. Suppressive effects of eugenol and ginger oil on arthritic rats. Pharmacology. 1994;49:314-318. [PubMed]

[24] Li EK, Tam LS, Wong CK, Li WC, Lam CW, Wachtel-Galor S, Benzie IF, Bao YX, Leung PC, Tomlinson B. Safety and efficacy of Ganoderma lucidum (lingzhi) and San Miao San supplementation in patients with rheumatoid arthritis: a double-blind, randomized, placebo-controlled pilot trial. Arthritis Rheum. 2007;57: 1143-1150. [PubMed]

[25] Spiller F, Alves MK, Vieira SM, Carvalho TA, Leite CE, Lunardelli A, Poloni JA, Cunha FQ, de Oliveira JR. Anti-inflammatory effects of red pepper (Capsicum baccatum) on carrageenan- and antigen-induced inflammation. J Pharm Pharmacol 2008;60: 473-478. [PubMed]

[26] Liu J. Pharmacology of oleanolic acid and ursolic acid. J Ethnopharmacol 1995;49 :57-68.

[27] Morita T, Jinno K, Kawagishi H, Arimoto Y, Suganuma H, Inakuma T, Sugiyama K Hepatoprotective effect of myristicin from nutmeg (Myristica fragrans) on lipopolysaccharide/d-galactosamine-induced liver injury. J Agric Food Chem 2003 ;51:1560-1565.

[28] Sharma S, Kulkarni SK, Chopra K. Curcumin, the active principle of turmeric (Curcuma longa), ameliorates diabetic nephropathy in rats. Clin Exp Pharmacol Physiol. 2006 ;33 : 940-945.

[29] Wongpa S, Himakoun L, Soontornchai S, Temcharoen P. Antimutagenic effects of piperine on cyclophosphamide-induced chromosome aberrations in rat bone marrow cells. Asian Pac J Cancer Prev 2007 ;8 : 623-627.

[30] Oyagbemi AA, Saba AB, Azeez OI. Molecular targets of [6]-gingerol: Its potential roles in cancer chemoprevention. Biofactors 2010 ;36 : 169-178.

[31] Al-Amin ZM, Thomson M, Al-Qattan KK, Peltonen-Shalaby R, Ali M. Anti-diabetic and hypolipidaemic properties of ginger (Zingiber officinale) in streptozotocin-induced diabetic rats. Br J Nutr 2006;96: 660–666. [PubMed]

[32] Ejaz A, Wu D, Kwan P, Meydani M. Curcumin inhibits adipogenesis in 3T3-L1 adipocytes and angiogenesis and obesity in C57/BL mice. J Nutr 2009;139: 919–925. [PubMed]

[33] Alwi I, Santoso T, Suyono S, Sutrisna B, Suyatna FD, Kresno SB, Ernie S. The effect of curcumin on lipid level in patients with acute coronary syndrome. Acta Med Indones 2008;40: 201–210. [PubMed]

[34] Alizadeh-Navaei R, Roozbeh F, Saravi M, Pouramir M, Jalali F, Moghadamnia AA. Investigation of the effect of ginger on the lipid levels. A double blind controlled clinical trial. Saudi Med J 2008;29: 1280–1284. [PubMed]

[35] Al-Yahya MA, Rafatullah S, Mossa JS, Ageel AM, Parmar NS, Tariq M. Gastroprotective activity of ginger zingiber officinale rosc., in albino rats. Am J Chin Med 1989;17: 51–56. [PubMed]

[36] Rafatullah S, Tariq M, Al-Yahya MA, Mossa JS, Ageel AM. Evaluation of turmeric (Curcuma longa) for gastric and duodenal antiulcer activity in rats. J Ethnopharmacol 1990;29: 25–34. [PubMed]

[37] Schmeda-Hirschmann G, Yesilada E. Traditional medicine and gastroprotective crude drugs. J Ethnopharmacol 2005 22;100 : 61-66.

[38] Graham DY, Smith JL, Opekun AR. Spicy food and the stomach. Evaluation by videoendoscopy. JAMA 1988;260: 3473–3475. [PubMed]

[39] Kivilaakso E. Pathogenetic mechanisms in experimental gastric stress ulceration. Scand J Gastroenterol Suppl 1985;110: 57–62. [PubMed]

[40] Nayeb-Hashemi H, Kaunitz JD. Gastroduodenal mucosal defense. Curr Opin Gastroenterol 2009;25: 537–543. [PubMed]

[41] Brzozowski T, Konturek PC, Konturek SJ, Brzozowska I, Pawlik T. Role of prostaglandins in gastroprotection and gastric adaptation. J Physiol Pharmacol 2005;56 Suppl 5: 33–55.

[42] Luo JC, Shin VY, Yang YH, Wu WK, Ye YN, So WH, Chang FY, Cho CH. Tumor necrosis factor-alpha stimulates gastric epithelial cell proliferation. Am J Physiol Gastrointest Liver Physiol 2005;288: G32–G38. [PubMed]

[43] Beales IL. Gastrin and interleukin-1beta stimulate growth factor secretion from cultured rabbit gastric parietal cells. Life Sci 2004;75: 2983–2995. [PubMed]

[44] Borelli F, Izzo AA. The plant kingdom as a source of anti-ulcer remedies Phytother Res 2000;14: 581–591.

[45] A. Jamal, Kalim Javed, M. Aslam, M.A. Jafri. Gastroprotective effect of cardamom, Elettaria cardamomum Maton. fruits in rats. J Ethnopharmacol 2006 :103, : 149-153.

[46] Badreldin H Ali, Gerald Blunden, Musbah O Tanira, Abderrahim Nemmar Some phytochemical, pharmacological and toxicological properties of ginger (Zingiber officinale Roscoe): a review of recent research. Food and chemical toxicology : an international journal published for the British Industrial Biological Research Association 03/2008; 46 : 409-420.

[47] Eswaran MB, Surendran S, Vijayakumar M, Ojha SK, Rawat AK, Rao ChVGastroprotective activity of Cinnamomum tamala leaves on experimental gastric ulcers in rats. J Ethnopharmacol. 2010 ;128 : 537-540. [PubMed]

[48] Al Mofleh IA. Spices, herbal xenobiotics and the stomach: friends or foes? World J Gastroenterol 2010 ;16 : 2710-2719. Editorial [PubMed]

[49] Jainu M, Vijai Mohan K, Shyamala Devi CS. Gastroprotective effect of Cissus quadrangularis extract in rats with experimentally induced ulcer. Indian J Med Res 2006;123: 799-806. [PubMed] .

[50] Baggio CH, Freitas CS, Otofuji Gde M, Cipriani TR, Souza LM, Sassaki GL, Iacomini M, Marques MC, Mesia-Vela S. Flavonoid-rich fraction of Maytenus ilicifolia Mart. ex. Reiss protects the gastric mucosa of rodents through inhibition of both H+,K+ - ATPase activity and formation of nitric oxide. J Ethnopharmacol 2007;113: 433-440. [PubMed]

[51] Baek SW, Kim NK, Jin HJ, Koh CW, Kim CK, Kwon OH, Kim JS, Cho MH, Park CK. Anti-ulcer actions of phytosphingosine hydrochloride in different experimental rat ulcer models. Arzneimittelforschung 2005;55: 461-465. [PubMed]

[52] Souccar C, Cysneiros RM, Tanae MM, Torres LM, Lima-Landman MT, Lapa AJ. Inhibition of gastric acid secretion by a standardized aqueous extract of Cecropia glaziovii Sneth and underlying mechanism. Phytomedicine 2008;15: 462-469. [PubMed]

[53] Zanatta F, Gandolfi RB, Lemos M, Ticona JC, Gimenez A, Clasen BK, Cechinel Filho V, de Andrade SF. Gastroprotective activity of alkaloid extract and 2-phenylquinoline obtained from the bark of Galipea longiflora Krause (Rutaceae) Chem Biol Interact 2009;180: 312-317. [PubMed]

[54] Olaleye SB, Owoyele VB, Odukanmi AO. Antiulcer and gastric antisecretory effects of Landolphia owariensis extracts in rats. Niger J Physiol Sci 2008;23: 23-26. [PubMed]

[55] Baggio CH, Freitas CS, Otofuji Gde M, Cipriani TR, Souza LM, Sassaki GL, Iacomini M, Marques MC, Mesia-Vela S. Flavonoid-rich fraction of Maytenus ilicifolia Mart. ex. Reiss protects the gastric mucosa of rodents through inhibition of both H+,K+ - ATPase activity and formation of nitric oxide. J Ethnopharmacol 2007;113 : 433-440.

[56] Alam S, Asad M, Asdaq SM, Prasad VS. Antiulcer activity of methanolic extract of Momordica charantia L. in rats. J Ethnopharmacol 2009;123 : 464-469.

[57] Kamath BS, Srikanta BM, Dharmesh SM, Sarada R, Ravishankar GA. Ulcer preventive and antioxidative properties of astaxanthin from Haematococcus pluvialis. Eur J Pharmacol 2008;590: 387-395. [PubMed]

[58] de Paula Ferreira M, Nishijima CM, Seito LN, Dokkedal AL, Lopes-Ferreira M, Di Stasi LC, Vilegas W, Hiruma-Lima CA.Gastroprotective effect of Cissus sicyoides (Vitaceae): involvement of microcirculation, endogenous sulfhydryls and nitric oxide. J Ethnopharmacol 2008 ;117 : 170-174.

[59] Naito Y, Yoshikawa T. Oxidative stress involvement and gene expression in indomethacin-induced gastropathy. Redox Rep 2006;11: 243-253. [PubMed]

[60] Srinivasan K. Black pepper and its pungent principle-piperine: a review of diverse physiological effects. Crit Rev Food Sci Nutr 2007;47: 735-748. [PubMed]

[61] Kanter M, Demir H, Karakaya C, Ozbek H. Gastroprotective activity of Nigella sativa L oil and its constituent, thymoquinone against acute alcohol-induced gastric mucosal injury in rats. World J Gastroenterol 2005;11: 6662–6666. [PubMed]

[62] Silva MI, Moura BA, Neto MR, Tomé Ada R, Rocha NF, de Carvalho AM, Macêdo DS, Vasconcelos SM, de Sousa DP, Viana GS, et al. Gastroprotective activity of isopulegol on experimentally induced gastric lesions in mice: investigation of possible mechanisms of action. Naunyn Schmiedebergs Arch Pharmacol 2009;380: 233–245. [PubMed]

[63] Bogdarin IuA, Potekhin PP, Kozlov DV, Shirokova NIu. [Efficacy of the new collection of herbs at stressful experimental sharp ulcer defects of the gastroduodenal zone] Eksp Klin Gastroenterol 2005: 74–78, 102. [PubMed]

[64] Cola M, Calvo TR, Barbastefano V, Ferreira AL, De Paula Michelatto D, Alves de Almeida AC, Hiruma-Lima CA, Vilegas W, Brito AR. Antioxidant activity of indigo and its preventive effect against ethanol-induced DNA damage in rat gastric mucosa. Planta Med 2007 ;73: 1241-1246. [PubMed]

[65] Fan TY, Feng QQ, Jia CR, Fan Q, Li CA, Bai XL. Protective effect of Weikang decoction and partial ingredients on model rat with gastric mucosa ulcer. World J Gastroenterol 2005;11: 1204–1209. [PubMed]

[66] I.A. Al-Mofleh, A.A. Alhaider, J.S. Mossa, M.O. Al-Sohaibani, S. Rafatullah, S. Qureshi. Inhibition of Gastric Mucosal Damage by Piper Nigrum (Black pepper) Pretreatment in Wistar Albino Rats. PHCOG MAG 2005; 1 : 64-68.

[67] I.A. Al-Mofleh, A.A. Alhaider, J.S. Mossa, M.O. Al-Sohaibani, S. Qureshi, S. Rafatullah. Pharmacological Studies on 'Clove' Eugenia caryophyllata. PHCOG MAG 2005; 1 : 105-109.

[68] Alhaider A.A., Al-Mofleh I.A., Mossa J.S., Al-Sohaibani M.O., Qureshi S. and Rafatullah S. Pharmacological and Safety Evaluation Studies on "Cardamon" Elettaria cardamomum: An Important Ingredient of Gahwa (Arabian Coffee). Arab Journal of Pharmaceutical Sciences 2005; 3 : 47-58.

[69] Alhaider, A.A., I.A. Al-Mofleh, J.S. Mossa, M.O. Al-Sohaibani, S. Rafatullah and S. Qureshi, 2006. Effect of Carum carvi on experimentally induced gastric mucosal damage in wistar albino rats. Int. J. Pharmacol 2006; 2: 309-315.

[70] I.A. Al-Mofleh, A.A. Alhaider, J.S. Mossa, M.O. Al-Sohaibani, S. Qureshi and S. Rafatullah. Antigastric Ulcer Studies on 'Saffron' Crocus sativus L. in Rats. Pakistan Journal of Biological Sciences 2006;9 : 1009-1013 .

[71] I.A. Al-Mofleh, A.A. Alhaider, J.S. Mossa, M.O. Al-Sohaibani, S. Rafatullah and S. Qureshi. Protection of gastric mucosal damage by Coriandrum sativum L. pretreatment in Wistar albino rats. Environmental Toxicology and Pharmacology 2006; 22 : 64-69.

[72] I.A. Al-Mofleh, A.A. Alhaider, J.S. Mossa, M.O. Al-Sohaibani, S. Qureshi and S. Rafatullah. Antisecretagogue, Antiulcer and Cytoprotective Effects of 'Peppermint' Mentha piperita L. In Laboratory Animals. J. Med. Sci 2006;6 : 930-936.

[73] Al Mofleh IA, Alhaider AA, Mossa JS, Al-Soohaibani MO, Rafatullah S. Aqueous suspension of anise "Pimpinella anisum" protects rats against chemically induced gastric ulcers. World J Gastroenterol 2007 ;13 : 1112-1118.

[74] Kushima H, Nishijima CM, Rodrigues CM, Rinaldo D, Sassá MF, Bauab TM, Stasi LC, Carlos IZ, Brito AR, Vilegas W, Hiruma-Lima CA. Davilla elliptica and Davilla

nitida: gastroprotective, anti-inflammatory immunomodulatory and anti-Helicobacter pylori action. J Ethnopharmacol 2009;123 : 430-438.

[75] Lima ZP, Calvo TR, Silva EF, Pellizzon CH, Vilegas W, Brito AR, Bauab TM, Hiruma-Lima CA. Brazilian medicinal plant acts on prostaglandin level and Helicobacter pylori. J Med Food 2008 ;11: 701-708. [PubMed]

[76] Gomes Rde C, Bonamin F, Darin DD, Seito LN, Di Stasi LC, Dokkedal AL, Vilegas W, Souza Brito AR, Hiruma-Lima CA. Antioxidative action of methanolic extract and buthanolic fraction of Vochysia tucanorum Mart. in the gastroprotection.. J Ethnopharmacol 2009; 121 : 466-471.

[77] Suleyman H, Albayrak A, Bilici M, Cadirci E, Halici Z. Different mechanisms in formation and prevention of indomethacin-induced gastric ulcers. Inflammation 2010 ;33: 224-234. [PubMed]

[78] Peskar BM, Maricic N, Gretzera B, Schuligoi R, Schmassmann A. Role of cyclooxygenase-2 in gastric mucosal defense. Life Sci. 2001;69: 2993-3003. [PubMed]

[79] Johansson C, Bergström S. Prostaglandin and protection of the gastroduodenal mucosa. Scand J Gastroenterol Suppl 1982;77: 21-46. [PubMed]

[80] Konturek SJ. Mechanisms of gastroprotection. Scand J Gastroenterol Suppl 1990;174: 15-28. [PubMed]

[81] Falalyeyeva TM, Samonina GE, Beregovaya TV, Andreeva LA, Dvorshchenko EA. Effect of glyprolines PGP, GP, and PG on homeostasis of gastric mucosa in rats with experimental ethanol-induced gastric ulcers. Bull Exp Biol Med 2010 ;149 : 699-701. [PubMed]

[82] Konturek SJ, Konturek PC, Brzozowski T. Prostaglandins and ulcer healing. J Physiol Pharmacol 2005;56 Suppl 5: 5-31. [PubMed]

[83] Gookin JL, Galanko JA, Blikslager AT, Argenzio RA. PG-mediated closure of paracellular pathway and not restitution is the primary determinant of barrier recovery in acutely injured porcine ileum. Am J Physiol Gastrointest Liver Physiol 2003;285: G967–G979. [PubMed]

[84] Hatazawa R, Ohno R, Tanigami M, Tanaka A, Takeuchi K. Roles of endogenous prostaglandins and cyclooxygenase isozymes in healing of indomethacin-induced small intestinal lesions in rats. J Pharmacol Exp Ther 2006;318: 691–699. [PubMed]

[85] Konturek PC, Brzozowski T, Konturek SJ, Taut A, Kwiecien S, Pajdo R, Sliwowski Z, Hahn EG. Bacterial lipopolysaccharide protects gastric mucosa against acute injury in rats by activation of genes for cyclooxygenases and endogenous prostaglandins. Digestion 1998;59: 284–297. [PubMed]

[86] Takayama C, de-Faria FM, Almeida AC, Valim-Araújo DD, Rehen CS, Dunder RJ, Socca EA, Manzo LP, Rozza AL, Salvador MJ, Pellizzon CH, Hiruma-Lima CA, Luiz-Ferreira A, Souza-Brito AR. Gastroprotective and ulcer healing effects of essential oil from Hyptis spicigera Lam. (Lamiaceae). J Ethnopharmacol 2011 135: 147-55. [PubMed]

[87] Mehrabani D, Rezaee A, Azarpira N, Fattahi MR, Amini M, Tanideh N, Panjehshahin MR, Saberi-Firouzi M. The healing effects of Teucrium polium in the repair of indomethacin-induced gastric ulcer in rats. Saudi Med J 2009;30: 494–499. [PubMed]

[88] Komoike Y, Nakashima M, Nakagiri A, Takeuchi K. Prostaglandin E receptor EP1 subtype but not prostacyclin IP receptor involved in mucosal blood flow response of mouse stomachs following barrier disruption. Digestion 2003;67: 186–194. [PubMed]

[89] Satyanarayana MN. Capsaicin and gastric ulcers. Crit Rev Food Sci Nutr 2006;46: 275–328. [PubMed]

[90] Rozza AL, Moraes Tde M, Kushima H, Tanimoto A, Marques MO, Bauab TM, Hiruma-Lima CA, Pellizzon CH.Gastroprotective mechanisms of Citrus lemon (Rutaceae) essential oil and its majority compounds limonene and β-pinene: involvement of heat-shock protein-70, vasoactive intestinal peptide, glutathione, sulfhydryl compounds, nitric oxide and prostaglandin E_2.Chem Biol Interact 2011 ;189: 82-89. [PubMed]

[91] Maity B, Banerjee D, Bandyopadhyay SK, Chattopadhyay S. Myristica malabarica heals stomach ulceration by increasing prostaglandin synthesis and angiogenesis. Planta Med 2008 ;74: 1774-1778. [PubMed]

[92] El-Abhar HS. Coenzyme Q10: a novel gastroprotective effect via modulation of vascular permeability, prostaglandin E , nitric oxide and redox status in indomethacin-induced gastric ulcer model. Eur J Pharmacol 2010; 649: 314-319. [PubMed]

[93] Tarnawski AS, Jones MK. The role of epidermal growth factor (EGF) and its receptor in mucosal protection, adaptation to injury, and ulcer healing: involvement of EGF-R signal transduction pathways. J Clin Gastroenterol 1998;27 Suppl 1: S12-20. [PubMed]

[94] Pai R, Tarnawski A.Signal transduction cascades triggered by EGF receptor activation: relevance to gastric injury repair and ulcer healing. Dig Dis Sci. 1998 ;43(9 Suppl): 14S-22S. [PubMed]

[95] Konturek PC, Brzozowski T, Konturek SJ, Ernst H, Drozdowicz D, Pajdo R, Hahn EG. Expression of epidermal growth factor and transforming growth factor alpha during ulcer healing. Time sequence study. Scand J Gastroenterol 1997;32: 6–15. [PubMed]

[96] Jones MK, Tomikawa M, Mohajer B, Tarnawski AS. Gastrointestinal mucosal regeneration: role of growth factors. Front Biosci 1999 ;4: D303-309. [PubMed]

[97] Sasaki E, Tominaga K, Watanabe T, Fujiwara Y, Oshitani N, Matsumoto T, Higuchi K, Tarnawski AS, Arakawa T. COX-2 is essential for EGF induction of cell proliferation in gastric RGM1 cells. Dig Dis Sci 2003;48: 2257-2262. [PubMed]

[98] Milani S, Calabrò A. Role of growth factors and their receptors in gastric ulcer healing. Microsc Res Tech 2001; 53 : 360-371. [PubMed]

[99] Szabo S, Vincze A. Growth factors in ulcer healing: lessons from recent studies. J Physiol Paris 2000 ;94 : 77-81. [PubMed]

[100] Konturek PC, Konturek SJ, Brzozowski T, Ernst H. Epidermal growth factor and transforming growth factor-alpha: role in protection and healing of gastric mucosal lesions. Eur J Gastroenterol Hepatol 1995 ;7: 933-937. [PubMed]

[101] Watanabe S, Hirose M, Wang XE, Kobayashi O, Nagahara A, Murai T, Iwazaki R, Miwa H, Miyazaki A, Sato N.Epithelial-mesenchymal interaction in gastric mucosal restoration. J Gastroenterol 2000;35 Suppl 12:65-68 [PubMed] .

[102] Tétreault MP, Chailler P, Rivard N, Ménard D. Differential growth factor induction and modulation of human gastric epithelial regeneration. Exp Cell Res 2005 ;306 : 285-297 [PubMed].

[103] Tétreault MP, Chailler P, Beaulieu JF, Rivard N, Ménard D. Epidermal growth factor receptor-dependent PI3K-activation promotes restitution of wounded human gastric epithelial monolayers. J Cell Physiol 2008 ;214 : 545-457. [PubMed]

[104] Ma L, Wang WP, Chow JY, Yuen ST, Cho CH. Reduction of EGF is associated with the delay of ulcer healing by cigarette smoking.Am J Physiol Gastrointest Liver Physiol 2000 ;278 : G10-17.

[105] Cao MB, Dong L, Chang XM, Zou BC, Qin B. Effect of Mexican tea herb and pilular adina herb on concrescence of gastric mucosa in experimental gastric ulcer rats. Chin J Integr Med 2007;13: 132-136. [PubMed]

[106] Ma L, Chow JY, Wong BC, Cho CH. Role of capsaicin sensory nerves and EGF in the healing of gastric ulcer in rats. Life Sci. 2000;66: PL213-PL220. [PubMed]

[107] Wang B, Zhao HY, Zhou L, Wang YF, Cao J. Effect of Kuiyangping on expressions of EGF and EGFR mRNA in gastric mucosa in rats with experimental gastric ulcer. Beijing Zhongyiyao Daxue Xuebao 2008;31: Abstract.

[108] Zheng XG, Zhang JJ, Huang YC. [Study on the effect of weitongning on epidermal growth factor and nitric oxide contents in tissue of stomach of rats with gastric ulcer] Zhongguo Zhongxiyi Jiehe Zazhi 2004;24: 549-551. [PubMed]

[109] Meng H, Guo J, Sun JY, Pei JM, Wang YM, Zhu MZ, Huang C. Angiogenic effects of the extracts from Chinese herbs: Angelica and Chuanxiong. Am J Chin Med 2008;36: 541-554. [PubMed]

[110] Ye YN, Koo MW, Li Y, Matsui H, Cho CH.Angelica sinensis modulates migration and proliferation of gastric epithelial cells. Life Sci 2001;68: 961-968. [PubMed]

[111] Debashish Banerjee,1 Biswanath Maity,1 Subrata K Nag,1 Sandip K Bandyopadhyay,1 and Subrata Chattopadhyay 2 Healing Potential of against indomethacin-induced gastric ulceration: a mechanistic exploration. BMC Complement Altern Med 2008; 8: 3. [PubMed]

[112] Banerjee D, Bauri AK, Guha RK, Bandyopadhyay SK, Chattopadhyay S. Healing properties of malabaricone B and malabaricone C, against indomethacin-induced gastric ulceration and mechanism of action. Eur J Pharmacol 2008;578: 300-312. [PubMed]

[113] Banerjee D, Maity B, Bandivdeker AH, Bandyopadhyay SK, Chattopadhyay S. Angiogenic and cell proliferating action of the natural diarylnonanoids, malabaricone B and malabaricone C during healing of indomethacin-induced gastric ulceration. Pharm Res 2008 ;25: 1601-1609. [PubMed]

[114] Seo JY, Yu JH, Lim JW, Mukaida N, Kim H. Nitric oxide-induced IL-8 expression is mediated by NF-kappaB and AP-1 in gastric epithelial AGS cells. J Physiol Pharmacol 2009 ;60 Suppl 7: 101-106.

[115] Li Ma, John L. Wallace. Endothelial nitric oxide synthase modulates gastric ulcer healing in rats. Am J Physiol Gastrointest Liver Physiol 2000 279: G341-G346.

[116] Wang L, Zhou Y, Peng J, Zhang Z, Jiang DJ, Li YJ. Role of endogenous nitric oxide synthase inhibitor in gastric mucosal injury. Clin Biochem 2007;40: 615-622. [PubMed]

[117] Reyes-Trejo B, Sánchez-Mendoza ME, Becerra-García AA, Cedillo-Portugal E, Castillo-Henkel C, Arrieta J. Bioassay-guided isolation of an anti-ulcer diterpenoid from Croton reflexifolius: role of nitric oxide, prostaglandins and sulfhydryls. J Pharm Pharmacol 2008;60: 931–936. [PubMed]

[118] Zayachkivska OS, Konturek SJ, Drozdowicz D, Brzozowski T, Gzhegotsky MR. Influence of plant-originated gastroproteciive and antiulcer substances on gastric mucosal repair. Fiziol Zh 2004;50: 118–127. [PubMed]

[119] Szabo S. Experimental basis for a role for sulfhydryls and dopamine in ulcerogenesis: a primer for cytoprotection—organoprotection. Klin Wochenschr 1986;64 Suppl 7: 116-122. [PubMed]

[120] Chen SH, Liang YC, Chao JC, Tsai LH, Chang CC, Wang CC, Pan S. Protective effects of Ginkgo biloba extract on the ethanol-induced gastric ulcer in rats. World J Gastroenterol 2005;11: 3746-3750. [PubMed]

[121] Chatterjee A, Chattopadhyay S, Bandyopadhyay SK. Biphasic Effect of Phyllanthus emblica L. Extract on NSAID-Induced Ulcer: An Antioxidative Trail Weaved with Immunomodulatory Effect. Evid Based Complement Alternat Med 2011;2011: 146808.

[122] M. A. Garcia-Gonzalez, A. Lanas2,S. Santolaria, J. B. A. Crusius , M. T. Serrano , A. S. Peña The polymorphic IL-1B and IL-1RN genes in the aetiopathogenesis of peptic ulcer. Clinical & Experimental Immunology 2001; 125 : 368–375.

[123] Toshio Watanabe, Kazuhide Higuchi, Masaki Hamaguchi, Masatsugu Shiba, Kazunari Tominaga, Yasuhiro Fujiwara, Takayuki Matsumoto, and Tetsuo Arakawa Monocyte chemotactic protein-1 regulates leukocyte recruitment during gastric ulcer recurrence induced by tumor necrosis factor-α Am J Physiol Gastrointest Liver Physiol 2004 287: G919-G928

[124] R Rad, A Dossumbekova , B Neu , R Lang , S Bauer , D Saur , M Gerhard , C Prinz Cytokine gene polymorphisms influence mucosal cytokine expression, gastric inflammation, and host specific colonisation during Helicobacter pylori infection. Gut 2004;53:1082-1089.

[125] T Watanabe, K Higuchi, K Tominaga, Y Fujiwara, T Arakawa Acid regulates inflammatory response in a rat model of induction of gastric ulcer recurrence by interleukin 1β. Gut 2001;48: 774-781.

[126] C.Lindholm, M. Quiding-Järbrink, H. Lönroth, A. Hamlet, βand A.-M. Svennerholm Local Cytokine Response in Helicobacter pylori-Infected Subjects Infection and Immunity 1998; 66 : 5964-5971.

[127] Carlo-F. Zambon , Daniela Basso , Filippo Navaglia , Claudio Belluco , Alessandra Falda , Paola Fogar , Eliana Greco , Nicoletta Gallo , Massimo Rugge , Francesco Di Mario and Mario Plebani.   Pro- and anti-inflammatory cytokines gene polymorphisms and Helicobacter pylori infection: interactions influence outcome Cytokine 2005;29: 141-152.

[128] Augusto AC, Miguel F, Mendonça S, Pedrazzoli J Jr, Gurgueira SA. Oxidative stress expression status associated to Helicobacter pylori virulence in gastric diseases. Clin Biochem 2007;40 : 615-622.

[129] Sugimoto M, Furuta T, Shirai N, Nakamura A, Xiao F, Kajimura M, Sugimura H, Hishida A.Different effects of polymorphisms of tumor necrosis factor-alpha and

interleukin-1 beta on development of peptic ulcer and gastric cancer. J Gastroenterol Hepatol 2007;22 : 51-59.

[130] Mitsushige Sugimoto, Yoshio Yamaoka, Takahisa Furuta. Influence of interleukin polymorphisms on development of gastric cancer and peptic ulcer. World J Gastroenterol 2010; 16 : 1188-1200.

[131] Mahattanadul S, Nakamura T, Panichayupakaranant P, Phdoongsombut N, Tungsinmunkong K, Bouking P. Comparative antiulcer effect of bisdemethoxycurcumin and curcumin in a gastric ulcer model system. Phytomedicine 2009;16 : 342-351.

[132] Alexa T. Smolinski and James J. Pestka. Modulation of lipopolysaccharide-induced proinflammatory cytokine production in vitro and in vivo by the herbal constituents apigenin (chamomile), ginsenoside Rb1 (ginseng) and parthenolide (feverfew). Food and Chemical Toxicology 2003; 41 : 1381-1390.

[133] Mahady GB, Pendland SL, Yun G, Lu ZZ. Turmeric (Curcuma longa) and curcumin inhibit the growth of Helicobacter pylori, a group 1 carcinogen. Anticancer Res 2002;22: 4179–4181. [PubMed]

[134] Salem EM, Yar T, Bamosa AO, Al-Quorain A, Yasawy MI, Alsulaiman RM, Randhawa MA Comparative study of Nigella Sativa and triple therapy in eradication of Helicobacter Pylori in patients with non-ulcer dyspepsia. Saudi J Gastroenterol 2010 ; 6 : 207-214.

[135] Ali SM, Khan AA, Ahmed I, Musaddiq M, Ahmed KS, Polasa H, Rao LV, Habibullah CM, Sechi LA, Ahmed N. Antimicrobial activities of Eugenol and Cinnamaldehyde against the human gastric pathogen Helicobacter pylori. Ann Clin Microbiol Antimicrob 2005;4: 20. [PubMed]

[136] O'Mahony R, Al-Khtheeri H, Weerasekera D, Fernando N, Vaira D, Holton J, Basset C. Bactericidal and anti-adhesive properties of culinary and medicinal plants against Helicobacter pylori. World J Gastroenterol 2005;11: 7499–7507. [PubMed]

[137] Shikov AN, Pozharitskaya ON, Makarov VG, Kvetnaya AS. Antibacterial activity of Chamomilla recutita oil extract against Helicobacter pylori. Phytother Res 2008 ;22 :252-253.

[138] Chun, S.-S., Vattem, D.A., Lin, Y.-T., Shetty K. Phenolic antioxidants from clonal oregano (Origanum vulgare) with antimicrobial activity against Helicobacter pylori. Process Biochemistry 2005;40 : 809-816.

[139] Zaidi SF, Yamada K, Kadowaki M, Usmanghani K, Sugiyama T. Bactericidal activity of medicinal plants, employed for the treatment of gastrointestinal ailments, against Helicobacter pylori. J Ethnopharmacol 2009 ;121: 286-291.

[140] Wang YC, Huang TLScreening of anti-Helicobacter pylori herbs deriving from Taiwanese folk medicinal plants. FEMS Immunol Med Microbiol 2005 ;43 : 295-300.

[141] Castillo-Juárez I, González V, Jaime-Aguilar H, Martínez G, Linares E, Bye R, Romero I. Anti-Helicobacter pylori activity of plants used in Mexican traditional medicine for gastrointestinal disorders. J Ethnopharmacol 2009 ;122 : 402-405.

[142] Stamatis G, Kyriazopoulos P, Golegou S, Basayiannis A, Skaltsas S, Skaltsa H. In vitro anti-Helicobacter pylori activity of Greek herbal medicines. J Ethnopharmacol 2003 ;88 : 175-179.

[143] J.B. Calixto Efficacy, safety, quality control, marketing and regulatory guidelines for herbal medicines (phytotherapeutic agents) Braz J Med Biol Res 2000; 33: 179-189.

[144] Balaji S, Chempakam B. Pharmacokinetics prediction and drugability assessment of diphenylheptanoids from turmeric (Curcuma longa L) Med Chem 2009;5: 130–138. [PubMed]

[145] Kandarkar SV, Sawant SS, Ingle AD, Deshpande SS, Maru GB. Subchronic oral hepatotoxicity of turmeric in mice--histopathological and ultrastructural studies. Indian J Exp Biol 1998;36: 675–679. [PubMed]

[146] Shah AH, Qureshi S, Ageel AM. Toxicity studies in mice of ethanol extracts of Foeniculum vulgare fruit and Ruta chalepensis aerial parts. J Ethnopharmacol 1991;34: 167–172. [PubMed]

[147] Shah AH, Al-Shareef AH, Ageel AM, Qureshi S. Toxicity studies in mice of common spices, Cinnamomum zeylanicum bark and Piper longum fruits. Plant Foods Hum Nutr 1998;52: 231–239. [PubMed]

[148] Teschke R. Kava hepatotoxicity--a clinical review. Ann Hepatol 2010;9: 251-265. [PubMed] .

[149] Nin Chau T, Cheung WI, Ngan T, Lin J, Lee KW, Tat Poon W, Leung VK, Mak T, Tse ML; Hong Kong Herb-Induced Liver Injury Network (HK-HILIN). Causality assessment of herb-induced liver injury using multidisciplinary approach and Roussel Uclaf Causality Assessment Method (RUCAM). Clin Toxicol (Phila) 2011;49: 34-39. [PubMed].

[150] Deshpande SS, Lalitha VS, Ingle AD, Raste AS, Gadre SG, Maru GB. Subchronic oral toxicity of turmeric and ethanolic turmeric extract in female mice and rats. Toxicol Lett 1998;95:183–193. [PubMed]

[151] Daware MB, Mujumdar AM, Ghaskadbi S. Reproductive toxicity of piperine in Swiss albino mice. Planta Med. 2000;66:231–236. [PubMed]) De Smet PA.Health risks of herbal remedies. Drug Saf 1995;13 : 81-93.

[152] De Smet PA.Health risks of herbal remedies. Drug Saf 1995 ;13: 81-93. [PubMed]

[153] Markowitz JS, DeVane CL. The emerging recognition of herb-drug interactions with a focus on St. John's wort (Hypericum perforatum). Psychopharmacol Bull 2001; 35: 53-64. [PubMed]

[154] Ioannides C. Pharmacokinetic interactions between herbal remedies and medicinal drugs. Xenobiotica 2002 ;32 : 451-478. [PubMed]

[155] Mannel M. Drug interactions with St John's wort: mechanisms and clinical implications.Drug Saf 2004;27 : 773-797. [PubMed]

[156] Borrelli F, Izzo AA. Herb-drug interactions with St John's wort (Hypericum perforatum): an update on clinical observations. AAPS J. 2009 ;11: 710-27.

[157] Izzo AA, Ernst E. Interactions between herbal medicines and prescribed drugs: an updated systematic review. Drugs 2009;69 : 1777-1798. [PubMed]

[158] Dasgupta A. Herbal supplements and therapeutic drug monitoring: focus on digoxin immunoassays and interactions with St. John's wort. Ther Drug Monit 2008 ;30 : 212-217. [PubMed]

[159] Dasgupta A, Tso G, Szelei-Stevens K. St. John's wort does not interfere with therapeutic drug monitoring of 12 commonly monitored drugs using immunoassays. Clin Lab Anal 2006;20: 62-67. [PubMed]

[160] Hafner-Blumenstiel V. [Herbal drug-drug interaction and adverse drug reactions]. Ther Umsch 2011;68: 54-57. [PubMed].

[161] Gurley BJ, Gardner SF, Hubbard MA, Williams DK, Gentry WB, Cui Y, Ang CY. Clinical assessment of effects of botanical supplementation on cytochrome P450 phenotypes in the elderly: St John's wort, garlic oil, Panax ginseng and Ginkgo biloba. Drugs Aging 2005;22 : 525-539. [PubMed]

[162] Dugo M, Gatto R, Zagatti R, Gatti P, Cascone C. [Herbal remedies: nephrotoxicity and drug interactions]. G Ital Nefrol 2010 ;27 Suppl 52: S5-9. [PubMed]

[163] Shaw D.Toxicological risks of Chinese herbs. Planta Med 2010;76: 2012-2018. [PubMed]

[164] Cuzzolin L, Francini-Pesenti F, Verlato G, Joppi M, Baldelli P, Benoni G. Use of herbal products among 392 Italian pregnant women: focus on pregnancy outcome. Pharmacoepidemiol Drug Saf 2010 ;19 : 1151-1158. [PubMed]

[165] Westfall RE. Use of anti-emetic herbs in pregnancy: women's choices, and the question of safety and efficacy. Complement Ther Nurs Midwifery 2004 ;10 : 30-36.

[166] Chattopandhyay I, Biswas K, Bandyyopadhyay U. Turmeric and curcumin: Biological actions and medicinal applications. Current Science 2004; 87: 44-53.

8

Herbal Treatment of Peptic Ulcer: Guilty or Innocent

Khaled A. Abdel-Sater

[1,2]*Department of Physiology, Faculty of Medicine for Boys*
[1]*Al-Azhar University Assiut branch, Assiut*
[2]*King Abdul-Aziz University Rabigh branch, Rabigh*
[1]*Egypt*
[2]*KSA*

1. Introduction

Normally there is a balance between the protective factors (e.g. mucus, bicarbonate, prostaglandins, nitric oxide and normal blood flow) and aggressive factors (e.g. acid plus pepsin, active oxidants, leukotrienes, endothelins, bile or exogenous factors including nonsteroidal anti-inflammatory drugs). Peptic ulcer develops when aggressive factors overcome the protective mechanisms (Borrelli & Izzo, 2000). *Helicobacter pylori*, nonsteroidal anti-inflammatory drugs and acid-pepsin hypersecretion are the major factors that disrupt this equilibrium. There is other type classified as idiopathic and may be related to defective mucosal defence mechanisms due to tobacco use, psychological stress (stress gastritis), rapid gastric emptying or genetics (Calam & Baron, 2001).

Drug treatment of peptic ulcers is targeted at either counteracting aggressive factors or stimulating the mucosal defences (Tepperman & Jacobson, 1994). The ideal aims of treatment of peptic ulcer disease are to relieve pain, heal the ulcer and delay ulcer recurrence (Borrelli & Izzo, 2000).

2. Aim of the work

The aims of this chapter are to review data about their herbs current usage by patients with peptic ulcer, evidence for their efficacy, the mechanisms by which they might act, and, lastly, their adverse effects on the body.

3. Herbal treatment of peptic ulcer

Tyler defines herbal medicines as "crude drugs of vegetable origin utilized for the treatment of disease states, often of a chronic nature, or to attain or maintain a condition of improved health (Tyler, 1994).

In spite of the progress in conventional chemistry and pharmacology in producing effective drugs, the herbal medicine might provide a source of treatment by many people in the world. In many cultures herbal knowledge was said to have been handed down from the gods. Herbs had been used by all cultures throughout history because patients are often unaware of the potential problems caused by herbal medicines. In addition, their physicians commonly lack knowledge about these compounds. This factor results in the perception by physicians that herbal drugs are ineffective placebos that can simply be ignored. Some physicians view use of these products as a threat to their paternalistic role and sternly admonish their patients or angrily label them as being crazy (Crone & Wise, 1998).

3.1 Examples of herbs used in treatment of peptic ulcer

Solanum nigrum (family: Solanaceae) commonly known as black nightshade, deadly nightshade, sunberry, makoy, fragrant tomato, duscle, Hound's berry , petty Morel , wonder berry, popolo or wonder cherry. It is effective in treatment of peptic ulcers. The raw juice of its leaves is given either separately or in conjunction with other beneficial juices (Akhtar & Munir, 1989).

A condensed tannin, polyflavonoid tannin, catechol-type tannin non-hydrolyzable tannin or flavolan has been isolated and their anti-peptic and anti-ulcer activity confirmed experimentally (Vasconcelos et al., 2010). When a low concentration of tannin is applied to the mucosa, only the outermost layer is tanned, becoming less permeable and affording an increased protection to the subjacent layers against the action of bacteria, chemical irritation, and, to a certain extent, against mechanical irritation. Tannins may promote a mechanic barrier that protects the stomach from ulcer formation and facilitates ulcer healing (Borrelli & Izzo, 2000).

Saponins (family: Sapindaceae) are so-called because of their soap-like effect, which is due to their surfactant properties. Saponins isolated from the rhizome of panax japonicas, the fruit of kochia scoparia (which contain approximately 20% of saponins) some oleanolic acid oligoglycosides extracted from P. japonicas, K. scoparia and a methanol extract of P. japonicus rhizome have been demonstrated to possess gastro-protective properties (Matsuda et al., 1998).

Licorice or glycyrrhiza glabra (family: Leguminosae) also known as lacrisse (German), licorice root, liquorice, reglisse (French), regolizia (Italian), suessholz, sweet licorice, sweet wood. It is one of the most widely used medicinal plants in the world, commonly used in European, Arabian and Asian traditional medicine systems. Licorice is very effective in the treatment of stomach ulcers. It soothes the irritation of the inner lining of the stomach caused due to excessive acids. Its root is taken, dried and then soaked overnight in water. This is taken in an infusion with rice gruel. This is such an effective treatment that it is used in conventional allopathic medicine also (Hayashi & Sudo, 2009).

Plants containing mucilages traditionally used in several countries in the treatment of gastric ulcer include althaea officinalis (marshmallow), cetraria islandica (Iceland moss), malva sylvestris (common mallow), matricaria chamomilla (chamomile) and aloe species (Capasso & Grandolini, 1999). Myrrh (meaning bitter), an oleo-gum-resin obtained from commiphora molmol, contains up to 60% gum and up to 40% resin (Newall et al., 1996). Myrrh pre-treatment produced a dose-dependent protection against the ulcerogenic effects of different necrotizing agents (Al-Harbi et al., 1997). The protective effect of myrrh is attributed to its effect on mucus production or increase in nucleic acid and non-protein sulphydryl concentration, which appears to be mediated through its free-radical scavenging, thyroid-stimulating and prostaglandin- inducing properties. Also aloe seems to be able to speed wound healing by improving blood circulation through the area and preventing cell death around a wound (Borrelli & Izzo, 2000).

3.2 Potential benefits and mechanism of action

Experimental studies have demonstrated that the herbs have gastroprotective activity against gastric mucosal injury induced by ethanol (Souza et al., 2007), ischemia reperfusion (El-Abhar et al., 2002), indomethacin (Souza et al., 2007), alcohol toxicity (Kanter et al., 2005) or stress (Khaled, 2009) in rat.

The mechanism of herb-induced gastroprotection varies according to the nature and chemical constituents of the herbs. The main functions including; inhibition of acid plus pepsin secretion (Baggio et al ., 2007), cytoprotective (by enhancement of epidermal growth factor content in gastric juice, nitric oxide and H+, K+-ATPase inhibitory activity in gastric tissue, PGE2 in plasma, inhibition of endothelin in plasma, an increase in mucosal thickness (Fan et al., 2007) and mucus content in the gastric mucosa) (Kamath et al., 2008), bactericidal activity, inhibition of the growth and activity of *helicobacter pylori* (Mahady et al., 2002) and antioxidant activities (and the ability to scavenge reactive oxygen species) (Souza et al., 2007), isolated or in combination, are responsible for gastric mucosal protection (Zaidi, et al., 2009). Moreover, plantextract- induced gastroprotection is probably related to the enhancing effect on NOS inhibitor expression, gastric microcirculation (Al Mofleh, 2010). Herbs could protect the gastric mucosa by increasing the bioavailability of arachidonic acid, resulting in biosynthesis of the cytoprotective prostaglandins in the stomach (Tsuji et al., 1990). Moreover, herbs have also been reported to produce a marked inhibition on the release of leukotrienes, which cause mucosal tissue injury and hypoxemia (Mansour, 1990).

3.3 Risks of herbal treatment of peptic ulcer

It is important to acknowledge that all conventional drugs have potential toxicities. However, in contrast to herbal products, conventional drugs undergo trials and postapproval surveillance that define these toxicities, giving practitioners data on that to weigh risks and benefits of treatment. The therapeutic window and dosage are also defined, as are the constituents of the medicine. Because of rigorous quality control, each pill has the same ingredients as another. Adverse reactions to herbal medicines are probably underrecognized and underreported (D'Arcy et al., 1991). Herbal medicines can produce unwanted side effects, toxicity and herbal drug interaction caused by their pharmacologic properties.

A-Side-effects and toxicity of herbal therapy

i.   Direct side-effects and toxicity of herbal therapy

Nausea, diarrhea, and skin reactions are common side effects of a wide variety of herbal medicines (tannins, mucilages, saponins and solanum nigrum). Also there is a serious side effects of herbal remedies on the liver (tannins and Licorice) include liver injury, acute and chronic hepatitis, hepatic failure and possibly hepatic tumours (Chandler, 1987). While most of the adverse effects on the digestive tube are self-limiting and relatively trivial, the same is not true of herb-induced hepatotoxicity, in which fatalities have been reported with alarming frequency (Chitturi & Farrell, 2000). More serious side effects of herbal medicines may include hypertension, heart failure (licorice), anaphylaxis (matricaria chamomilla), and lupus-like symptoms (D'Arcy et al., 1991). Ventricular arrhythmias, intravascular hemolysis, hemorrhage, renal failure, and pulmonary hypertension have all been linked to the active chemical components found in herbal remedies (Larrey et al., 1992). Psychoactive effects in several herbal medicines have produced behavioural, cognitive, mania and emotional disturbances (Capwell, 1995). Most of these herbs are not recommended for woman with pregnancy or breast feeding (Roulet et al., 1988).

Black nightshade is UNSAFE. It contains a toxic chemical called solanin. At higher doses, it can cause severe poisoning. Signs of poisoning include irregular heartbeat, trouble breathing, dizziness, drowsiness, twitching of the arms and legs, cramps, diarrhea, paralysis, trembling, paralysis, coma, and death (Duke, 1985).

In sensitive individuals, a large intake of tannins may cause bowel irritation, kidney irritation, liver damage, irritation of the stomach and gastrointestinal pain. A correlation has been made between esophogeal or nasal cancer in humans and regular consumption of certain herbs with high tannin concentrations (Lewis, 1977). Tannins interfere with iron absorption through a complex formation with iron when it is in the gastrointestinal lumen which decreases the bioavailability of iron. There is an important difference in the way in which the phenolic compounds interact with different hydroxylation patterns (gallic acid, catechin, chlorogenic acid) and the effect on iron absorption. The content of the iron-binding galloyl groups may be the major determinant of the inhibitory effect of phenolic compounds. However, condensed tannins do not interfere with iron absorption (Brune et al., 1989).

Saponins are harmful if swallowed or inhaled. They cause irritation to skin, eyes and respiratory tract. Symptoms include redness, itching, and pain. Saponin inhalation causes sneezing and may irritate the respiratory tract. They cause haemolysis of RBC's if reach the blood. Frequent ingestion of small amounts of saponin results in chronic githagism (a disease, similar to lathyrism, that results in pain, burning and prickling sensations in lower extremities, and increasing paralysis) (Hostettmann and Marston, 2005).

Excessive consumption of licorice is known to be toxic to the cardiovascular system and may produce oedema (van Uum, 2005). Comparative studies of pregnant women suggest that licorice can also adversely affect both IQ and behaviour traits of offspring (De Smet, 2002). In large amounts, licorice containing glycyrrhizin can cause high blood pressure, salt and water retention, and low potassium levels, which could lead to heart failure (Blumenthal et al., 2000).

Mucilage side effects include bloating, abdominal pain, flatulence and oesophageal obstruction. Matricaria chamomilla (chamomile) causes symptoms of an allergic reaction such as rash, itching, swelling, dizziness and trouble breathing (Andres et al., 2009). Althaea officinalis is generally regarded as safe. However, the potential for marshmallow to cause allergic reactions or low blood sugar, genotoxicity, carcinogenicity and/or reproductive and developmental toxicity has been noted anecdotally (Büechi et al., 2005). Taking aloe by mouth is unsafe, especially at high doses. There is some concern that some of the chemicals found in aloe latex might cause cancer. Additionally, aloe latex is hard on the kidneys and could lead to serious kidney disease and even death (Poppenga, 2002).

ii.   Indirect Side-Effects and Toxicity of Herbal Therapy

The use of herbal therapy may be complicated by several indirect adverse effects. People initially consulting herbal practitioners may suffer from misdiagnosis and consequent delay in obtaining effective conventional treatment (Angell & Kassirer, 1998). Others may delay or forego appropriate conventional options in favour of ineffective unconventional ones. When expectations of alternative therapy are high, failure to obtain relief from symptoms, particularly if treatment has been expensive, could also be construed as an adverse effect (Langmead & Rampton, 2001).

B-Drug–herb Interactions

A pharmacodynamic interaction occurs when substances act at the same receptor, site of action or physiologic system. Pharmacodynamic interactions result in an antagonistic or additive drug effect (Anastasio et al., 2000). A drug or substance that accentuates or interferes with the absorption, distribution and elimination of a second drug or substance produces a pharmacokinetic interaction. This mechanism is the most frequent cause of adverse interactions, commonly caused by altered drug elimination. Induction of elimination can result in a decreased therapeutic benefit whereas inhibition of drug elimination can produce excessively increased dose related toxicity (Nicole & Mitchell, 2003).

Saponins and mucilage can interfere with the absorption of other medicines within the gut if they are taken at the same time (Mohammed, 2009).

Several medications may cause potentially negative drug interactions with licorice. Some of these medications include blood pressure medications (beta blockers, calcium channel blockers, and nervous system inhibitors), certain diuretics (such as bumetanide, chlorothiazide, chlorthalidone, ethacrynic acid, furosemide, hydrochlorothiazide, metolazone and torsemide), hypoglycemics and corticosteroids (D'Arcy et al., 1991). These licorice drug interactions can result in serious problems, such as low blood potassium and low blood calcium (Blumenthal et al., 2000). Licorice should not be taken concurrently with corticosteroid treatment (Poppenga, 2002). Concurrent use of furosemide may potentiate development of acute renal failure. Potassium loss due to other drugs, e.g. thiazide diuretics, can be increased. With potassium loss, sensitivity to digitalis glycosides increases (D'Arcy et al., 1991).   Licorice should not be administered in conjunction with spironolactone or amiloride (Poppenga, 2002).

It is mentioned in some literature sources (Barnes et al. 2002, Poppenga, 2002) that absorption of concomitantly administered medicines can be delayed due to mucilage protecting layer. Potential risks of chamomile include interference with warfarin and infant botulism in very young children (Biancoa et al., 2008).   Aloe may increase K + loss and potentiate cardiac glycosides and antiarrhythmic agents such as quinidine. Increased K + loss when used with other drugs, such as diuretics, with similar effect on K +. Laxative effect may reduce absorption of other drugs (Poppenga, 2002).

4. Conclusion

Herbal medicine is prescribed by the herbalists symptomatically — based on signs and symptoms alone — rather than as a result of a full understanding of the underlying disease. Proper diagnosis is totally absent. As any plant, medicinal herbs contain many chemicals that are subjected to change with changing conditions of the environment, especially storage. The discriminate and proper use of some herbal products is safe and may provide some therapeutic benefits, but the indiscriminate or excessive use of herbs can be unsafe and even dangerous (Borrelli & Izzo, 2000).

There is an urgent need for further scientific assessment of the potential benefits and dangers of the huge range of herbal medications available. Herbal preparations used for medicinal purposes should require licensing by an independent national body in order to improve their quality and safety, and to ensure that claims of efficacy are validated by randomized controlled trials.

The general public, as well as pharmacists, general practitioners and hospital doctors, should be aware, particularly, of the risks associated with the use of herbal remedies, whether on their own or in combination with other herbal or conventional medicines. The incorporation of a short course on alternative and complementary therapy in medical school curricula would help achieve this end.

Lastly, because of the potential for side effects, toxic reactions, and unwanted drug-drug interactions, it is essential for physicians to ascertain if their patients are taking herbal medications. So if you are thinking about using herbal medicine it would be a good idea to check with your physician about possible adverse reactions and interactions with medications you may be taking before starting (D'Arcy et al., 1991).

IF YOU NEED ONE WORD "Do not take herbs internally except under the supervision of a qualified professional".

Herbs you're guilty until proven innocent by researchers!

5. References

Akhtar, M. & Munir, M. (1989). Evaluation of the Gastric Antiulcerogenic Effects of Solanum Nigrum, Brassica Oleracea and Ocimum Basilicum in Rats. *J. Ethnopharm.*, Vol.27, No. 1, pp.163-176. ISSN 0378-8741

Al Mofleh, I. (2010). Spices, herbal xenobiotics and the stomach: Friends or foes? *World J Gastroenterol*, Vol.16, No. 22, pp. 2710-2719. ISSN 1007-9327

Al-Harbi, M., Quereshi, S, Raza, M, Ahmed, MM, Afzal, M, Shah, AH. (1997). Gastric Antiulcer and Cytoprotective Effect of Commiphora Molmol in Rats. *J Ethnopharmacol*, Vol.55, pp. 141- 150. ISSN 0378-8741

Anastasio, G., Cornell, K., Menscer, D. (1997). Drug Interactions: Keeping it Straight. *Am Fam Phys*; Vol.56, pp. 883–894. ISSN 0002-838X

Andres C, Chen WC, Ollert M, Mempel M, Darsow U, Ring J. (2009). Anaphylactic Reaction to Chamomile Tea. *Allergology International*, Vol.58, pp.135-136. ISSN 1323-8930

Angell, M. & Kassirer, J. (1998). Alternative Medicine—The Risks of Untested and Unregulated Remedies. *N Engl J Med*; Vol.339, pp. 839–41(Editorial; Comment). ISSN 0028-4793

Arslan, O., Ethem, G., Ferah, A., Omer, C., Ahmet, G., Hale, S. & Levent, C. (2005). The Protective Effect of Thymoquinone on Ethanol-Induced Acute Gastric Damage in the Rat. *Nutrition Research*, Vol.25, pp. 673–680. ISSN 0271-5317

Baggio, C., Freitas, C., Otofuji Gde, M., Cipriani, T., Souza, L., Sassaki, G., Iacomini, M., Marques, M., Mesia-Vela, S. (2007). Flavonoid-Rich Fraction of Maytenus Ilicifolia Mart. Ex. Reiss Protects the Gastric Mucosa of Rodents Through Inhibition of Both H+,K+ -Atpase Activity and Formation of Nitric Oxide. *J Ethnopharmacol*; Vol.113, pp. 433-440. ISSN 0378-8741

Barnes, J., Anderson, L. & Phillipson J. (2002). Herbal Medicines. A Guide for Healthcare Professionals. 2nd ed. Pharmaceutical Press, x- London, Chicago, part 1. pp. 47–50.

Biancoa, M., Carolina, L., Laura, I. & Rafael A. (2008). Presence of Clostridium Botulinum Spores in Matricaria Chamomilla (Chamomile) and its Relationship with Infant Botulism. *International Journal of Food Microbiology*, Vol.121, No.3, pp. 357-360. ISSN 0168-1605

Blumenthal, M., Goldberg, A. & Brinckman, J. (2000). Licorice Root. In: Herbal Medicine: Expanded Commission E Monographs. Newton, MA: Lippincott Williams & Wilkins; pp. 233–239.

Borrelli, F. & Izzo, A. (2000). The Plant Kingdom as a Source of Anti-ulcer Remedies. *Phytother Res*, Vol. 14, pp.581–591. ISSN 0951-418X.

Brune, M., Rossander, L. & Hallberg, L. (1989). Iron Absorption and Phenolic Compounds: Importance of Different Phenolic Structures. *Eur J Clin Nutr,* Vol.43, No. 8, pp. 547–57. ISSN: 0954-3007.

Büechi, S., Vögelin, R., von Eiff, M., Ramos, M. & Melzer, J. (2005). Open Trial to Assess Aspects of Safety and Efficacy of A Combined Herbal Cough Syrup With Ivy and Thyme. *Forsch Komplementarmed Klass Naturheilkd;* Vol. 12, No. 6, pp. 328-32.

Calam, J. & Baron. J. (2001). ABC of the Upper Gastrointestinal Tract: Pathophysiology of Duodenal and Gastric Ulcer and Gastric Cancer. *B.M.J.,* Vol. 323, pp. 980-982. ISSN 09598138.

Capasso, F. & Grandolini G. (1999). Fitofarmacia Impiego Razionale Delle Droghe Vegetali,. Springer Verlag Italia: Milan. 2nd ed.

Capwell, R. (1995). Ephedrine-Induced Mania from An Herbal Diet Supplement. *Am J Psychiatry;* Vol. 152, pp. 647. ISSN 0002-953X

Chandler, R. (1987). Herbs As Foods and Medicines. Drugs and therapeutics for maritime practitioners; Vol. 10, pp. 22-30.

Chitturi, S. & Farrell, G. (2000). Herbal hepatotoxicity: An Expanding but Poorly Defined Problem. *J Gastroenterol Hepatol;* Vol. 15, pp. 1093-9. ISSN 0954-691X

Crone, C. & Wise. T. (1998). Use of Herbal Medicines Among Consultation-Liaison Populations. *Psychosomatics,* Vol. 39, No. 1, pp. 3–13. ISSN 0033-3182

D'Arcy, P. (1991). Adverse Reactions and Interactions with Herbal Medicines, I: Adverse Reactions. *Adverse Drug React Toxicol Rev.,* Vol. 10, pp.189-208. ISSN 1176-2551

De Smet, P. (2002). Herbal Remedies. *N Engl J Med.;* Vol. 347, No. 25, pp.2046-56. ISSN 0028-4793

Duke, J. (1985). Handbook of Medicinal Herbs. CRC Press, Boca Raton, FL.

El-Abhar, H., Abdallah, D. & Saleh, S. (2002). Gastroprotective, Activity of Nigella sativa Oil and its Constituent, Thymoquinone, Against Gastric Mucosal Injury Induced by Ischemia/Reperfusion in Rats. *J Ethnopharmacol;* Vol. 84, pp. 251-258. ISSN 0378-8741

Fan, T., Feng, Q., Jia, C., Fan, Q., Li, C., Bai, X. (2005). Protective Effect of Weikang Decoction and Partial Ingredients on Model Rat with Gastric Mucosa Ulcer. *World J Gastroenterol;* Vol. 11, pp. 1204-1209. ISSN 1007-9327

Hayashi, H., Sudo, H. Economic Importance of Licorice (2009). *Plant Biotechnology,* Vol. 26, pp. 101–104. ISSN 1467-7652

Hostettmann, K. & Marston, A. (2005). Saponins First edition. Cambridge University Press.

Kamath, B., Srikanta, B., Dharmesh, S., Sarada, R. & Ravishankar, G. (2008). Ulcer Preventive and Antioxidative Properties of Astaxanthin from Haematococcus Pluvialis. *Eur J Pharmacol;* Vol. 590, pp. 387-395. ISSN 0014-2999

Kanter, M., Halit, D., Cengiz, K. & Hanefi, O. (2005). Gastroprotective Activity of Nigella Sativa Oil and its Constituent, Thymoquinone Against Acute Alcohol-Induced Gastric Mucosal Injury in Rats, *World J Gastroenterol;* Vol. 11, No. 42, pp. 6662-6666. ISSN 1007-9327

Khaled, A. (2009). Gastroprotective effects of Nigella Sativa Oil on the Formation of Stress Gastritis in Hypothyroidal rats. *Int J Physiol Pathophysiol Pharmacol;* Vol. 1 pp. 143-149. ISSN 1944-8171

Langmead, L. & Rampton, D. S. (2001) Review article: herbal treatment in gastrointestinal and liver disease - benefits and dangers. *Aliment Pharmacol Ther;* Vol. 15, pp. 1239-1252. ISSN 1365-2036

Larrey, D., Vial, T., Pauwels, A., Castot, A., Biour, M., David, M. & Michel, H. (1992). Hepatitis after Germander Administration: Another Instance of Herbal Medicine Hepatotoxicity. *Ann Intern Med.;* Vol. 117, pp. 129–132. ISSN 0003-4819

Lewis, W. (1977). Medical Botany: Plants Affecting Man's Health. New York: Wiley. ISBN 0-471-53320-3.

Mahady, G., Pendland, S., Yun, G. & Lu, Z. (2002). Turmeric (Curcuma Longa) and Curcumin Inhibit the Growth of *Helicobacter Pylori*, A Group 1 Carcinogen. *Anticancer Res;* Vol. 22, pp. 4179-4181. ISSN 0250-7005

Mansour, M. (2000). Protective Effects of Thymoquinone and Desferrioxamine Against Hepatotoxicity of Carbon Tetrachloride in Mice. *Life Sci;* Vol. 66, pp. 2583-2591. ISSN: 0024-3205

Matsuda, H., Li, Y., Murakami, T., Yamahara, J. & Yoshikawa, M. (1998). Protective Effects of Oleanolic Acid Oligoglycosides on Ethanol- or Indomethacin-Induced Gastric Mucosal Lesions in Rats. *Life Sci.,* Vol. 63, pp. PL245–PL250.

Mohammed, Y. (2009). Drug Food Interactions and Role of Pharmacist. *Asian Journal of Pharmaceutical and Clinical Research,* Vol. 2, No.4, pp.1-10. ISSN 0974-2441

Newall, C., Anderson, L. & Phillipson J. (1996). Herbal Medicines. The Pharmaceutical Press: London.

Nicole, C. & Mitchell A. (2003). Levine Understanding Drug–Herb Interactions. *Pharmacoepidemiology and drug safety;* Vol. 12, pp. 427–430. ISSN 1099-1557

Poppenga, R. (2002). Herbal Medicine: Potential for Intoxication and Interactions with Conventional Drugs Clinical Techniques in Small Animal Practice, Vol. 17, No. 1, pp. 6-18

Roulet, M., Laurini, R., Rivier L. & Calame A. (1988). Hepatic Venoocclusive Disease in Newborn Infant of A Woman Drinking Herbal Tea. *J Pediat,* Vol. 112, pp. 433–436. ISSN: 0022-3476

Souza, S., Aquino, L., Milach Jr, A. , Bandeira, M., Nobre, E. & Viana, G. (2007). Antiinflammatory and Antiulcer Properties of Tannins from Myracrodruon Urundeuva Allemão (Anacardiaceae) in Rodents. *Phytother. Res.* Vol. 21, pp.220–225. ISSN 0951-418X

Tepperman, B. & Jacobson, E. (1994): Circulatory Factors in Gastric Mucosal Defense and Repair. In Physiology of the Gastrointestinal Tract, Johnson LR (ed.). Raven Press: New York; pp.1331-1352.

Tsuji, S., Kawano, S., Sato, N. & Kamada, T. (1990). Mucosal Blood Flow Stasis and Hypoxemia as the Pathogenesis of Acute Gastric Mucosal Injury: Role of Endogenous Leukotrienes and Prostaglandins. *J Clin Gastroenterol;* Vol. 12, No.1, pp. S85-S9137. ISSN 0192-0790

Tyler V. (1994). Herbs of Choice: The Therapeutic Use of Phytomedicinals. Binghampton, NY, Pharmaceutical Products Press.

van Uum, S.(2005). Liquorice and Hypertension Editorial in *The Netherlands Journal of Medicine.* ISSN 0300-2977

Vasconcelos, P., Andreob, M., Vilegasb, W., Hiruma-Limaa, C. & Pellizzon, C. (2010). Effect of Mouriri Pusa Tannins and Flavonoids on Prevention and Treatment Against Experimental Gastric Ulcer. *Journal of Ethnopharmacology;* Vol. 131, pp. 146–153. ISSN 0378-8741

Zaidi, S., Yamada, K., Kadowaki, M., Usmanghani, K. & Sugiyama, T. (2009). Bactericidal Activity of Medicinal Plants, Employed for The Treatment of Gastrointestinal Ailments, Against Helicobacter Pylori. *J Ethnopharmacol;* Vol. 121, No.2, pp.286-91. ISSN 0378-8741

9

In Vitro and In Vivo Anti-Helicobacter pylori Activity of Natural Products

Maria do Carmo Souza
Federal University of Mato Grosso,
Brazil

1. Introduction

Since old times plants have been a resource used by human beings an important sources of biologically active products. Recently, efforts have been made in order to identify new antiulcerogenic drugs from natural sources, having as the main target the *Helicobacter pylori*, a bacterium considered as the most important etiological agent of the human peptic ulcer. It has been shown to be a rich source of bioactive substances, having antifungal, gastroprotective, analgesic, anti-HIV, antibacterial, antitumoral properties and inhibitor of gastric H+,K+-ATPase and angeotensin-converting enzyme. This chapter aims to demonstrate methods anti-*Helicobacter pylori in vitro* and *in vivo* for screening of plant extracts.

Helicobacter pylori was identified in 1982 by Marshall and Warren (1984) and quickly became the subject of countless microbiological, histological, epidemiological, immunological, ecological and clinical studies (Vaz, 2005). This organism has its nomenclature revised, starting with Campylobacter pyloridis, and a correction of the name was originally Greek to Latin, Campylobacter pylori (Marshall and Goodwin, 1987) and organisms like Campylobacter. Taxonomic studies have led to reclassification, resulting in the name Helicobacter pylori (Goodwin and Armstrong, 1990).

H. pylori is a bacillus, Gram negative, microaerobic, spiral and curved (Dunn et al. 1997). It has two to six flagella that provide motility to it to resist the rhythmic contractions of stomach and penetrate the gastric mucosa. It has 2.4 to 4.0 mm in length and 0.5 to 1.0 mm in width (Brown, 2000).

The identification and isolation of *Helicobacter pylori* allowed for a considerable development of knowledge about peptic ulcer (Marshall and Warren, 1984). This pathogen is considered the main etiological agent of human peptic ulcer, with a worldwide prevalence rate of about 40% in developed countries and over 80% in developing countries (Shi et al., 2008).

H. pylori produces a number of virulence factors that may have different associations with the disease. The establishment of chronic infection may be influenced by host genetic factors as well as the blood group ABO and Lewis-blood group antigen and differences in susceptibility to particular strains of *H. pylori* (Brown, 2000).

To establish and maintain the infection, H. pylori expresses a variety of different types of maintenance factors that allow bacteria to colonize and remain within the host and virulence factors, which contributes to the pathogenic effects of bacteria, with emphasis on gastric inflammation, mucosal barrier disruption gastric and changes in gastric physiology (Dunn et al. , 1997). *H. pylori* is a genetically highly diverse bacterium, featuring several genotypes which have been associated with virulence factors and risk of gastric disease and other outcomes of infection. Among these, the vacA gene, which encodes a cytotoxin of vacuolization, is present in all types of *H. pylori*. This gene is also strongly associated with high levels of inflammation and epithelial damage in the gastric mucosa, caused by cagA gene is a marker for the presence of PAI pathogenicity (cag pathogenicity island) (Ladeira et al., 2003).

In previous studies, infection with different types of Helicobacter, as H. mustela, H. felis, H. heilmanii, and H. pylori in mice, cats, pigs, monkeys and gerbils have been described suggesting its relevance to human infection, but these animal models do not mimic the infection of H. pylori in humans because of the lack of virulence factors of infecting organisms, such as vacA and cagA encoded cytotoxins, required for the mucosal damage, inflammation and ulcer formation (Konturek et al., 2000). Moreover, some of these animals are large and unwieldy, there is a need to test commonly used in animal models such as mice, which could be used to study various aspects of infection by H. pylori, ulcer healing and therapy of infection (Ross et al., 1992).

Results in experimental studies in animal models using rodents, concluded that H. pylori alone causes little or no effect on the gastric mucosa of intact rats. However, this organism can cause persistence of pre-existing ulcers and chronic active inflammation. Presence of predisposing factors leading to disruption of the integrity of the gastric mucosa may be necessary for the H. pylori enhancement inflammation and tissue damage to the stomach of these animals (Konturek et al 2000). Whereas peptic ulcer is generally a disease which results from the circumscriptive loss of tissue in regions of the digestive tract that may come into contact with the stomach's chloride peptic secretion (Coelho, 2003). In general, it is caused by an imbalance between aggressive and defensive factors of the gastric mucosa (Rao et al., 2000). It seems that the Helicobacter pylori takes advantage of this situation to colonize and settle in the gastric mucosa.

2. Experimental protocols

2.1 Animals
Male Wistar albino rats (160-210 g) and male Swiss-Webster mice (25-30 g), can be used. The animals should be kept in propylene cages at 26±2°C under 12h light-dark cycle, with free access to water and restricted access to food, 2 hours/day (9-10a.m. and 6-7p.m.).

2.2 Microorganism
The strain of *Helicobacter pylori* ATCC 43504 (vacA and cagA positives) can be used to express the factors that determine their virulence. Stock cultures can be maintained in Mueller-Hinton broth at -20°C.

2.3 Botanical material
Plants should be carefully collected and treated to prevent fungal contamination. The plants should be deposited, registered and taxonomically verified.

2.4 Extract preparation and phytochemical analysis
Plants should be cleaned, dried at room temperature and shredded in an electric mill with a sieve with a mesh size of 40μm, until powder be obtained. The dried powder should be

successively macerated (1:5, w/v), with hexane, dichloromethane, ethyl acetate, methanol and water-ethanol 75%, for 7 days each. Every extract should be separated by filtration and concentrated under reduced pressure at, approximately, 40°C, with the residual solvent being eliminated in an incubator at 40°C. To prepare the dichloromethanic fraction (Fig. 1), the crude dichloromethanic extract should be submitted to silica filtration using dichloromethane. The preliminary phytochemical analyses of the hydroethanolic extract and the dichloromethanic fraction may follow the methodology described by Matos (1998).

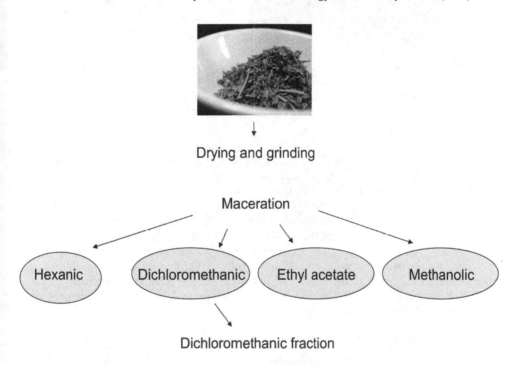

Fig. 1. Scheme of preparation of extracts and fractions

2.5 In-vitro assays
2.5.1 Disk diffusion

For the disk diffusion assay, serial dilutions of the hexanic, ethyl acetate, dichloromethanic, methanolic and hydroethanolic extracts from plants, should be prepared, in order to obtain the following doses: 0.0625; 0.125; 0.25; 0.5 and 1 mg/disk. The sterile disks utilized (6 mm - CECON®) should be imbibed in 25μL of each dose of extract and fraction. The extract- or fraction-imbibed disks should be deposited on the surface of the plate inoculated with *H. pylori*, in a suspension of 6×10^8 CFU/mL (McFarland turbidity standard 2), using clarithromycin (15μg - CECON®) as the standard drug, incubated at 37°C under microaerophilic conditions in an atmosphere of 5 to 15% O_2 and 5 to 10% CO_2 for 3-5 days. After this period, the growth inhibition halos should be quantified with a digital pachymeter. The diameters of inhibitory zones should be measured in duplicate and mean values ≥10 mm are considered active (Fig. 2).

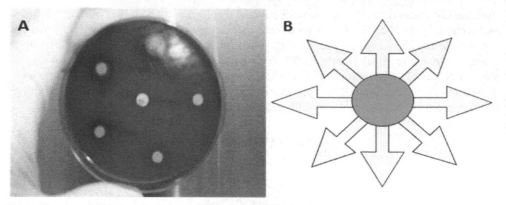

Fig. 2. Photograph (A) and scheme (B) of a disk diffusion

2.5.2 Broth microdilution

The broth microdilution assay allows the determination of the Minimum Inhibitory Concentration (MIC). To each well in the microplate should be added 100µL of Mueller-Hinton broth, supplemented with 10% foetal calf serum inoculated with 6×10^8 *H. pylori* (McFarland turbidity standard 2), 100µL of the hexanic, ethyl acetate, dichloromethanic, methanolic and hydroethanolic extracts from plants, should be also added to reach the final concentrations of 0.0625; 0.125; 0.25; 0.5 and 1 mg/mL. Clarithromycin (5 mg/mL) is used as the standard drug for growth inhibition. Next, the microplate (Fig. 3), should be incubated at 37°C under microaerophilia in an atmosphere of 5 to 15% O_2 and 5 to 10% CO_2, for 3-5 days. After incubation, the plates should be visually examined and each well should be replicated in blood agar (Mueller-Hinton agar with 5% sheep blood), to determine whether growth had occurred, with the MIC defined as the lowest concentration to cause complete bacterial growth inhibition (bactericidal activity).

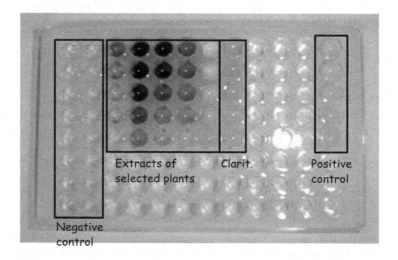

Fig. 3. Photograph of a microdilution plate

2.6 In-vivo assays
2.6.1 Acute toxicity evaluation

The acute toxicity evaluation of each extract of plant should be performed in mice (n = 4). The animals should be treated orally (p.o.) with extract at 250, 500, 1000, 3000 and 5000 mg/kg doses. A control animal should be used for each dose, having received the vehicle (distilled water, 10 mL/kg). After the administration of the extract or vehicle, the animals should be observed individually in appropriate cages (open field) at 0, 15 and 30 minutes; 1, 2, 4 and 8 hours and, once every day, for 14 days. The results for the general behavioural observations should be recorded in a table adapted from Malone (1977).

2.6.2 Ulcer induction and colonization by *H. pylori*

Rats should be ulcerated by acetic acid according to method described by Takagi et al. (1969), with modifications. After ulcer induction, the animals should be kept in propylene cages, with daily access to commercial food restricted to the time periods of 9-10 a.m. and 5-6 p.m., allowing for adequate fasting for administration of *H. pylori*, and of extract at 50, 100 and 200mg/kg doses of preparations, as well as of the standard drugs (amoxicillin 50mg/kg + clarithromycin 25mg/kg + omeprazole 20mg/kg).

According to the method described by Konturek et al. (1999), with modifications, 24h after ulcer induction by acetic acid, the animals should be inoculated intragastrically with 1 mL of *H. pylori* ATCC 43504 (9x10⁸) suspended in Mueller-Hinton broth, by using a cannula appropriate for orogastric gavage. For the animals in the control, Sham and acetic acid-induced ulcer groups without *H. pylori* infection, only Mueller-Hinton broth should be orally administered. The orogastric inoculation of *H. pylori* should be maintained twice a day for 7 days, whereas the administration of extracts from plants and of the standard drugs, twice a day, for 14 consecutive days, starting from the third day after ulcer induction by acetic acid. After treatment, the animals should be sacrificed by cervical dislocation; blood can be collected from the inferior vena cava. The stomachs should be removed for evaluation of gastric lesions, the ulcerated area (mm²) should be measured and the healing rate (%) and then determined according to method described by Takagi et al. (1969). Prostaglandin E2 (PGE2) levels should be measured from gastric mucosal scrapings and a fragment from each stomach can be used for the histopathological exam and for the urease determination.

2.6.3 Determination of PGE₂ concentration

The concentration of PGE_2 in scrapings of gastric mucosa should be quantified by ELISA using a commercial kit (Parameter®, R&D Systems). The mucosal scrapings (100 mg) should be homogenized with 1 mL phosphate buffer and centrifuged at 3,000 RPM at 4°C for 10 min. The PGE_2 levels should be determined according to the manufacturer's instructions.

It has been demonstrated that PGE_2, derived from COX-1 and COX-2, is involved in the regulation of gastric mucosa inflammation and also contributes to maintaining its integrity during infection by *H. pylori* through several mechanisms, including augmentation of the gastric mucosal flow, synthesis of mucus and bicarbonate, inhibition of gastric motility, and the release of enzymes, free radicals from neutrophils and gastric secretion (Chao et al., 2004).

2.6.4 Urease production determination

With the aid of tweezers, a fragment of gastric tissue should be inserted in the centre of a minitube containing urease gel (NEWPROV®). Inoculation times should be recorded, the minitubes should be kept at room temperature and the change in colour should be evaluated after 1 hour, and whenever it is negative, a final reading should be taken after 24 hours. A urease test should be considered positive if an alkaline reaction has developed (red or dark pink colour), and negative when there are no changes in the medium's colour (yellow or light orange).

Urease, an enzyme produced by *H. pylori*, acts by promoting the hydrolysis of urea, a substrate that is present in gastric juice under physiological conditions, leading to the production of ammonium, that behaves as a receptor for H^+ ions and generates a neutral pH inside the bacteria, thus contributing to the survival of these organisms in the highly acidic environment of the stomach (Ladeira et al., 2003). The rapid urease test is considered one of the most useful and cheapest tests among the invasive assays, with a 100% sensitivity and 89.5% specificity (Ogata et al., 2002), although false positive results may occur given the other bacterial species that might be isolated from the oral and/or gastric cavities (*Proteus mirabilis*, *Citrobacter freundii*, *Klebsiella pneumoniae*, *Enterobacter cloacae* and *Staphylococcus aureus*) and that also produce urease (Osaki et al., 2008).

2.6.5 Determination of cytokines IL-1β, TNF-α, IL-10 and VEGF

Total blood should be collected from the inferior vena cava, in tubes containing 5% EDTA, centrifuged at 3000 RPM for 10 min., and the plasma should be separated and frozen at -20°C until the assay. For measuring plasma levels of IL-1β, TNF-α, IL-10 and VEGF, a plex kit for rat cytokines and chemokines (RCYTO-80K) should be used according to the manufacturer's instructions, and the fluorescence should be determined through a Luminex ® device.

The literature refers to IL-1β as being the most potent among the known gastroproctective agents (Kondo et al., 1994; El-Omar, 2004). TNF-α also inhibits gastric secretion, although to a lesser extent than IL-1β and is found, together with IL-10, elevated in patients with chronic gastritis associated with *H. pylori* infection (El-Omar, 2004). VEGF has been mentioned as a cicatrisation-promoting factor in gastric ulcer (Okabe and Amagase, 2005).

2.6.6 Histopathological analysis

After their removal, half of each stomach should be fixated in 10% buffered formalin and embedded in paraffin. From each block, two 5μm sections should be made, one being stained by hematoxilin and eosin (HE) and the other by a modified Giemsa stain for H. pylori detection.

All tissues should be examined by a pathologist, according to criteria established by Dixon et al. (1996), and the following parameters should be analyzed:

- Inflammation - presence of lymphocytes and plasmocytes in the lamina propria;
- Activity – characterized by the presence of neutrophils inside the superficial and glandular epithelial layers;
- Regeneration - characterized by a proliferative response to epithelial lesion, in which epithelial cells presenting larger hyper-stained / excessively stained nuclei, with an increase in the nucleus-cytoplasm ratio, and observation of occasional mitotic figures;
- Atrophy – reduction of glandular structures;

- Metaplasia - presence of caliciform cells with an intestinal morphology.

2.6.7 Statistical analyses

Results for the parametric tests should be expressed as mean ± standard error of the mean (S.E.M.). Statistical significance should be determined by one-way analysis of variance (ANOVA), followed by Tukey-Kramer or Dunnett's post-test. For frequency comparisons, Fisher's exact test should be used, and p values <0.05 should be considered significant.

3. Some considerations

Gastrointestinal diseases are one of the most important causes of the previously high morbidity rates in non-industrialized countries, which have been lowered, in part, by the many drugs employed for treatment of peptic ulcers. However, such drugs may have several side effects, on top of their high financial cost for underprivileged populations (Borrelli and Izzo, 2000). Therefore, the use of medicinal plants and the development of phytotherapies, at a low cost, would represent an alternative for treatment of gastrointestinal problems for a large population segment that does not have access to medication (Sartori 1997). In Brazil, numerous plant extracts are used in conventional medicine to treat many digestive disorders (Falcão et al., 2008).

With respect to the *in vitro* assays, it is important to emphasize that the disk diffusion method is recommended for studying polar substances, given that it allows the evaluation of different compounds against a microorganism and, therefore, establishes its antibacterial spectrum. For non-polar extracts the employment of diffusion techniques seems inadequate, since they do not readily diffuse in agar. In the broth microdilution method, the compound to be tested is mixed into the proper liquid medium that had been previously inoculated with the microorganism, allowing determination as to whether the compound is bacteriostatic (minimum bacteriostatic concentration) or bactericidal (minimum bactericidal concentration - MBC). It presents a higher sensitivity to drugs than the disk diffusion method because it permits direct contact between the drug and the microorganism and is, therefore, appropriate for assays assessing either polar or nonpolar substances (Rios and Recio, 2005).

With respect to the *in vivo* assays, the establishment of a persistent infection by *H. pylori* in laboratory animals that completely reproduces the basic characteristics of human infections (an intense active chronic gastritis, either antral or diffuse), their complications (mucosa atrophy and intestinal metaplasia) and their associated pathologies (peptic ulcer, gastric adenocarcinoma and lymphoma) is not easy to accomplish. Chronic ulcer by acetic acid injection into the gastric subserosa area, differently from acute ulcers, penetrates the muscle layer of the glandular area and, occasionally, relapses after wound healing, and is highly similar to the human gastric ulcer in light of its pathological characteristics and healing process (Okabe and Pfeiffer, 1972).

Previous results indicate that Wistar rats with pre-existing gastric ulcers, experimentally produced by acetic acid injection, developed active ulcers when exposed to *H. pylori*, similar to the results of Konturek et al. (1999), which were obtained with a different species (Souza *et al*, 2009).

In order to evaluate the *in vivo* anti-*H. pylori* activity and to verify the presence of this bacteria in the gastric mucosa of ulcerated infected rats, the urease test and histopathological analysis should be carried out and monitored by the degree of cicatrisation of the gastric lesion.

The histopathological exam is considered one of the most specific tests for diagnosing *H. pylori* infections, presenting 98% sensitivity and 97% specificity (Lin et al., 1996; Ogata et al., 2002). The histopathological findings confirm the results found in the urease test, in which treatment of animals, ulcerated and inoculated with *H. pylori*. Moreover, parameters such as inflammation, ulcer persistency and neutrophilic activity, which are characteristics of *H. pylori* infection.

4. References

Borrelli, F., Izzo, A.A., 2000. The plant kingdom as a source of anti-ulcer remedies. Phytotherapy Research 14, 581-591.

Brown LM. *Helicobacter pylori*: Epidemiology and Routes of Transmission. *Epidemiologic Reviews* 2000; 22(2): 283-297.

Chao, J.C-J., Hung, H-C., Chen, S-H., Fang, C-L., 2004. Effects of Ginkgo biloba extract on cytoprotective factors in rats with duodenal ulcer. World Journal of Gastroenterology 10 (4), 560-566.

Coelho, L.G.V., 2003. Ulcera Péptica – Projeto Diretrizes. Associação Médica Brasileira e Conselho Federal de Medicina, Brasil.

Dixon, M.F., Genta, R.M., Yardley, J.H., Correa, P., 1996. Classification and grading of gastritis. The updated Sydney System. American Journal of Surgical Pathology, 20, 1161-1181.

Dunn BR, Cohen H, Blasé MJ. 1997. *Helicobacter pylori*. Clinical Microbiology Reviews; 10; 720-41.

El-Omar, E.M., 2004. The role of Interleukin-l beta in *Helicobacter pylori*-associated disease. The Netherlands Journal of Medicine 62 (3), 47-54.

Falcão, H.S., Mariath, I.R., Diniz, M.F.F.M., Batista, L.M., Barbosa-Filho, J.M., 2008. Plants of the American continent with antiulcer activity. Phytomedicine. 15, 132-146.

Goodwin CS and Armstrong JA. 1990. Microbiological aspects of Helicobacter pylori (Campylobacter pylori). European *Journal of Clinical Microbiology & Infections Diseases*; 9 (1): 1-13.

Kondo, S., Shinomura, Y., Kanayama, S., Kawabata, S., Miyazaki, Y., Imamura, I., Fukui, H, Matsuzawa, Y., 1994. Interleukin-I beta inhibits gastric histamine secretion and synthesis in the rat. American Journal of Physiology 267 (6), G966-71.

Konturek, P.C., Brzozowski, T., Konturek, S.J., Satchura, J., Karczewska, E., Pajdo, R., Ghiara, P., Hahn, E.G., 1999. Mouse model of *Helicobacter pylori* infection: studies of gastric function and ulcer healing. Alimentary Pharmacology & Therapeutics 13, 333-346.

Konturek SJ, Brzozowski T, Konturek PC, Kwiecien S, Karczewska E, Drozdowicz D, et al.. 2000. *Helicobacter pylori* infection delays healing of ischemia-reperfusion induced gastric ulcerations: new animal model for studying pathogenesis and therapy of H. pylori infection. *European Journal of Gastroenterology & Hepatology*; 12: 1299-1313.

Ladeira, M.S.P., Salvadori, D.M.F, Rodrigues, M.A.M., 2003. Biopatologia do *Helicobacter pylori*. Jornal Brasileiro de Patologia e Medicina Laboratorial, Rio de Janeiro, v. 39, n.4, 335 – 342.

Lin, S.Y., Jeng, Y.S., Wang, C.K., Ko, F.T., Lin, K.Y., Wang, C.S., Liu, J.D., Chen, P.H., Chang, J.G., 1996. Polymerase chain reaction diagnosis of *Helicobacter pylori* in gastroduodenal diseases: comparison with culture and histopathological examinations. Journal of Gastroenterology and Hepatology 11(3), 286-289.

Malone, M.H., 1977. Pharmacological approaches to natural products and evaluating. In: Wayner, H., Wolff, P. Jr. (Eds.), New Natural Products and Plant Drugs with Pharmacological, Biological or Therapeutically Activity. Springer, Berlim, pp. 23-56.

Marshall, B.J., Warren, J.R., 1984. Unidentified curve bacilli the stomach of patients with gastritis and peptic ulceration. Lancet 1(8390), 1311-1315.

Marshall BJ and Goodwin CS. 1987. Revised nomenclature of Campylobacter pyloridis. *International Journal of Systematic Bacteriology*; 37 (1): 68.

Ogata, S.K., Kawakami, E., Reis, F.P.S., 2002. Evaluation of invasive methods to diagnosis *Helicobacter pylori* infection in children and adolescents with dyspepsia invasive methods to diagnose *Hp* infection. Medicina, Ribeirão Preto 35, 24-29.

Okabe, S., Amagase, K., 2005. An Overview of Acetic Acid Ulcer Models – The History and State of Art of Peptic Ulcer Research. Biological & Pharmaceutial Bulletin. 28 (8), 1321-1341.

Okabe, S., Pfeiffer, C.J., 1972. Chronicity of acetic acid ulcer in the rat stomach. The American Journal of Digestive Diseases 14: 619-629.

Osaki, T., Mabe, K., Hanawa, T., Kamiya, S., 2008. Urease-positive bacteria in the stomach induce a false-positive reaction in a urea breath test for diagnosis of Helicobacter pylori infection. Journal of Medical Microbiology 57(Pt 7), 814-919

Rao, C.V., Saíram, K., Goel, R.K., 2000. Experimental evaluation of Bacopa monniera on rat gastric ulceration and secretion. Indian Journal of Physiology & Pharmacology 44, 335-441.

Rios, J.L., Recio, M.C., 2005. Medicinal plants and antimicrobial activity. Journal of Ethnopharmacology, 100, 80-84.

Ross JS, Bui HX, Rosario Ad, Sonbati H, George M, Lee CY. 1992. *Helicobacter pylori*: Its role in the pathogenesis of peptic ulcer disease in a new animal model. *American Journal of Pathology*; 141 (3): 721-727.

Sartori, N.T., Canepelle, D., Sousa, P.T., Martins, D.T.O., 1997. Gastroprotective effect from *Calophyllum brasiliense* Camb. Bark on experimental gastric lesions in rats and mice. Journal of Ethnopharmacology, 67, 149-156.

Shi, R., Xu, S., Zhang, H., Ding, Y., Sun, G., Huang. X., Chen ,X., Li, X., Yan, Z., Zhang, G., 2008. Prevalence and risk factors for *Helicobacter pylori* infection in Chenese Populations. Helicobacter 13, 157-165.

Souza MC, Beserra AM, Martins DC, Real VV, Santos RA, Rao VS,Silva RM, Martins DT, 2009. In vitro and in vivo anti-Helicobacter pylori activity of Calophyllum brasiliense Camb. Journal of Ethnopharmacology. 25;123(3):452-8.

Takagi, K., Okabe, S., Saziki, R., 1969. A new method for the production of chronic gastric ulcer in rats and the effect of several drugs on its healing. Japanese Journal of Pharmacology 19, 418-426.

Vaz, C. L. G. Zaterka, S. 2005. II Consenso Brasileiro sobre Helicobacter pylori. *Arquivos de Gastroenterologia*; 42(2): 128-132.

10

Anti-Ulcerative Potential of Some Fruits and the Extracts

Yasunori Hamauzu
Shinshu University
Japan

1. Introduction

Concern about the effects of various foods on human health has risen significantly in recent years. Plant-based foods, including fruit and vegetables, are regarded as important for human health. It is believed that plant-based diets have positive effects on health due to their phytochemical components. Plant extracts that contain various phytochemicals have been used in a numbers of studies to assess their biological effect on health, but the precise roles of phytochemicals in human health are still unclear in many cases.

There are many reports indicating that various plant extracts and related phytochemicals can act as ulcer preventing agents. Studies have shown that extracts of plants used in ayurvedic medicine (traditional medicine native to India) display a certain level of efficiency on gastric ulcer prevention in animals (Ajaikumar et al., 2005; Bhatnagar et al., 2005; Mishra et al., 2009). Moreover, extracts from vegetables, such as artichoke (*Cynara Scolymus*) leaf (Ishida et al., 2010), rocket or arugula (*Eruca sativa*) (Alqasoumi et al., 2009), Indian cluster bean 'Guar' (*Cyamopsis tetragonoloba*) (Rafatullah et al., 1994), cabbage (*Brassica oleracea*) (Akhtar & Munir, 1989) and basil (*Ocimum basilicum*) (Akhtar & Munir, 1989), also have been reported to have certain effect on gastric ulcer prevention in rats.

Studies on fruit extracts using experimental gastric ulcer in rodents, have revealed antiulcerative activity, for banana (*Musa* species) (Pannangpetch et al., 2001), pomegranate (*Punica granatum*) (Ajaikumar et al., 2005), dates (*Phoenix dactylifera*) (Al-Qarawi et al., 2005), cluster fig (*Ficus glomerata*) (Rao et al., 2008), prickly pear (*Opuntia ficus indica*) (Galati et al., 2003), Indian cherry (*Cordia dichotoma*) (Kuppast t al., 2009), dried papaya (*Carica Papaya*) (Rajkapoor et al., 2003) etc.

There are various experimental models for gastric ulcers such as ethanol-, aspirin-, indomethacin- or stress-induced gastric ulcers. We have used ethanol-induced gastric ulcer (or gastric mucosal injury) in rats to find effective extracts from underutilized fruits, including immature fruits. Among these underutilized fruits, we have found that Chinese quince (*Pseudocydonia sinensis* (Thouin) C. K. Schneider) extracts were the most effective against gastric mucosal injury. Extracts from European (normal) quince (*Cydonia oblonga* Miller) fruit also showed activity, but in our experiments, Chinese quince extracts were superior to the quince (cv. Smyrna) extracts on a same weight basis.

Chinese quince and quince fruits have been used in traditional medicines in Asian and western countries, respectively. Chinese quince is believed to be native of China (Zhejiang province) and is now widely planted in Japan, China, and Korea. As for quince, the primary area of natural growth seems to be the eastern Caucasus and Transcaucasus, and it is cultivated in all countries with worm-temperate to temperate climates (Khoshbakht and Hammer, 2006).

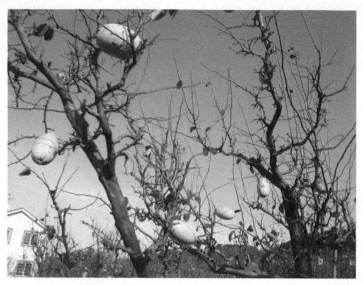

Fig. 1. Chinese quince (*Pseudocydonia sinensis* Schneid.) fruits on tree.

The Chinese quince fruit is inedible when raw because of its hard flesh, strong astringency, and high acidity. This characteristics are similar to those of the quince fruit, but Chinese quince has numerous stone cells that are larger than those in the quince fruit, making the flesh more unpleasant to eat. Therefore, these fruits, especially the Chinese quince fruit, are usually consumed as processed food products such as concentrated juice extracts, liquor, jam, jelly, glutinous starch syrup, crystallized fruit, and throat lozenges. The dried fruit has also been used in traditional medicine in the form of hot water extracts, for its antitussive and/or expectorant properties. Thus homemade medicines from Chinese quince fruit (including fruit liquor, decoction, syrup, and paste) have been said to have antitussive, expectorant, antispasmodic, and antidiuretic actions, and have been used for combating respiratory infections, intestinal dysregulation, and diuresis, and for treating people with a weak constitution. On the other hand, European quince fruits have been used as traditional medicines to treat cough (Kültür, 2007), constipation (Khoshbakht and Hammer, 2005) and also as stomach's comforter (Wilson, 1999).

In this chapter, studies on extracts of Chinese quince are presented and the efficacy of other fruit extracts and some of their chemical components on ulcer is also discussed.

2. Efficacy of fruit extracts and fruit products against HCl/ethanol induced mucosal injury in rats

2.1 Hot-water extracts from underutilized fruits and byproducts
2.1.1 Introduction

Attempts to find a use for underutilized fruits, including immature fruits picked through fruit thinning during fruit growth, have been made because those fruits have been known to be rich in various phytochemicals. Moreover, there is an interest in residue of fruits (or pomace), by-products in the food industry, because it has become a big problem of waste disposal. For these reasons, a research project to discover a use for under-utilized fruits and industrial by-products of fruit processing has been carried out. In this research project, over 30 plant materials including underutilized fruits and horticultural by-products were collected and hot-water extracts were made to assess their biological activities. We investigated the antiulcerative potential of hot-water extracts from selected plant materials using an HCl/ethanol-induced ulcer model in rats for screening purpose. In addition, some chemical components and free radical scavenging activity were also measured.

2.1.2 Materials and methods

Plant materials were collected at various places in the Nagano prefecture, Japan. Hot-water extracts were obtained by boiling each plant material in four times its volumes of water for 1 hour. The suspended solution was filtered using two layers of cheesecloth and a filter paper, concentrated, then lyophilized. For determination of antiulcerative activity, male Wistar rats were orally administered 2.5 ml of water (control) or sample suspention containing 200 mg of extracts 30 min before gastric ulcer induction. The gastric mucosal lesions that lead to acute gastric ulcer were induced by oral administration of 1.5 ml of 150 mM HCl/ethanol (40:60, v/v) solution (Mizui & Doteuchi, 1983). Animals were sacrificed under anesthesia 60 min after the HCl/ethanol administration. Stomachs were removed, opened along the greater curvature, rinsed with physiological saline solution and stretched on balsa boards. The degree of gastric mucosal damage was evaluated from digital pictures using a computerized image analysis system. Percentage of the total lesion area (hemorrhagic sites) to the total surface area of the stomach except the forestomach was defined as the ulcer index. For chemical component analysis in the hot-water extracts, total polyphenol and polyuronide contents were determined using Folin-Ciocalteu method (Singleton & Rossi, 1965) and 3,5-dimethylphenol assay (Schott, 1979), respectively. Proanthocyanidin content was determined using butanol-HCl assay. Free radical scavenging activity (RSA) was determined using the 1,1-diphenyl-2-picrylhydrazyl (DPPH) method (Brand-Williams et al., 1995).

2.1.3 Results and discussion

In our experiment, many fruit extracts tested displayed some level of efficacy against gastric mucosal injury (antiulcerative activity) induced by HCl/ethanol in rats (Fig. 2). Among the fruit extracts, Chinese quince fruit extracts showed the strongest activity on the same weight basis although quince fruit, immature apple and apple pomace extracts also had a significant activity. Lack of clear activity in liquor residues of Chinese quince fruit suggests that the active ingredients were eliminated by dissolution in the alcoholic solution. Because boiling-water can extract polyphenolic compounds and cell wall polysaccharides effectively, the fruit extracts contained these components at various concentrations (4.4–106 mg/gDW for total polyphenols; 7.9–46 mg/gDW for total polyuronides). Study of the relationship between ulcer index and the presence of chemical components or radical scavenging activity indicated that total polyphenol and proanthocyanidin content tended to have a negative relation to the ulcer intensity induced by HCl/ethanol. Meanwhile, polyuronide content and radical scavenging activity do not seem to bear any relation with the ulcer index. However, it has been reported that antioxidant capacity is related to prevention of gastric ulcer because oxygen radicals generated from neutrophils have an important role in formation of gastric lesions (Matsumoto et al., 1993). Our results indicate that not only radical scavenging activity, but also composition of antioxidants or other components were strongly related to the antiulcerative property of the fruit extracts. Hot-water extracts from Chinese quince fruit that were rich in procyanidins seemed to have a significant potential as an antiulcer agent. The effect of polyphenols and polysaccharides on experimental gastric ulcer is described later (in section 3). Additionally, it is not negligible that hot-water extracts from quince fruit or apple by-products also had moderate activity of ulcer prevention.

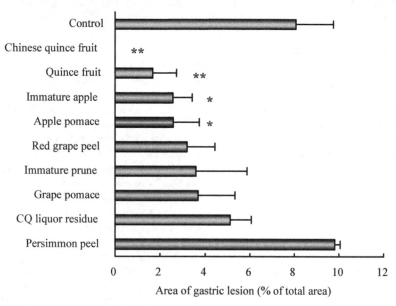

Fig. 2. Antiulcerative activity of hot (boiling)-water extracts from underutilized fruits or by-products. Rats were orally administered 2.5 ml of water (control) or a solution containing 200 mg of fruit extract 30 min before ulcer induction by 150 mM HCl/ethanol (40:60, v/v). Data are mean ± SE (n=7 for control; n=5 for Chinese quince and quince fruits group; n=3 for other study group). * $P< 0.05$; ** $P< 0.01$ vs control (Student-t test). CQ, Chinese quince.

2.2 Boiling-water extracts and jelly of Chinese quince fruits
2.2.1 Introduction
Chinese quince and quince fruit are normally consumed after being processed into jam, jelly, fruit paste (quince cheese), or fruit liquor. During processing, the fruits are often heated or boiled for extended periods of time. Moreover, quince juice and jelly have been traditionally used as folk medicine for treating stomach illness (Kloss, 1999; Wilson, 1999). Quince marmalade has been believed to help digestion, to comfort or strengthen the stomach (Wilson, 1999). Although it is unclear whether the antiulcerative properties of the fruits was part of the folk medicine knowledge, study of food function including the antiulcerative properties of boiling-water extracts of these fruits is interesting and meaningful. Therefore, we investigated the chemical characteristics and preventive efficacy of boiling-water extracts and jelly made from the Chinese quince and quince fruits on HCl/ethanol induced gastric lesions in rats.

2.2.2 Materials and methods

Commercial ripe fruits of the Chinese quince 'Kegai' and quince 'Smyrna' were obtained at a local orchard in the Nagano prefecture, Japan. For boiling water extraction, fruit were cut into small pieces, put into 3 times their volumes of boiling water, and boiled for up to 4 hr. An small volume of boiling water was added every hour to make up for evaporation. The boiled fruit extract was filtered using 2 layers of cheesecloth and gently squeezed, brought to a volume of 800 ml (from 200 g fruit) and stored in a freezer until use. Fruit jelly was made using the boiled fruit extract as follows: 200 mL of extract (from 50 g of fruit) was mixed with 50 g of superfine sugar and reduced by boiling for 50 min to make 70 g of jelly. The procedure to determine antiulcerative activity and chemical components was as described above.

2.2.3 Results and discussion

In the experiment with Chinese quince extracts, administration of 2.5 ml of fruit extracts obtained by boiling for 2 hr significantly prevented the gastric mucosal lesions induced by HCl/ethanol but extracts obtained by boiling for 1 hr did not show significant activity (Fig. 3). Because boiling for extended periods of time has the advantage of breaking cell wall polysaccharides and to extract chemical components from the fruit tissue, the extracts obtained by boiling for 2 hr had more phytochemicals such as antioxidants than that obtained by boiling for 1 hr. In fact, amount of polyphenols extracted from 100 g of the fruit tissue after 1 hr and 2 hr of boiling was 791 mg (62.3%) and 985 mg (77.6%), respectively. Likewise, the amount of pectic polysaccharides extracted from 100 g of tissue after boiling for 1 hr and 2 hr was 291 mg (34.6%) and 365 mg (43.5%), respectively. Therefore, prolonged heating (boiling) in processing of Chinese quince fruit may be beneficial from a viewpoint of antiulcerative activity in HCl/ethanol induced ulcer.

Because the boiling water extracts of Chinese quince and quince fruits are rich in pectic polysaccharides and organic acids, they can easily form gels by addition of sugar and brief heating. To determine whether the gelling products (fruit jelly) retain the antiulcerative activity, Chinese quince and quince jellies made from the extract obtained by boiling for 2 hr were used for the study. The administration of jelly made from extracts of either fruits strongly prevented the development of gastric lesions (Table 1). This indicates that the preventive effect was retained even after jelly manufacturing. The antiulcerative activity of Chinese quince jelly was stronger than that of quince jelly. This may be due to the difference of polyphenolic content and radical scavenging activity in the jellies. The actual polyphenolic composition is currently being analyzed, but procyanidins (the major component in Chinese quince and quince fruit) in the jellies may be an important factor.

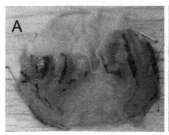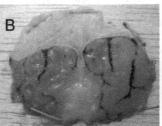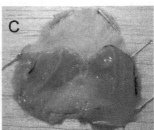

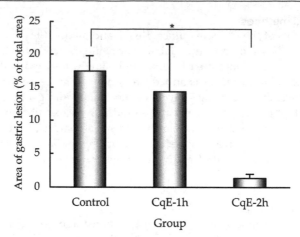

Fig. 3. Antiulcerative properties of boiling-water extracts of Chinese quince fruits on gastric legions induced by HCl/ethanol in rats. Photographs shows mucosal surface of rat stomach. Rats were administered 2.5 ml of water (A; control) or fruit extracts obtained by boiling for 1 h (B) and 2 h (C) then gastric ulcer was induced by administration of 1.5 ml of HCl/ethanol. Histogram shows percentage of area of gastric lesion to total surface area of stomach. Data are mean ± SE (n=19 for the controls; n=3 for each extract). * $P < 0.05$. CqE, Chinese quince extracts.

	Chinese quince	Quince
Reddish color (A458)	0.61 ± 0.02	0.56 ± 0.12
pH	2.9	3.2
Brix (%)	83 ± 3.3	79 ± 2.4
Viscosity (Pa·s)	66.2 ± 24	33.1 ± 11
Polyphenol content [a] (mg/100 g)	704 ± 18	166 ± 2.5
Polyuronide content [b] (mg/100 g)	33.3 ± 1.6	41.0 ± 0.8
Radical scavenging activity (EC_{50}[c])	132 ± 3.9	23.6 ± 9.1
Antiulcerative activity [d]		
Area of gastric legion [e]	0.04 ± 0.01	0.47 ± 0.22
Inhibition ratio (%)	99.5 ± 0.16	93.5 ± 3.1

[a] (-)-epicatechin equivalent (Folin-Ciocalteu assay).
[b] α-D-galacturonic acid equivalent (Dimethylphenolic assay).
[c] Expressed as the dilution factor needed to decrease the initial DPPH concentration by 50%.
[d] Rats (n = 5) were administered 2 ml of a diluted jelly solution (1 g jelly + 1 ml of water). Control rats (n = 19) were administered with water.
[e] Percentage of legion area in total surface area of stomach. The value for the control rats was 17.5 ± 2.3 (%).

Table 1. Characteristics of Chinese quince and quince fruit jellies made from the extracts obtained by boiling for 2 hours.

2.3 Juice extracts of Chinese quince and apple fruits
2.3.1 Introduction
There are some commercial juice extracts of Chinese quince fruit available, but the production is very limited in Japan. Unlike other fruits such as apple, it is difficult to separate the juice of Chinese quince fruit from the pulp after homogenization using a blender. This is because their large amounts of fiber absorb the juice such that almost no liquid remains. Therefore, merely squeezing the mealy homogenate is not an effective means of juice extraction; hence, large quantities of sugar are often added to create a sucrose osmotic gradient, and then the juice is extracted. Practically, the crushed fruit obtained using a hammer crusher is added to a quantity of sugar approximately equal to 80% of the fruit weight and macerated for about three months. The mushy pulp is then squeezed in a pressing machine to obtain the juice extracts that contain approximately 60% sugar. This is the simplest method to obtain juice extracts from Chinese quince fruit. Because boiling-water extracts of Chinese quince fruit have a strong antiulcerative potential, we tried to see the effect of the juice extracts of Chinese quince fruit on prevention of the gastric mucosal lesions. In addition, the effect of apple juice was also investigated a comparison.

2.3.2 Materials and methods
Chinese quince fruit extract (juice extracted by using osmotic pressure as described above) and apple juice (cloudy type) were purchased from a local market affiliated to a juice factory in Nagano prefecture, Japan. The Chinese quince extract contained 60% (w/w) of sugar and had a pH of 3.4. The apple juice was made from 'Fuji' apples and contained >12% Brix and 0.25% organic acid. Treatment of rats including the induction of gastric mucosal injury was as described above except that the volume of sample solution administered was 3 ml. In addition to measurement of lesion area, myeloperoxidase (MPO) activity of mucosa was also measured because this enzyme indicates amount of infiltrating leukocytes. For this experiment, a crude enzyme solution was prepared from homogenized mucosa randomly collected with a razor blade from the inner surface of the frozen stomach. MPO activity was measured spectrophotometrically using 3,5,3',5'-tetramethylbenzidine (TMB) and 0.3% H_2O_2 in acetate buffer (pH 5). Free radical scavenging activity of the extract and juice was measured using DPPH radical. Polyphenolic composition was analyzed using PDA-HPLC.

2.3.3 Results and discussion
The HCl/ethanol-induced gastric lesions were strongly suppressed in rats that were given Chinese quince extracts and apple juice but the effect was stronger in those given Chinese quince extract (Fig. 4). The intensity of the gastric lesions, as quantified by the percentage of the injury surface area, was 20% in control rats versus 0.002% and 2.1% in rats given Chinese quince extract and apple juice, respectively. MPO activity in gastric mucosa (22.3 U/mg protein in controls) also was suppressed significantly ($P < 0.05$) in rats given Chinese quince extract (10.5 U/mg protein), and the activity tended to be suppressed in rats given apple juice (11.6 U/mg protein) as well.

The free radical scavenging activity of Chinese quince extract, expressed as the volume (ml) that can scavenge 50% of DPPH, was 4 times stronger than that of apple juice (Table 2). From these results, it appeared that the preventative effect of Chinese quince extract or apple juice might be due to the radical scavenging capacity and the suppression of leukocyte

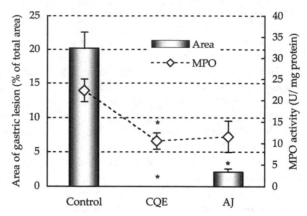

Fig. 4. Antiulcerative property of commercial Chinese quince extract and apple juice in rats.

Rats were administered 3 mL of water (control) or test solution (extract or juice) 30 min before gastric ulcer induction by HCl/ethanol. Vertical bars indicate SE (n=5). * $P < 0.05$ vs control. (from Hamauzu et al., 2008)

	Chinese quince extract	Apple juice
Free radical scavenging activity (EC_{50}) [a]	0.03 ± 0.001	0.12 ± 0.01
Soluble pectin (mg/100 mL) [b]	1.3 ± 0.07	4.9 ± 0.2
Total phenolics (mg/100 mL) [c]	342.2 ± 21.5	85.0 ± 6.4
Phenolic composition [d]		
(+)-Catechin	nd	0.57 ± 0.07
(–)-Epicatechin	3.7 ± 0.6	3.1 ± 0.09
Procyanidin B1 [e]	2.3 ± 0.2	1.3 ± 0.03
Procyanidin B2 [e]	7.3 ± 1.9	4.1 ± 0.07
Oligomeric procyanidins [e]	11.9 ± 3.2	tr
Polymeric procyanidins [e]	106.1 ± 38.8	nd
3-Caffeoylquinic acid [f]	4.9 ± 0.7	nd
5-Caffeoylquinic acid	5.5 ± 0.5	17.0 ± 0.2
Phloretin derivative [g]	nd	0.86 ± 0.01
Phlorizin	nd	0.70 ± 0.01

Data are mean ± SE. Abbreviations: nd, not detected; tr, trace.
[a] Values are volume (mL) of sample that can scavenge 50% of DPPH.
[b] Values are expressed as α-galacturonic acid equivalent.
[c] Values are expressed as (–)-epicatechin equivalent in Folin–Ciocalteu method.
[d] Values are results of HPLC analysis and expressed as mg/100 mL.
[e] Values were calculated using standard curve for (–)-epicatechin.
[f] Values were calculated using standard curve for 5-caffeoylquinic acid.
[g] Values were calculated using standard curve for phlorizin.

Table 2. Free radical scavenging activity, soluble pectin content, total phenolic content and phenolic composition of Chinese quince extract and apple juice (from Hamauzu et al., 2008)

migration to the gastric mucosa, which could be indicated by lowered activity of MPO, a marker enzyme of leukocytes. It has been thought that leukocytes migrate to the site of inflamed mucosa after injury by HCl/ethanol and subsequently expand the lesion area by producing reactive oxygen species, including free radicals (Osakabe et al., 1998). Therefore, suppression of leukocyte migration may be an important mechanism of action in the antiulcerative activity as well as radical scavenging capacity of the fruit extract and juice. There was a remarkable difference not only in polyphenolic content but also in the chemical composition of Chinese quince extract and apple juice (Table 2). The major polyphenols in Chinese quince extract were polymeric procyanidins, whereas predominant component in apple juice was 5-caffeoylquinic acid (chlorogenic acid). This difference might be the cause of the different strength of the two fruit extracts in terms of antiulcerative activity. Although apple juice had relatively weaker activity than Chinese quince extracts, the preventive effect of apple juice against HCl/ethanol-induced gastric lesions is also worth noting.

3. Effect of fruit components on the experimental gastric ulcer in rats

3.1 Polyphenolic compounds

Some polyphenolic compounds have been reported to have antiulcerative activity and are believed to be the main factor of the beneficial effects of medicinal plants in some cases. Extracted polyphenols or particular polyphenols belonging to the flavonoids family of compounds (such as quercetin, rutin, naringenin) (de Lira Mota et al., 2009), catechin and proanthocyanidins (Saito et al., 1998; Iwasaki et al., 2004) and phenolic acids (such as caffeic, ferulic, p-coumaric acids) (Barros et al., 2008) were reported to have certain efficacy in animal models. For example, Alarcón de la Lastra et al. (1994) reported that oral pretreatment with the highest dose of quercetin (200 mg/kg), 120 min before absolute ethanol administration, was most effective in necrosis prevention. Moreover, flavonoids such as quercetin, flavone and flavanone have been shown to inhibit growth of *Helicobacter pylori* in a dose-dependent manner *in vitro* (Beil et al., 1995). (+)-Catechin has been reported to protect gastric mucosa against ischaemia-reperfusion-induced gastric ulcers by its antioxidant activity and mucus protection (Rao et al., 2008). Proanthocyanidins (condenced tannins) are polymers of a variable number of flavan-3-ol (catechins) units. The most abundant of proanthocyanidins are procyanidins which are widely distributed in the plant kingdom. Saito et al. (1998) studied the antiulcer capacity of pure procyanidin oligomers and showed that the antiulcer activity of a series of procyanidins increased as the degree of polymerization of the catechin unit increased. Oligomers longer than three catechin units showed a strong protective effect against stomach mucosal injury. In our research, we have shown that administration of highly polymerized procyanidins isolated from pear fruit (cv. Winter Nélis) with 60%(v/v) acetone after washing with 80%(v/v) methanol strongly suppressed the induction of gastric mucosal lesion (Hamauzu et al., 2007). The preventative effect of these molecules was clearly in histological sections (Fig. 5).

Moreover, semi-purified Chinese quince polyphenols that mainly consist of polymeric procyanidins also showed strong antiulcerative activity in a dose-dependent manner (Fig. 6). The effect was observed in the ulcer index (area of gastric lesion) and myeloperoxidase activity. Apple polyphenols also showed antiulcerative activity but it was not dose-dependent. This may be due to the presence of chlorogenic acid, the predominant component in apple polyphenols (see below).

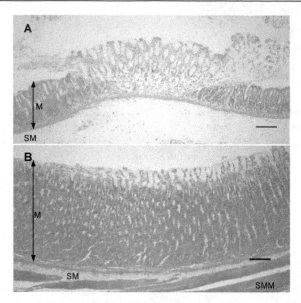

Fig. 5. Histological section analysis of rat gastric mucosa after treatment of HCl/ethanol. (A) Water was administered before induction of gastric mucosal lesions by HCl/ethanol. (B) Pear procyanidins, in an aqueous solution, were administered before induction of the lesion. M, mucosal layer; SM, submucosal layer; SMM, smooth muscle layer. Bar: 100 μm.

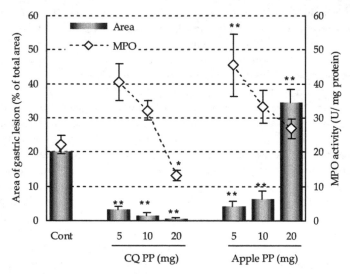

Fig. 6. Intensity of gastric lesions and mucosa myeloperoxidase activity (MPO) in rats that were administered 1.5 ml of water (control) or a solution of semi-purified Chinese quince polyphenols (CQ PP) or apple polyphenols (Apple PP) before treatment with HCl/ethanol. Bars indicate SE (n=15 for control group; n=5 for CQ PP and Apple PP group). * $P < 0.05$; ** $P < 0.01$ vs control.

The efficacy of procyanidins that have a high mDP may be due to both radical scavenging activity and affinity to the gastric mucosa. Procyanidins have affinity to protein (because they are a kind of tannin) and the affinity is known to depend in their degree of polymerization. Saito et al. (1998) reported that procyanidins such as pentamers and hexamers strongly bound to BSA. The highly polymerized procyanidins isolated from 'Winter Nélis' pear had a very high value of mean degree of polymerization (mDP = 89). Moreover, the mDP of procyanidins contained in semi-purified polyphenols from Chinese quince fruit was approximately 19, whereas that in apple polyphenols was 3-4. Their affinity to protein was actually affected by the mDP (Fig. 7 upper panel). Because of their high affinity to protein, fruit procyanidins having high mDP may have potential to bind to the mucosa. Additionally, radical scavenging activity of semi-purified Chinese quince polyphenols was stronger than that of apple polyphenols (Fig. 7 lower panel). Therefore, Chinese quince polyphenols may be superior to apple polyphenols in gastric protection because of the radical scavenging activity and its continuance on the gastric mucosa.

Thus, the mechanism of protection of the mucosa by fruit procyanidins may be both physical and chemical. By binding strongly to the mucosa, procyanidins build a protective layer against ethanol, reducing leukocyte migration, and then deploying a local antioxidant protection against free radicals. The real chemical pathway for activation and migration of leukocytes is not well understood, and it is difficult to say at which level procyanidins prevent this migration.

In our research, we have observed that chlorogenic acid-rich phenolic extract or chlorogenic acid standard showed a negative effect on prevention of gastric lesions when it was administered in excess dose.

Chlorogenic acid (5-caffeoylquinic acid) is a phenolic compound and is widely distributed in plant kingdom. It is observed in coffee beverage, blueberries, apples and ciders (Clifford, 1999). Coffee beans are one of the richest dietary sources of chlorogenic acid and for many consumers must be the major dietary source for this molecule. Chlorogenic acid has been reported to have a series of biological effects in vitro and in vivo, such as antioxidant capacity, radical scavenging activity, antimutagenic/anticarcinogenic effect, inflammation inhibiting and endothelial protective properties, etc. (Chang & Li, 2005), and thought that the compound might contribute to body health promotion to some extent. Zhao et al. (2008) has reported that chlorogenic acid has the down-regulative effects on the H_2O_2- or TNF-α-induced secretion of interleukin (IL)-8, a central pro-inflammatory chemokine involved in the pathogenesis of inflammatory bowel diseases, in human intestinal Caco-2 cells. In relation to the gastric ulcer prevention, Graziani et al. (2005) reported that chlorogenic acid was equally effective as apple extracts in preventing oxidative injury to gastric cells.

However, in some cases, chlorogenic acid seems to be ineffective in preventing gastric ulcers in animal models. Ishida et al. (2010) reported that oral administration of chlorogenic acid (4 mg/kg or 16 mg/kg, respectively) was ineffective to prevent absolute ethanol-induced or restraint plus water immersion stress-induced gastric ulcer in male Sprague-Dawley strain rats.

In our experiment, administration of a high dose (20 mg/rat; approx. 80 mg/kg b.w.) of chlorogenic acid tended to enhance the gastric lesion induced by HCl/EtOH in male Wistar rats. We also observed that a high dose (20 mg/rat) of semi-purified apple polyphenols (rich in chlorogenic acid) enhanced the ethanol-induced gastric lesions in rats. These findings suggest that chlorogenic acid has potential to increase some factors that progress gastric lesions in ethanol-induced ulcer model when it administered at high dose. The actual mechanism is unclear, but chlorogenic acid seems to stimulate gastric acid secretion. It has been reported that chlorogenic acid affects the expression of gastric acid secretion-related proteins in human gastric cancer cell (Rubach et al., 2008). The excessive secretion of hydrochloric acid, the main constituent of gastric acid, in the stomach is considered an important factor in the formation of peptic ulcer (Welgan, 1974).

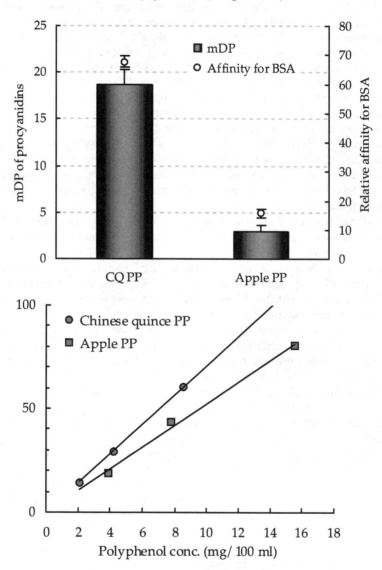

Fig. 7. Mean degree of polymerization (mDP) of procyanidins, relative affinity for bovine serum albumin and free radical scavenging activity of semi-purified Chinese quince polyphenols (CQ PP) and apple polyphenols (Apple PP).

Although high dose of chlorogenic acid or apple polyphenols have the potential to promote gastric mucosal lesions, normal consumption of apple polyphenol has been shown to prevent gastric ulcer in rats (Graziani et al., 2005). We also have confirmed that administration of cloudy apple juice suppressed gastric mucosal lesions induced by HCl/ethanol (section 2.3). Therefore, it should be emphasized that the natural concentration of phenolics in both apple fruit and juice may not cause any deteriorating effect on HCl/ethanol-induced gastric lesions and, in fact, may have some health benefit. This may indicate that excessively purified compounds may have adverse effects on health under particular conditions, even though they are known as health-promoting components.

3.2 Dietary fiber

Fruits contain high amount of soluble- and insoluble-fiber components. Soluble-fiber, such as pectic polysaccharides (pectin), might be an effective ingredient in gastric ulcer prevention because some soluble polysaccharides or mucilage were reported to have antiulcerative activity. For example, a galactomannoglucan with an estimated weight–average molar mass of 415,000 g/mol, obtained from an aqueous extract of the mesocarp of fruits of catolé palm (*Syagrus oleracea*), significantly inhibited gastric lesions induced by ethanol in mice, showing a gastroprotective property (da Silva & Parente, 2010). Lemnan, a pectic polysaccharide of duckweed *Lemna minor*, was also reported to be a potent gastroprotective agent for chemical and emotional stress models in animals (Khasina et al., 2003); it enhanced resistance of the stomach tissue to various ulcerogenic factors (emotional stress, indomethacin, pesticide 2,4-D).

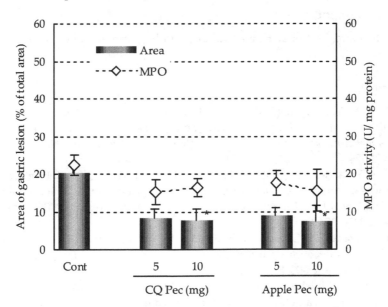

Fig. 8. Intensity of gastric lesions and myeloperoxidase (MPO) activity of mucosa of rats that were administered water (control), soluble pectin from Chinese quince fruit (CQ Pec) or commercial apple pectin (Apple Pec) before treatment with 150 mM HCl/ethanol (40:60, v/v). * $P < 0.05$ vs control.

In our research, soluble pectin extracted from Chinese quince fruit and commercial apple pectin both showed antiulcerative activity (Fig. 8). However, the effect seemed weaker than that of extracted polyphenols, especially in case of Chinese quince fruit. Therefore, pectic polysaccharides may partly contribute to antiulcerogenic activity together with polyphenols.

4. Conclusions

Many fruits, especially medicinal fruits, have been reported to have antiulcerative activity in animal experiment. Chinese quince fruit extract show strong activity for the prevention of gastric mucosal lesions induced by HCl/ethanol in rats. The effect is probably due to a high content of procyanidins that exhibit antioxidant activity and affinity to proteins. The preventative effect of fruit extracts on gastric mucosal lesions is retained even after prolonged heating (as observed in the effect of fruit jelly). Moreover, pectin, a cell wall polysaccharide, may enhance the effect of polyphenols on the prevention of gastric lesions. Meanwhile, some other fruit products such as apple juice and hot-water extract of quince also have a significant effect. However, a high dose of chlorogenic acid may promote the ethanol-induced gastric lesions. This indicates that excess intake of purified compounds should be avoided even if it is a natural antioxidant. Future research to elucidate the mechanisms of action of fruit polyphenols that prevent or increase the gastric lesions that lead to ulcer will be needed.

5. Acknowledgment

The author thank to Dr. Kohzy Hiramatsu for providing histological data and the technical support.

6. References

Akhtar, M. S. & Munir, M. (1989). Evaluation of the gastric antiulcerogenic effects of *Solanum nigrum*, *Brassica oleracea* and *Ocimum basilicum* in rats. *Journal of Ethnopharmacology*, Vol. 27, No. 1-2 (November 1989), pp. 163–176, ISSN: ISSN 0378-8741

Ajaikumar, K.B.; Asheef, M.; Babu, B.H. & Padikkala, J. (2005). The inhibition of gastric mucosal injury by *Punica granatum* L. (pomegranate) methanolic extract. *Journal of Ethnopharmacology*, Vol. 96, No. 1-2 (January 2005), pp. 171–176, ISSN 0378-8741

Alarcón de la Lastra, C.; Martin, M. J. & Motilva, V. (1994). Antiulcer and gastroprotective effects of quercetin: a gross and histologic study. *Pharmacology*, Vol. 48, No. 1, pp. 56-62, ISSN 1423-0313

Al-Qarawi, A.A.; Abdel-Rahman, H.; Ali, B.H.; Mousa, H.M. & El-Mougy, S.A. (2005). The ameliorative effect of dates (*Phoenix dactylifera* L.) on ethanol-induced gastric ulcer in rats. *Journal of Ethnopharmacology*, Vol. 98, No. 3 (April 2005), pp. 313–317, ISSN 0378-8741

Alqasoumi, S.; Al-Sohaibani, M.; Al-Howiriny, T.; Al-Yahya, M. & Rafatullah, S. (2009). Rocket "*Eruca sativa*": A salad herb with potential gastric anti-ulcer activity. *World Journal of Gastroenterology*, Vol. 15, No. 16 (April 2009), pp. 1958–1965, ISSN 1007-9327

Barros, M.P.; Lemos, M.; Maistro, EL.; Leite, M.F.; Sousa, J.P.; Bastos, J.K. & Andrade, S.F. (2008). Evaluation of antiulcer activity of the main phenolic acids found in Brazilian Green Propolis. *Journal of Ethnopharmacology*, Vol. 120, No. 3 (December 2008), pp. 372–377, ISSN 0378-8741

Beil, W.; Birkholz, C. & Sewing, K.F. (1995). Effects of flavonoids on parietal cell acid secretion, gastric mucosal prostaglandin production and *Helicobacter pylori* growth. *Arzneimittelforschung*, Vol. 45, No. 6 (June 1995), pp. 697–700, ISSN 0004-4172

Bhatnagar, M.; Sisodia, S.S. & Bhatnagar, R. (2005). Antiulcer and antioxidant activity of *Asparagus racemosus* Willd and *Withania somnifera* Dunal in rats. *Annals of the New York Academy of Sciences*, Vol. 1056, No. 1 (January 2005), pp. 261–278, ISSN 0077-8923 (Print); 1749-6632 (Online)

Brand-Williams, W.; Cuvelier, M.E. & Berset, C. (1995). Use of a free radical method to evaluate antioxidant activity. *Lebensmittel-Wissenschaft und-Technologie*, Vol. 28, No. 1 (1995), pp. 25-30, ISSN 0023-6438

Chang, C.Q. & Li, S.Y. (2005). Biological effects of chlorogenic acid and body health (Article in Chinese). *Wei Sheng Yan Jiu / Journal of Hygiene Research*, Vol. 34, No.6 (November 2005), pp. 762–764, ISSN 1000-8020

Clifford, M. N. (1999). Chlorogenic acids and other cinnamates – nature, occurrence and dietary burden. *Journal of the Science of Food and Agriculture*, Vol. 79, No. 3 (May 1999), pp. 362–372, ISSN 1097-0010 (Online)

da Silva, B.P. & Parente, J.P. (2010). Chemical properties and antiulcerogenic activity of a galactomannoglucan from *Syagrus oleracea*. *Food Chemistry*, Vol. 123, No. 4 (December 2010), pp. 1076–1080, ISSN 0308-8146

de Lira Mota, K.S.; Dias, G.E.N.; Pinto, M.E.F.; Luiz-Ferreira, Â.; Souza-Brito, A.R.M.; Hiruma-Lima, C.A.; Barbosa-Filho, J.M. & Batista, L.M. (2009). Flavonoids with gastroprotective activity. *Molecules*, Vol. 14, No. 3 (March 2009) pp. 979-1012, ISSN 1420-3049

Galati, E.M.; Mondello, M.R.; Giuffrida, D.; Dugo, G.; Miceli, N.; Pergolizzi, S. & Taviano, M.F. (2003). Chemical characterization and biological effects of Sicilian *Opuntia ficus indica* (L.) Mill. Fruit juice: antioxidant and antiulcerogenic activity. *Journal of Agricultural and Food Chemistry*, Vol. 51, No. 17 (August 2003), pp. 4903–4908, ISSN 0021-8561 (Print); 1520-5118 (Online)

Graziani, G.; D'Argenio, G.; Tuccillo, C.; Loguercio, C.; Ritieni, A.; Morisco, F.; Del Vecchio Blanco, C.; Fogliano, V. & Romano, M. (2005). Apple polyphenol extracts prevent damage to human gastric epithelial cells in vitro and to rat gastric mucosa in vivo. *Gut*, Vol. 54, No. 2 (February 2005), pp. 193–200, ISSN 0017-5749

Hamauzu, Y.; Irie, M.; Kondo, M. & Fujita, T. (2008). Antiulcerative properties of crude polyphenols and juice of apple, and Chinese quince extracts. *Food Chemistry*, Vol. 108, No. 2 (May 2008), pp. 488–495, ISSN 0308-8146

Hamauzu, Y.; Forest, F.; Hiramatsu, K. & Sugimoto, M. (2007). Effect of pear (*Pyrus communis* L.) procyanidins on gastric lesions induced by HCl/ethanol in rats. *Food Chemistry*, Vol. 100, No. 1, pp. 255-263, ISSN 0308-8146

Ishida, K.; Kojima, R.; Tsuboi, M.; Tsuda, Y. & Ito, M. (2010). Effects of artichoke leaf extract on acute gastric mucosal injury in rats. *Biological & Pharmaceutical Bulletin*, Vol. 33, No. 2 (February 2010) pp. 223–229, ISSN 0918-6158 (Print) 1347-5215 (Online)

Iwasaki, Y.; Matsui, T. & Arakawa, Y. (2004). The protective and hormonal effects of proanthocyanidin against gastric mucosal injury in Wistar rats. *Journal of Gastroenterology*, Vol. 39, No. 9 (October 2004), pp. 831–837, ISSN 0944-1174 (Print) 1435-5922 (Online)

Khasina, E.I.; Sgrebneva, M.N.; Ovodova, R.G.; Golovchenko, V.V. & Ovodov, Y.S. (2003). Gastroprotective effect of lemnan, a pectic polysaccharide from *Lemna minor* L. *Doklady Biological Sciences*, Vol. 390, No. 3 (May-June 2003), pp. 204–206, ISSN 0012-4966 (Print); 1608-3105 (Online)

Khoshbakht, K. & Hammer, K. (2006). Savadkouh (Iran) – an evolutionary centre for fruit trees and shrubs. *Genetic Resources and Crop Evolution*, Vol. 53, No. 3 (May 2006), pp. 641–651, ISSN 0925-9864 (Print); 1573-5109 Online)

Kloss, J. (1999). *Back to Eden*, Back to Eden Books, ISBN 0-940985-10-1, Twin Lakes, Wisconsin, USA

Kültür, Ş. (2007). Medicinal plants used in Kırklareli Province (Turkey). *Journal of Ethnopharmacology*, Vol. 111, No. 2 (May 2007) pp. 341–364, ISSN: 0378-8741

Kuppast, I.J.; Vasudeva Nayak, P.; Chandra Prakash, K. & Satsh Kumar, K.V. (2009). Anti-ulcer effect of Cordia dichotoma Forst .f. fruits against gastric ulcers in rats. *The Internet Journal of Pharmacology*, Vol. 1, No. 7, ISSN 1531-2976, Available from: http://www.ispub.com/journal/the_internet_journal_of_pharmacology/volum e_7_number_1_27/article_printable/anti-ulcer-effect-of-cordia-dichotoma-forst-f-fruits-against-gastric-ulcers-in-rats.html

Matsumoto, T.; Moriguchi, R. & Yamada, H. (1993). Role of polymorphonuclear leukocytes and oxygen-derived free radicals in the formation of gastric lesions induced by HCl/ethanol, and a possible mechanism of protection by anti-ulcer polysaccharide. *Journal of Pharmacy and Pharmacology*, Vol. 45, No. 6 (June 1993), pp. 535–539, ISSN 0022-3573

Mishra, A.; Arora, S.; Gupta, R.; Manvi; Punia, R.K. & Sharma, A. K. (2009). Effect of *Feronia elephantum* (Corr) fruit pulp extract on indomethacin-induced gastric ulcerin albino rats. *Tropical Journal of Pharmaceutical Research*, Vol. 8, No. 6 (December 2009), pp. 509–514, ISSN 1596-5996 (print); 1596-9827 (electronic)

Mizui, T. & Doteuchi, M. (1983). Effect of polyamines on acidified ethanol-induced gastric lesions in rats, *Japanese Journal of Pharmacology*, Vol. 33, No. 5, pp. 939–945, ISSN 0021-5198 (Print); 1347-3506 (Online)

Osakabe, N.; Sanbongi, C.; Yamagishi, M.; Takizawa, T. & Osawa, T. (1998). Effects of polyphenol substances derived from *Theobroma cacao* on gastric mucosal lesion induced by ethanol. *Bioscience, Biotechnology and Biochemistry*, Vol. 62, No. 8 (August 1998), pp. 1535–1538, ISSN 0916-8451 (Print); 1347-6947 (Online)

Pannangpetch, P.; Vuttivirojana, A.; Kularbkaew, C.; Tesana, S.; Kongyingyoes, B. & Kukongviriyapan, V. (2001). The antiulcerative effect of Thai *Musa* species in rats. *Phytotherapy research*, Vol. 15, No. 5 (June 2001), pp. 407–410, ISSN: 1099-1573 (Online)

Rafatullah, S.; Al-Yahya, M.A.; Al-Said, M.S.; Abdul Hameed Taragan, K.U. & Mossa, J. S. (1994). Gastric anti-ulcer and cytoprotective effects of *Cyamopsis tetragonoloba* ('Guar') in rats. *International Journal of Pharmacognosy*, Vol. 32, No. 2, pp. 163–170, ISSN 0925-1618

Rajkapoor, B.; Jayakar, B.; Anandan, R. & Murugesh, N. (2003). Antiulcer effect of dried fruits of *Carica papaya* Linn in rats. *Indian Journal of Pharmaceutical Sciences*, Vol. 65, No. 6, pp. 638–639, ISSN 0250-474X (Print); 1998-3743 (Online)

Rao, C.V.; Verma, A.R.; Vijayakumar, M. & Rastogi, S. (2008). Gastroprotective effect of standardized extract of *Ficus glomerata* fruit on experimental gastric ulcers in rats. *Journal of Ethnopharmacology*, Vol. 115, No. 2 (January 2008), pp. 323–326, ISSN 0378-8741

Rubach, M.; Lang, R.; Hofmann, T. & Somoza, V. (2008). Time-dependent component-specific regulation of gastric acid secretion-related proteins by roasted coffee constituents. *Annals of the New York Academy of Sciences*, Vol. 1126, No. 1 (April 2008), pp. 310–314, ISSN 1749-6632 (Online)

Saito, M.; Hosoyama, H.; Ariga, T.; Kataoka, S. & Yamaji, N. (1998). Antiulcer activity of grape seed extract and procyanidins. *Journal of Agricultural and Food Chemistry*, Vol. 46, No. 4 (April 1998), pp. 1460–1464, ISSN 0021-8561 (Print); 1520-5118 (Online)

Scott, R.W. (1979). Colorimetric determination of hexuronic acids in plant materials. *Analytical Chemistry*, Vol. 51, No. 7 (June 1979), pp.936–941, ISSN 0003-2700 (Print); 1520-6882 (Online)

Singleton, V.L. & Rossi, J. (1965). Colorimetry of total phenolics with phosphomolybdic-phosphotungstic acid reagents. *American Journal of Enology and Viticulture*, Vol. 16, No. 3 (September 1965), pp. 144–158, ISSN 002-9254 (Print)

Welgan, P.R. (1974). Learned control of gastric acid secretions in ulcer patients. *Psychosomatic Medicine*, Vol. 36, No.5 (September-October 1974), pp. 411–419, ISSN 0033-3174 (Print); 1534-7796 (Online)

Wilson, C.A. (1999). *The Book of Marmalade*. (Revised Edition), University of Pennsylvania Press, ISBN 0-8122-1727-6, Philadelphia, Pennsylvania, USA

Zhao, Z.; Shin, H.S.; Satsu, H.; Totsuka, M. & Shimizu, M. (2008). 5-Caffeoylquinic acid
    and caffeic acid down-regulate the oxidative stress- and TNF-α-induced secretion
    of interleukin (IL)-8 from Caco-2 cells. *Journal of Agricultural and
    Food Chemistry*, Vol. 56, No. 10 (May 2008), pp. 3863–3868, ISSN 0021-8561 (Print);
    1520-5118 (Online)

11

Prevention of Gastric Ulcers

Mohamed Morsy and Azza El-Sheikh
Pharmacology Department, Minia University
Egypt

1. Introduction

Upper gastrointestinal tract integrity is dependent upon the delicate balance between naturally occurring protective factors as mucus or prostaglandins and damaging factors as hydrochloric acid present normally in the digestive juices. An imbalance causes peptic ulcer formation and destruction of gastrointestinal tract mucosal lining. Ulcer may develop in the esophagus, stomach, duodenum or other areas of elementary canal. In women, gastric ulcers are more common than duodenal ulcers, while in men the opposite is true.

The ulcer irritates surrounding nerves and causes a considerable amount of pain. Obstruction of the gastrointestinal tract may occur as a result of spasm or edema in the affected area. The ulcer may also cause the erosion of major blood vessels leading to hemorrhage, hematemesis and/or melena. Deep erosion of the wall of the stomach or the intestine may cause perforation and peritonitis, which is a life-threatening condition needing emergency intervention. Duodenal ulcers are almost always benign but stomach ulcers may turn malignant. Although mortality rates of peptic ulcer are low, the high prevalence of the disease, the accompanying pain and its complications are very costly.

The ongoing rapidly expanding research in this field provides evidence suggesting that, with therapeutic and dietetic advances, gastric ulcer may become preventable within the next decade. This could be achieved by strengthening the defense mechanisms of the gastric mucosa and, in parallel, limiting the aggression of predisposing factors causing gastric ulceration. The defenses of the gastric mucosa are incredibly efficient under normal mechanical, thermal or chemical conditions. These defenses can endure insults from food, gastric enzymes and acid secretion. Even trauma caused by a biopsy wound is dealt with and can heal relatively fast, within hours.

However, under certain condition, some risk factors may contribute to mucosal injury and initiation of gastric ulcer, as psychological stress, increased hydrochloric acid secretion, Zollinger Ellison syndrome and family history of gastric ulcer. Conditions associated with increased risk of gastric ulcer include also chronic disorders as liver cirrhosis, chronic obstructive pulmonary disease, renal failure, organ transplantation and rheumatoid arthritis. In addition, severe physical stress as in case of burns, major surgery or head trauma may also contribute as risk factors.

Avoidable risk factors that may predispose to gastric ulcer include smoking, high consumption of alcohol and intake of some medications as non-steroidal anti-inflammatory drugs. Some factors are thought to aggravate already established gastric ulcer, but are no longer considered risk factors predisposing to it, as ingestion of too hot or cold foods or drinks, eating spicy food and intake of caffeine. The key cause of gastric ulcer is now known to be the infection by a certain gram negative bacterium called Helicobacter pylori. Although the mechanism by which the infection by this bacterium leads to ulcer formation is not yet fully understood, it is believed that infection decreases the normal immunity of the gastrointestinal tract wall, which in turn weakens the mucosa and makes it vulnerable to ulceration under the acidic effect of gastric secretions.

Avoiding risk factors is the first line in prevention of gastric ulcer. Smoking cessation and alcoholic consumption minimization may help in reducing the risk of ulcer formation. In addition, sanitary food and drinking habits to avoid infection with Helicobacter pylori may help in ameliorating the initiation of gastric ulcer and its recurrence. Therapeutic interventions to eradicate Helicobacter pylori can also prevent ulcer formation and its transformation into gastric cancer, one of the major complications of chronic gastric ulcer. Avoiding unnecessary intake of ulcer-inducing over-the-counter medications may help in reducing the prevalence of gastric ulcers.

Active therapeutic measures can aid in preventing gastric ulcers in predisposed groups and in patients with healed gastric ulcer to avoid its recurrence. Such therapeutic interventions may be of natural herbal sources or medicinal drugs. A number of traditional anti-ulcer drugs may be used in prevention as well as in treatment of gastric ulcer. Proton pump inhibitors, histamine H_2 receptor antagonists and mucosal protective agents can thus all be used as protective drugs against initiation of gastric ulcer in predisposed groups as well as prevention of remittent attacks. Recent investigations showed that a number of drugs, other than traditional anti-ulcer medications, can help in prevention of gastric ulcer formation. Herbal compounds can also protect against gastric ulcer and they have the advantage of being safer, cheaper and usually having limited, if any, side effects.

In this chapter, a collection of updated recent information published about gastric ulcer protection is gathered. Information in this chapter can be considered as guidelines for clinical practice to direct medical personnel perception to preferred approaches to prevent gastric ulcer as established by scientifically valid research. Making such information available may also increase public awareness of preventive means of gastric ulcer, which may aid in decreasing the suffering of a large number of populations exposed to the disease worldwide.

2. Avoidance of gastric ulcer risk factors

The best and cheapest method to prevent gastric ulceration is the avoidance of risk factors resulting in the occurrence of the disease. Avoiding Helicobacter pylori infection, alternation of life style and substitution of ulcer-inducing medications with less harmful drugs can thus contribute largely to prevent gastric ulcer disease (Fig. 1). Unfortunately, some risk factors are unavoidable. One of the strongest risk factors for initiation of a gastric ulcer is the presence of prior ulcer disease with history of ulcer complications as previous perforation or hemorrhage.

Zollinger-Ellison Syndrome is another unavoidable cause of gastric ulceration. In this syndrome, tumors producing gastrin hormone (gastrinomas) in the pancreas and duodenum stimulate gastric acid secretion. The large amounts of excess acid produced cause gastro-intestinal ulceration. Ulcers may form in the stomach, duodenum, jejunum or other atypical sites in the elementary tract. The incidence of this disease is less than 1% and men are more affected than women. The syndrome is suspected in patients with ulcers who are not infected with Helicobacter pylori and who have no history of non-steroidal anti-inflammatory drugs use. Diagnosis is confirmed by measurement of serum gastrin hormone

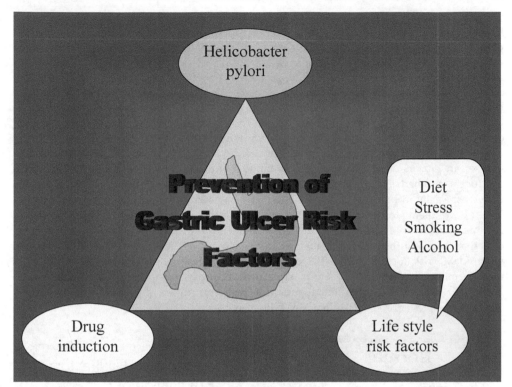

Fig. 1. Methods of prevention of gastric ulcer: Avoiding risk factors as Helicobacter pylori, drug-induced ulcer by medications as non-steroidal anti-inflammatory drugs and performance of life style changes.

levels which is usually very high, reaching above 1000 pg/ml (normal level is < 100 pg/ml). Diarrhea may occur before ulcer symptoms. Gastro-esophageal reflux disease may occur and its complications may include narrowing due to strictures of the esophagus. Ulcers associated with this syndrome are usually persistent and difficult to treat. In the past, removing the stomach was the only option for treatment. Nowadays, treatment includes removing the tumors only and therapeutic suppression of acid secretion.

Other unavoidable factors associated with higher incidence of gastric ulcer include sex, as there is higher prevalence of the disease among women then men. People over age 60 years old are also more prone to gastric ulcer disease. In addition, ethnic backgrounds as African-Americans or Hispanics have 2-fold higher risk in developing gastric ulcer. Furthermore, patients suffering from other diseases as congestive heart failure have higher incidence of having gastric ulcer as well. Type O blood group has also been associated with increased incidence of the disease. Genetics is another unavoidable risk factor of gastric ulcer. Pepsinogen C gene polymorphism, for example, is significantly associated with development of gastric ulcer (Sun et al., 2009). Other relatively rarer predisposing factors to development of gastric ulcer includes Crohn's disease of the stomach, eosinophilic gastritis, systemic mastocytosis, radiation damage and viral infections by cytomegalovirus or herpes simplex (Malfertheiner et al., 2009).

2.1 Helicobacter pylori as a risk factor for gastric ulcer

Infection with Helicobacter pylori is the most well-defined risk factor for the development of peptic ulcers. The two Australian scientists who identified Helicobacter pylori as the main cause of stomach ulcers in 1982 were awarded the Nobel Prize in Medicine in 2005 for this discovery. Helicobacter pylori bacteria are found in about 50% of people with gastric ulcer disease. Inflammation of the stomach and stomach ulcers result from the infection by these bacteria, as their corkscrew shape enables them to penetrate the mucus layer of the stomach so that they can attach themselves to the lining. The surfaces of the cells lining the stomach contain a protein, called decay-accelerating factor, which acts as a receptor for the bacterium.

Helicobacter pylori can survive in the highly acidic medium of the stomach by producing urease, an enzyme that generates ammonia to neutralize the acid. These bacteria then produce a number of toxins causing inflammation and damage to the stomach, leading to ulcers especially in predisposed individuals. The bacteria also alter certain immune factors that allow them to evade detection by the immune system and cause persistent inflammation. Even if ulcers do not develop, the bacterium is considered to be a major cause of active chronic inflammation in the stomach (gastritis). Helicobacter pylori together with unavoidable risk factors as genetics and concomitant diseases may contribute in gastric ulcer formation and the subsequent metaplasia and dysplasia leading to gastric cancer (Fig. 2). Avoidance of risk factors, therapeutic intervention and some protective herbs can be employed to prevent the initiation of this sequence.

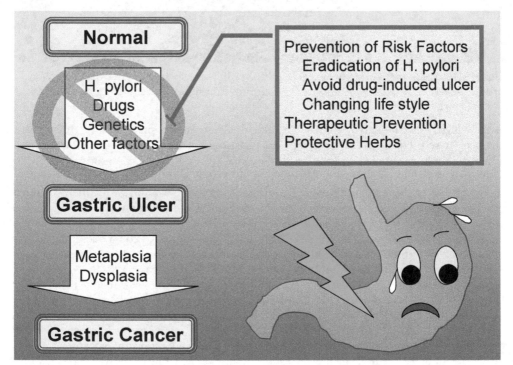

Fig. 2. Prevention of gastric ulcer formation is a step in preventing the development of gastric cancer.

Less than 15% of people infected with Helicobacter pylori develop gastric ulcer. Factors that trigger gastric ulcers in Helicobacter pylori carriers include genetic factors, which explain the higher incidence of development of ulcers in certain ethnicity. Another factor is abnormal immune response, which allows the bacteria to injure the stomach lining. Lifestyle factors as chronic stress, drinking coffee and smoking were long believed to be primary causes of gastric ulcer; it is now thought that they only increase susceptibility to ulcers in some Helicobacter pylori carriers. Interrupted sleep may be another trigger as people who work at night shifts have a significantly higher incidence of ulcers than day workers. Frequent interruption of sleep is thought to weaken the immune system's ability to protect against harmful bacterial substances.

Using certain medications as non-steroidal anti-inflammatory drugs or corticosteroids may contribute to higher infection rates of Helicobacter pylori. Patients with prior gastric ulcer, Zollinger-Ellison syndrome, congenital stomach malformations, malignant diseases such as mastocytosis and basophilic leukemia, head trauma, severe traumatic injuries, burns, radiation, or recently had major surgery are also more prone to Helicobacter pylori infection. Increased risk of Helicobacter pylori infection is seen among people who live in crowded places with unsanitary conditions. Some genetic predispositions for Helicobacter pylori infection cure rate may exist. One example is cytochrome P450-2C19 polymorphism that seems to predict the cure of Helicobacter pylori infection and predisposition to gastric ulcer (Lay and Lin, 2010). Another example is cytokine genes polymorphism that was significantly associated with persistent infection (Abdiev et al., 2010). Polymorphism of multidrug resistance protein 1 also was reported to influence Helicobacter pylori-induced gastric inflammation (Tahara et al., 2011). Such genetic predisposition gives us hope that the infection predisposing to peptic ulcer and gastric cancer may some day be a target for preventive gene therapy in the near future.

Therapeutic interventions to eradicate Helicobacter pylori are needed to prevent ulcer formation and its transformation to gastric cancer, one of the major complications of chronic gastric ulcer. Helicobacter pylori eradication therapy comprises a combination of two or more drugs including antimicrobials, proton pump inhibitors and gastro-protective agents. Several eradication methods were suggested. Dual eradication therapy using proton pump inhibitor with amoxicillin was tried (Graham et al., 2010). Triple eradication therapy employing 2 antimicrobials together with proton pump inhibitor also showed some success, but not enough to be considered first-line treatment. Quadruple Helicobacter pylori eradication was also successfully tried and consisted of 2 antimicrobials, proton pump inhibitor and the gastro-protective agent colloidal bismuth subcitrate (Zheng et al., 2010).

Nowadays, the first line of Helicobacter pylori eradication therapy is a regimen of 7 or 14 days consisting of a proton pump inhibitor as omeprazole (20 mg 12 hourly), in combination with clarithromycin (500 mg 12 hourly) and metronidazole (400 mg 12 hourly). A second regimen that is equally effective is by using omeprazole as previously mentioned, together with less dose of clarithromycin (250 mg 12 hourly) and substituting metronidazole with amoxicillin (1 g 12 hourly). Omeprazole can be replaced with other proton pump inhibitors. Despite that the prevalence of Helicobacter pylori is decreasing in developed countries, as a result of improvements in living standards and hygiene, Helicobacter pylori is still a common cause of gastric ulcer in developing countries. Attempts to develop effective vaccination against this bacterium reached phase I and II clinical trials, and may present effective preventive strategy in preventing gastric ulcer formation and, more importantly, preventing gastric cancer in the future (Majumdar et al., 2011).

2.2 Avoidance of drug-induced gastric ulcers

Patients receiving medications as non-steroidal anti-inflammatory drugs, the anticoagulant drug warfarin, corticosteroids or the anti-osteoporotic drug alendronate may be more prone to gastric ulcer. Non-steroidal anti-inflammatory drugs are valuable therapeutics that act not only as anti-inflammatory, but also as analgesics and antipyretics. They are used in a wide variety of clinical scenarios, including arthritis and other musculoskeletal disorders. Unfortunately, their use has been limited by their gastric ulcer-inducing effects. Nearly 25 % of chronic users of these drugs develop gastric ulcer disease (Lanza et al., 2009).

The rate of non-steroidal anti-inflammatory drugs-induced gastric ulcers is increasing, as more people are taking these drugs regularly as over-the-counter self-therapy. In general, the possibility of gastric ulcer initiation of a non-steroidal anti-inflammatory drug with non-selective cyclooxygenase inhibition actions correlates with its anti-inflammatory activity. Non-steroidal anti-inflammatory drugs with a high analgesic effect at doses with low anti-inflammatory activity, such as ibuprofen, are less ulcerogenic than those that have adequate analgesic effects only at doses with high anti-inflammatory activity, as in case of piroxicam. Ibuprofen appears safer compared to other members of this drug group in part because it is frequently prescribed for short durations in a low dose to control temporary mild painful conditions. However, when full anti-inflammatory doses of ibuprofen are given, the risk of gastric ulceration with ibuprofen is comparable with other non-steroidal anti-inflammatory drugs.

One member of this group is indomethacin, which is a frequently clinically used and is also applied to induce experimental animal model of acute gastric ulcer. Indomethacin induces gastric injury by suppressing the formation of prostaglandins, which control many of the components of mucosal defense system, as they stimulate mucus and bicarbonate secretion, elevate mucosal blood flow, increase the resistance of epithelial cells to injury induced by cytotoxins and suppress the recruitment of leucocytes into the mucosa. Prostaglandins can also inhibit the release of a number of inflammatory mediators, such as tumor necrosis factor-α from macrophages and interleukin-8 from neutrophils. Tumor necrosis factor-α promotes gastric epithelial cell apoptosis and triggers activation of adhesion molecules and leucocyte recruitment, leading to microvascular perturbations. Other mechanisms by which indomethacin induce gastric injury involves gastric hypermotility and the increased production of reactive oxygen species, as well as lipid peroxidation (Morsy et al., 2010).

Physicians prescribing these drugs face two problems; one problem is identification of high-risk patients and the second is selection of appropriate strategies to prevent gastric ulcer. Risk factors of these drugs-induced gastric ulcers include older age, concomitant use of anticoagulants, corticosteroids, other non-steroidal anti-inflammatory drugs including low-dose aspirin, and chronic debilitating disorders, especially cardiovascular diseases. Helicobacter pylori infection increases the risk of this drugs-induced gastric ulcer. Eradication of Helicobacter pylori infection, if present, in patients requiring long-term therapy by these drugs is recommended.

Patients who require long-term non-steroidal anti-inflammatory drug therapy can reduce their risk of inducing ulcers by concomitantly taking conventional anti-ulcer therapy. Proton pump inhibitors and/or histamine H_2 receptor antagonists can significantly reduce these drug-induced gastric ulcers. The synthetic prostaglandin E_1 analog, misoprostol, is also very effective in preventing the development of gastric ulcers in patients taking these medications. Unfortunately, its use is limited by its gastrointestinal adverse effects.

Avoiding unnecessary intake of ulcer-inducing over-the-counter medications may help in reducing the prevalence of gastric ulcers. When it is mandatory to use such therapeutics, their replacement with less irritating drugs may reduce ulcer formation. Non-steroidal anti-inflammatory drugs which are selective cyclooxygenase-2 inhibitors show similar anti-inflammatory, analgesic and antipyretic efficacy compared to non-selective inhibitors. However, these selective drugs are associated with lower incidence of gastric ulcers. Unfortunately, there use is limited due to their association with myocardial infarction and thrombosis. Unexpectedly, experiments using cyclooxygenase-1 knockout mice showed that these animals do not develop gastric ulceration at higher rate and have some reduced inflammatory response.

Some studies tried to find a safer replacement for non-steroidal anti-inflammatory drugs as regards their gastric ulcerogenic effect. In one study, a safer anti-inflammatory drug as regards its gastric toxicity was developed (Shoman et al., 2009). A number of nitric oxide donating pyrazoline derivatives were synthesized and they showed equivalent anti-inflammatory effect to the anti-inflammatory drug indomethacin, with significantly less development of gastric ulceration. Other similar trials have been made by other investigators, for example testing the effect of cyclodextrin combination with non-steroidal anti-inflammatory drugs on gastric ulcer formation which resulted in gastro-protective effect (Alsarra et al., 2010).

2.3 Life style risk factors

Several studies implied that modulating life style factors as dietary factors, controlling stress, reducing smoking and alcohol intake may directly prevent the initiation of gastric ulcers, especially in predisposed people. Some even suggested certain physical exercises to reduce the risk of ulcer formation or recurrence. Such exercises were seen to directly improve psychological and cardiovascular conditions and thus may be indirectly related to decreasing gastric ulcer development.

2.3.1 Diet

Diet rich in fibers may decrease the risk of developing gastric ulcers by about 50%. Fiber found in fruits and vegetables is particularly protective, as vitamin A contained in many of these foods may increase the benefit. Milk, previously thought to aid in decreasing ulcer symptoms, actually encourages the production of acid in the stomach, although moderate amounts (2-3 cups/day) appear to do no harm. However, yogurt may protect against gastric ulcer, as it contains probiotics. Coffee (caffeinated and decaffeinated), soft drinks and fruit juices with citric acid increase stomach acid production. Although no studies have proven that any of these drinks contribute to ulcers, consuming more than 3 cups of coffee per day may increase susceptibility to Helicobacter pylori infection (University of Maryland Medical Center website).

Studies conducted on spices and peppers have yielded conflicting results. In general, these substances should be used moderately, and should be avoided if they irritate the stomach. Some studies suggest that high amounts of garlic may have some protective properties against stomach cancer, although a recent study concluded that garlic offered no benefits against Helicobacter pylori and, in large amounts, can cause considerable gastrointestinal distress. Studies have shown that phenolic compounds in virgin olive oil may be effective against Helicobacter pylori infection. Although no vitamins have been shown to protect against Helicobacter pylori-induced ulcers, Helicobacter pylori appears to impair the absorption of vitamin C, which may play a role in the higher risk of stomach cancer.

2.3.2 Psychological factors: stress

As a body response to stress, many diseases may develop. There is debate as to whether psychological stress can influence the development of gastric ulcers. Some studies still suggest that stress may predispose a person to ulcers or prevent existing ulcers from healing. Some even believe that the relationship between stress and ulcers is so strong that people with ulcers should be treated for psychological conditions. Stress causes the digestive tract to slow down and more gastric acid is allowed to accumulate in the stomach. Increased stomach acidity may predispose to or aggravate an already present ulcer. Stress can also cause change in appetite, leading to over-eating or lack of appetite. Overeating causes the stomach to produce more acid while lack of appetite will subject the stomach mucosa to the acid produced in an empty stomach. Although psychological stress is no longer considered a direct cause of ulcers, it surely can delay the healing and aggravate already existing gastric ulcers. Physical stress, however, is definitely a risk factor for developing gastric ulcers, as in patients with injuries such as severe burns or patients undergoing major surgeries.

2.3.3 Smoking

Cigarette smoking appears to be a risk factor for the development and recurrence of gastric ulcer. The incidence of gastric ulcer is higher among smokers than non-smokers. Compared with non-smokers, people who smoke cigarettes are twice as likely to develop gastric ulcer. Smoking may lead to initiation of ulceration, slow ulcer healing and an increased risk of gastric ulcer recurrence. Smoking may have an inconsistent effect on gastric acid secretion; however it reduces prostaglandin and bicarbonate production, reduces mucosal blood flow, interferes with the action of histamine H_2 receptor antagonists and accelerates gastric emptying of liquids. Cessation of smoking or reducing it is usually associated with the prompt relief of already existing gastric ulcer symptoms.

2.3.4 Excess alcohol intake

Alcohol increases the production of acid in the stomach, which may irritate an existing ulcer. Alcohol also relaxes the lower esophageal sphincter, allowing stomach contents to reflux back up into the esophagus, increasing the discomfort associated with gastric ulcer. Patients suffering of gastric ulcer should, thus, avoid taking alcohol. People predisposed to gastric ulcer may dilute alcoholic beverages to reduce their concentration, restrict the number of drinks to one or two a day, replace red wine with white wine of less toxic content, or better, have drinks which are non-alcoholic.

3. Endogenous protection against gastric ulcer

Astonishingly, despite of the presence of one or more risk factors as smoking, alcohol intake, non-steroidal anti-inflammatory drugs consumption and/or Helicobacter pylori infection, some people still do not develop gastric ulcer. For example, non-steroidal anti-inflammatory drugs induce clinically significant gastric ulceration in 17% of patients receiving these drugs. This is due to the strong natural endogenous gastric cyto-protection that spares the vast majority of patients at risk. Gastric mucosal barrier together with endogenous mediators comprise a strong defense mechanism against gastric ulceration. Understanding these naturally occurring defense mechanisms is crucial to try to enhance them to prevent gastric damage and ulceration in more vulnerable patients.

3.1 Physiological gastric mucosal barrier

The gastric mucosal barrier is considered the main defense system against gastric ulcer formation. Several luminal factors contribute to this barrier (Fig. 3). These factors include secretion of bicarbonates, mucus, phospholipids and immunoglobulins. The gastric epithelial barrier also represents part of the defense system that is remarkably resistant to acids or irritants and has the capability of rapid repair. The mucosal microcirculation, together with sensory innervations, harmonically defends the mucosal barrier. Sensing acidic diffusion into the gastric mucosa results in neural system-mediated induced endogenous mediator release and hormonal responses leading to increase in mucosal blood flow, which is a critical step in preventing damage and facilitating repair of gastric mucosa. The mucosal immune system represents another gastric mucosal protective method. Mast cells and macrophage generate immune signals of inflammatory response that contributes to prevention of gastric damage.

3.1.1 Luminal gastric protection

The mucus-bicarbonate-phospholipid barrier comprises the first line of mucosal defense mechanism. This barrier is formed of mucus, bicarbonate and phospholipids. Mucus presents a layer that contains secreted bicarbonate and surfactant phospholipids. Mucus that acts as a physical barrier against luminal digestive enzymes, bicarbonate that maintains an almost neutral pH at the epithelial surface, together with phospholipids of high hydrophobic properties can naturally protect against mucosal damage. Disruption of this mucus-bicarbonate-phospholipid barrier by ulcerogenic substances, as bile salts or non-steroidal anti-inflammatory drugs causes elevated diffusion of acid into the mucosa and mucosal damage (Allen and Flemstrom, 2005). Helicobacter pylori release phospholipase enzymes and ammonium ions that can reduce the strength of this single and only barrier existing between the epithelium and the lumen. Other protective mechanisms may then interfere to protect against this bacterial induced injury.

3.1.2 Gastric epithelial barrier

Mucosal surface is formed of a continuous layer of surface epithelial cells that secrete components of the mucus barrier as well as endogenous protective mediators as prostaglandins, heat shock proteins and cathelicidins (see below; section 3.2). These surface epithelial cells form a physical barrier preventing back-diffusion of gastric acid and digestive enzymes. Basolateral membrane of epithelial parietal cells, that secrete hydrochloric acid in high concentrations into the lumen of the stomach, contains transporters responsible for maintaining intracellular homeostasis. These transporters efflux large amounts of bicarbonate to prevent cell alkalinization. The effluxed bicarbonate, known as alkaline tide, is an integral constituent of mucus-bicarbonate barrier (Tulassay and Herszenyi, 2010). Continuous and rapid cell renewal enhances the resistance of epithelial barrier to damage. Mucosal progenitor cells in gastric epithelium promote cell renewal by continuously replacing surface cells that undergo apoptosis. Proliferation of progenitor cells is controlled by endogenous growth factors' mediators.

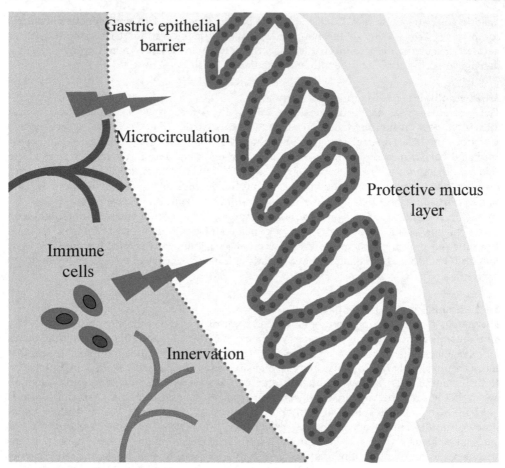

Fig. 3. Physiological gastric mucosal barrier. It is composed mainly of protective luminal mucus layer, gastric epithelial barrier, immune cells, gastric microcirculation and sensory gastric innervation.

3.1.3 Mucosal microcirculation

Mucosal ischemia triggers gastric ulcer by inducing tissue necrosis, free radical formation and cessation of nutrient transport, all resulting from vascular and microvascular injury such as thrombi, constriction or other occlusions. Mucosal blood flow thus provides gastric lining with adequate vascular perfusion that prevents epithelial damage from progressing to necrosis of deeper layers of the mucosa. Increase in mucosal blood flow occurs as a response to gastric mucosal exposure to an irritant or when acid back-diffusion occurs. Potent vasodilators such as nitric oxide and prostaglandin I_2 generated by endothelial cells protect the gastric mucosa against injury and damaging action of vasoconstrictors such as leukotriene C_4, thromboxane A_2 and endothelin. These potent vasodilators prevent platelet and leucocyte adherence to endothelial cells, maintain the integrity of the gastric epithelium and the mucus barrier and protect the gastrointestinal tract by inhibiting gastric acid secretion from parietal cells. Endogenous mediators that affect mucosal microcirculation as nitric oxide and hydrogen sulfide are further discussed below (section 3.2).

3.1.4 Gastric sensory innervation

Gastric mucosal defense is also regulated by the central nervous system innervation. Gastric mucosa and submucosal vessels are innervated by primary afferent sensory neurons. When gastric mucosa gets exposed to damage by gastric acid or other irritating chemicals, afferent neurons are activated and directly start controlling the tone of the submucosal arterioles, which regulate mucosal blood flow. When sensory afferent nerves of the superficial mucosa detect gastric acid, they respond by releasing neurotransmitters as substance P and calcitonin gene-related peptide. These mediators cause relaxation of smooth muscle surrounding gastric mucosal arterioles, resulting in an elevation of mucosal blood flow. In addition, vagal activation increase mucus secretion, while nervous response to stress control central corticotropin-releasing factor signaling pathways. Furthermore, the transient receptor potential vanilloid 1 agonists are effective in protecting gastric mucosa against various experimentally induced ulcer models (Morsy and Fouad, 2008).

3.1.5 Mucosal immune system

The mucosal immune system is a key factor of mucosal defense against exogenous and endogenous irritants. Impairment of this immune system can lead to mucosal injury and to impairment of endogenous cyto-protective repair mechanisms. The mucosal immune system is coordinated by innate and adaptive immune response regulated by several mediators released from immuno-regulating cells. Neutrophils and macrophages infiltrate into the gastric mucosa as a response to Helicobacter pylori infection. These cells release lysosomal enzymes, leukotrienes and reactive oxygen species which impairs mucosal defense and drives the immunopathogenetic process of ulcerogenesis. T and B lymphocytes activated by bacterial antigens and pro-inflammatory cytokines regulate the local and systemic immune response with release of further cytokines and antibodies. The type of T-cell response can change the outcome of this infection, as more mucosal damage results from T-helper predominant response, whereas a high regulatory T-cell response with interleukin-10 release confers gastric ulcer protection (Malfertheiner et al., 2009).

3.2 Endogenous gastro-protective mediators

Some endogenous mediators can work through cyto-protective mechanisms reducing gastrointestinal injury induced by topical irritants, thus preventing the initial steps of gastric inflammation. These endogenous mediators may be inhibited by causative risk factors, leading to gastric ulceration and thus provide a mechanism through which these risk factor contribute in gastric damage. On the other hand, therapeutic modulation of endogenous gastric mediators can provide a target to improve gastric protection against ulceration.

3.2.1 Mediators of cyclooxygenase pathway: prostaglandins and lipoxins

Prostaglandins are fatty acids produced from arachidonic acid via cyclooxygenase enzyme. It is known that suppression of prostaglandin synthesis is a major mechanism of action of aspirin and other non-steroidal anti-inflammatory drugs, which is probably one of the mechanisms by which these drugs cause gastric ulcers. Prostaglandins modulate a number of components of mucosal defense as they stimulate mucus and bicarbonate secretion, promote mucosal blood flow, increase the resistance of epithelial cells to cytotoxins-induced injury and suppress the recruitment of leukocytes into gastric mucosa. Prostaglandins can also down regulate the release of a number of other inflammatory mediators that may contribute to the generation of gastric ulcer (Martin and Wallace, 2006). Prostaglandin E receptors have a prominent role in mucosal protection and gastric ulcer healing (Takeuchi, 2010). Prostaglandin E_2 has been shown to be a potent inhibitor of tumor necrosis factor-α and interleukin-1 release from macrophages and of leukotriene B4 and interleukin-8 release from neutrophils.

Lipoxins are the resultant of consequent conversion of arachidonic acid by cyclooxygenase-2 and 5-lipoxygenase enzymes. Lipoxin-A_4 is an endogenous mediator contributing to resolution of the inflammatory state and, thus, has an important role in mucosal defense. Lipoxin A_4 protects the stomach from aspirin-induced damage via suppressing leukocyte adherence within gastric micro-circulation. In addition, Lipoxin A_4 can inhibit inflammatory pain processing and regulate trans-epithelial electrical resistance. Antagonism of Lipoxin A_4 receptor can significantly exacerbate gastric ulcer (Lim et al., 2009).

3.2.2 Nitric oxide

Oxidization of arginine by nitric oxide synthase yields the volatile gas nitric oxide, which has numerous physiologic properties including regulation of inflammation. Nitric oxide is an important factor in modulating gastrointestinal mucosal defense mechanisms. Some of nitric oxide actions overlaps with that of prostaglandins, as it modulate the activity of mucosal immunocytes and reduce leukocytic endothelial adhesion. In addition, it modulates mucosal blood flow and reduces epithelial permeability, resulting in enhanced mucosal resistance to ulceration. Nitric oxide also prevents adherence of leukocytes to the vascular endothelium. This gaseous mediator has a role also in modulating gastric mucus and bicarbonate secretion. Suppression of nitric oxide synthesis renders the gastric mucosa more susceptible to injury, while administration of nitric oxide donors can protect the stomach from injury. Agents that release nitric oxide in small amounts over a prolonged period have been shown to greatly reduce inflammation and to accelerate ulcerative healing (Martin and Wallace, 2006).

Some studies showed that dietary nitrate and pretreatment with nitric oxide donor protected against drug-induced gastric ulcer. Furthermore, the use of nitric oxide-donating agents concomitantly with non-steroidal anti-inflammatory drugs as aspirin also resulted in reduced risk for gastric ulceration and bleeding. This lead to the development of cyclo-oxygenase inhibiting/nitric oxide donating drugs, in which nitric oxide is chemically linked to a non-steroidal anti-inflammatory drug, which showed effective anti-inflammatory capabilities together with less gastric injury. Examples of such drugs include nitric oxide-flurbiprofen, nitric oxide-ketoprofen, nitric oxide-diclofenac and nitric oxide-naproxen. These drugs are suitable therapeutic options for patients with diseases requiring long-term non-steroidal anti-inflammatory drugs therapy (Lanas, 2008).

Despite all evidence that nitric oxide contribute in mediating mucosal defense under normal conditions, under different circumstances, as in case of already inflamed mucosa, it is suggested that nitric oxide may contribute to tissue injury. In this case, nitric oxide reacts with superoxide anion, produced by activated neutrophils, to form peroxynitrite, which is another potent oxidant. Peroxynitrite is known to produce widespread gastrointestinal injury and inflammation. Although the role of nitric oxide is still controversial, most studies suggest a net protective effect of this molecule in the gastrointestinal tract.

3.2.3 Hydrogen sulfide

Hydrogen sulfide is another gaseous mediator generated endogenously that causes vasodilatation, decreases adhesion of leukocyte to vascular endothelium, inhibits non-steroidal anti-inflammatory drugs-induced gastric mucosal injury and inhibit tumor necrosis factor-α expression (Tulassay and Herszenyi, 2010). The enzymes responsible for hydrogen sulfide generation in the gastric mucosa are cystathionine β-synthase and cystathionine γ-lyase.

Despite the protective role of this gas against mucosal injury, it suspected that hydrogen sulphide may contribute to the pro-inflammatory actions in Helicobacter pylori infection. Nevertheless, with non-steroidal anti-inflammatory drugs, hydrogen sulfide provide gastric protection by inducing up-regulation of anti-inflammatory and cyto-protective genes, including hemeoxygenase-1, vascular endothelial growth factor, insulin-like growth factor receptor and several genes associated with the transforming growth factor-β receptor signaling pathway (Lim et al., 2009).

A number of therapeutic possibilities combining hydrogen sulfide with non-steroidal anti-inflammatory drugs are considered in early stages of development. This new class of combination is based on that non-steroidal anti-inflammatory drugs reduce hydrogen sulphide production in gastric mucosa, which may contribute to these drugs' inducing mechanisms of gastric ulcer. In return, sodium hydrogen sulfide prevents the reduction of mucosal blood flow induced by non-steroidal anti-inflammatory drugs. Furthermore, this gaseous mediator reduces non-steroidal anti-inflammatory drugs-induced leukocyte adhesion to vascular endothelial cell. The combination causes reversal of the increased expression of tumor necrosis factor-α and improvement prostaglandin E_2 synthesis impaired by non-steroidal anti-inflammatory drugs (Lim et al., 2009).

3.2.4 Cytokines

Cytokines are important in mucosal defense and play a pivotal role in the regulation of the mucosal immune system. Interleukin-1β and tumor necrosis factor-α release comprise the early inflammatory systemic response to inflammation or infection. Various types of cells produce interleukin-1β, including monocytes, macrophages, neutrophils, endothelial cells and fibroblasts. Interleukin-1β increases the resistance of gastric mucosa to injury and reduces the severity of ulcerative damage. This is through its action as a potent inhibitor of gastric acid secretion, stimulator of prostaglandins and nitric oxide release and inhibitor of ulcer-promoting mediators as platelet-activating factor from mast cells (Tulassay and Herszenyi, 2010). Tumor necrosis factor-α is another key cytokine that contribute in producing gastric mucosal injury. Still, by stimulating cell proliferation, tumor necrosis factor-α may also promote mucosal repair after damage associated with Helicobacter pylori infection and the use of non-steroidal anti-inflammatory drugs. Tumor necrosis factor-α reverses gastric mucosal injury via stimulation of epithelial cell proliferation.

3.2.5 Proteinase-activated receptors

Proteinase-activated-2 receptors are expressed throughout the gastrointestinal tract, especially in the epithelial cells and sensory afferent neurons. In the stomach, the activation of these receptors triggers mucus secretion and reduces the extent of stomach endothelial damage induced by non-steroidal anti-inflammatory drugs. This may be through modulating sensory afferent nerves and regulating the release of vascular endothelial growth factor from platelets, which affect new blood vessel angiogenesis that promote ulcer healing (Yoshida and Yoshikawa, 2008).

3.2.6 Proteolytic enzymes

Proteolytic enzymes have important functions in gastric ulcer prevention and healing. It has been shown that impaired fibrinolysis occurs due to alteration of the proteolytic enzymes formed through tissue-type plasminogen activator-inhibitor system. Intramucosal proteases; as cathepsins, are also involved in protection against gastric ulcer initiation and promotion of healing. Cathepsins act as antimicrobial peptides expressed by the gastric epithelium preventing bacterial colonization and accelerate ulcer healing. The proteolytic enzymes urokinase-type plasminogen activator and plasminogen activator-inhibitor type-1 are involved in angiogenesis process, and thus has a direct role in cell proliferation, inflammation and ulcer healing. Matrix metalloproteases are involved in extracellular matrix reconstitution and tissue remodeling and thus may have an impact in gastric ulcer healing (Tomita et al., 2009). Secretory leucocyte protease inhibitor exerts antimicrobial and anti-inflammatory effects. Its expression is induced during inflammation. However, the expression is significantly decreased during Helicobacter pylori-mediated gastritis. This is due to local down-regulation of this proteolytic enzyme in gastric mucosa in response to Helicobacter pylori infection (Tulassay and Herszenyi, 2010).

3.2.7 Heat shock proteins

Heat shock proteins are important mediators of cellular homeostasis during normal cell growth. They also promote cell survival during various cellular stresses, as they are generated by gastric epithelial cells in response to oxidative stress, cytotoxicity and high temperature. Heat shock proteins generated play an important role in cellular recovery. This is done through acting on enzymes related to cyto-protection, gastric inflammation and gastric ulcer healing. Heat shock proteins act by refolding these partially damaged functional enzymes or increasing delivery of their precursor proteins to important organelles such as mitochondria and endoplasmic reticulum. This results in improvement of mucosal defense, protection against gastric ulcer and promotion of healing of existing damage (Choi et al., 2009).

3.2.8 Growth factors

Growth factors are considered a pivotal stimulus for cell proliferation, division, migration and re-epithelization. Cell proliferation and repair of injured gastric mucosal epithelium are controlled by a number of these growth factors activated as a response to tissue injury. Growth factors such as epidermal growth factor, hepatocyte growth factor, platelet derived growth factor and basic fibroblast growth factor activate epithelial cell migration and proliferation and accelerate ulcer healing by binding to their specific receptors on the cell surface, triggering a number of intracellular signaling events that result in cell migration and proliferation.

In the stomach, epidermal growth factor triggers mitogenic response and is important for epithelial cell proliferation, migration, re-epithelization and reconstruction of gastric glands. Vascular endothelial growth factor is important for angiogenesis, vascular remodeling and mucosal regeneration. Transforming growth factor-α protects against gastric mucosal injury and promotes wound healing. Receptors for epidermal and transforming growth factors are expressed in gastric progenitor cells and are trans-activated by gastrin and prostaglandin E_2 that trigger cell proliferation and repair of gastric mucosa (Tulassay and Herszenyi, 2010). These growth factors are mainly derived from platelets, macrophages and injured tissue. Ulceration also triggers induction of genes encoding these growth factors in cells lining mucosa of the ulcer margin. These locally produced growth factors activate epithelial cell migration and proliferation via actions on autocrine and/or paracrine systems.

3.2.9 Peroxisome proliferation-activated receptor
Peroxisome proliferation-activated receptors (α, β and γ) are members of the nuclear response family of transcription factors. These receptors are expressed in the gastrointestinal tract, liver, skeletal muscle, heart, adipose tissue, breast and skin. Stimulation of peroxisome proliferation-activated receptors plays an important role in the mechanism of non-steroidal anti-inflammatory drugs action. Peroxisome proliferation-activated receptors cause subsequent inhibition of nuclear factor-κB and other transcription factors. These receptors regulate transcription of target genes involved in lipid and lipoprotein metabolism, glucose homeostasis and cell differentiation. In addition, peroxisome proliferation-activated receptors inhibit the activation of certain inflammatory response genes. Thus, activation of peroxisome proliferation-activated receptors during non-steroidal anti-inflammatory drugs administration blocks the production of inflammatory response markers, such endothelin-1, vascular cell adhesion molecule-1 in endothelial cells and tissue factors as matrix metalloproteinase-3 and tumor necrosis factor-α in macrophages. These anti-inflammatory actions are mediated by inhibition of pro-inflammatory transcription pathways as nuclear factor-κB, activator protein-1 and nuclear factor of activated T cells (Lim et al., 2009).

3.2.10 Neuropeptides
Several neuropeptides as cholecystokinin, gastrin 17, bombesin, corticotrophin-releasing factor, peptide YY and intragastric peptone are involved in gastro-protection. Ghrelin is also a neuropeptide associated with gastro-protective effects with important effects on energy homeostasis and gastrointestinal motility. Ghrelin is effective against ethanol-induced gastric ulcers. This protective effect is dependent on cyclooxygenase-1-derived prostaglandin E_2. Ghrelin mediates its gastro-protective effects also via stimulation of nitric oxide production and calcitonin gene related peptide release from sensory afferent nerves, enhancing gastric mucosal blood flow. Orexins are another family of neuropeptides having gastro-protective role, especially orexin-A. Orexin-A prevents mucosal injury and gastric ulceration through several mechanism including increasing gastric blood flow, elevating luminal nitric oxide, reducing lipid peroxidation, generating prostaglandin E_2 and enhancing vagal and sensory nerve activity (Nayeb-Hashemi and Kaunitz, 2009).

3.2.11 Hemeoxygenase-1 enzyme
Hemeoxygenase-1 is the rate-limiting enzyme of heme catabolism that catalyzes the breakdown of heme into carbon monoxide, iron and biliverdin. Hemeoxygenase isoform 1 is a phase II drug detoxifying enzyme. It is highly inducible as a response to stress, as oxidative stressors, ultraviolet irradiation, inflammatory cytokines, heavy metals and non-steroidal anti-inflammatory drugs. Up-regulation of hemeoxygenase-1 infers anti-apoptotic resistance to the cells due to potent antioxidant effect of bilirubin, biliverdin and carbon

monoxide formed. Hemeoxygenase was shown to protect gastric mucosal cells against non-steroidal anti-inflammatory drugs (Aburaya et al., 2006).

4. Therapeutic interventions in prevention of gastric ulcer

Several therapeutic interventions may aid in preventing gastric ulcer. Enhancement of normal physical barriers and physiological protective factors can aid in prevention of gastric ulcer. Some endogenous gastro-protective factors (see above) may be enhanced to decrease the risk of gastric ulcer formation. Conventional medications used in treatment of gastric ulcer can also be used in prevention as well, especially in predisposed people. Several investigations also tested drugs not conventionally used in treatment of gastric ulcer for having possible ulcerogenic protective effects. The main aim of most of these studies is to decide which drug to preferentially use in treating conditions presenting concomitantly with high risk of development gastric ulcer.

4.1 Prevention of gastric ulcer by conventional anti-ulcer drugs

Most anti-ulcer drugs target gastric acid secretion and mucosal defense mechanisms (Table 1). Successful classes in treating gastric ulcer include Helicobacter pylori eradication therapy, prostaglandin analogs, cyto-protective drugs, histamine H_2 receptor antagonist and proton pump inhibitor groups. In terms of acid inhibition, proton pump inhibitors possess higher acid inhibitory potency. Histamine H_2 receptor antagonists have, thus, been gradually replaced with the more potent class of acid inhibitory drugs, the proton pump inhibitors. Current ulcer therapy consists of Helicobacter pylori eradication in Helicobacter pylori-positive gastric ulcer and proton pump inhibitors for healing and preventing peptic ulcers induced by drugs.

Proton pump inhibitors selectively block the H^+/K^+ ATPase of the parietal cells. These proton pump inhibitors are the most popular group of drugs used in Helicobacter pylori eradication regimens (see before; section 2.1). Misoprostol, a prostaglandin analog, has been the most widely used but its application is limited by abdominal side-effects as abdominal cramps and diarrhea. Sucralfate and bismuth salts improve mucosal repair. Sucralfate also acts by reducing acid secretion and suppressing Helicobacter pylori infection. Bismuth salts, having mild anti-Helicobacter pylori activity, are used in treatment of gastric ulcer therapy in combination with antibiotics (Malfertheiner et al., 2009).

All of these drugs have been used successfully to treat gastric ulcers and prevent remittent attacks. Nevertheless, their efficiency in prevention of gastric ulcers in individual predisposed groups is still controversial. Histamine H_2 receptor antagonist is one example, as their standard dosage succeeded only in reducing the risk of duodenal ulcer, but not gastric ulcer induced by non-steroidal anti-inflammatory drugs. The benefit from histamine H_2 receptor antagonists was limited to preventing the risk of ulcers induced by Helicobacter pylori infection (Chan and Graham, 2004). Contrarily, in another study, histamine H_2 receptor antagonists were effective for prevention of low dose aspirin-induced ulcers and showed similar potency as proton pump inhibitors (Nakashima et al., 2009). Another example is the use of cyto-protective drugs (as in Table 1) for prevention of gastric ulcer, whose efficacy is still controversial.

Using these conventional anti-ulcer drugs in prevention of gastric ulceration is, thus, dependent on the type of predisposing risk factor. Risk factors used in assessment are old age, presence of cardiovascular diseases, use of high dose or multiple non-steroidal anti-inflammatory drugs, concomitant use of low-dose aspirin and other anti-platelet drugs, corticosteroids or warfarin. When one or two of these factors are present, presenting a moderate risk, an anti-secretory agent or misoprostol may be used. If three or more risk factors are combined, presenting a high risk, switching from non-selective, to selective cyclooxygenase inhibitors is recommended. In addition, misoprostol can be used for prevention of aspirin- or warfarin-induced gastric ulcers. In very high risk patients, who have been subjected to previous ulcer complications, avoidance of non-steroidal anti-inflammatory drugs and intake of proton pump inhibitor and/or misoprostol is recommended.

Drug group	Examples	Mechanism of action
Helicobacter pylori eradication therapy	Proton pump inhibitor with two antibiotics	Treatment of Helicobacter pylori infection and prevention of ulcer formation
Proton pump inhibitors	Omeprazole, pantoprazole, lansoprazole, rabeprazole, esomeprazole	Most potent acid inhibition
Histamine H$_2$ receptor antagonists	Cimetidine, ranitidine, famotidine, nizatidine, roxatidine, lafutidine	Less potent acid inhibition
Prostaglandin analogs	Misoprostol	Weak acid inhibition and increase mucosal resistance
Cyto-protective drugs	Rebamipide, azulensulfonate, teprenone, polaprezinc, sofalcone, alginate sodium	Very weak effect in cyto-protection and enhancement of natural defense mechanisms
Bismuth salts	Subcitrate, subsalicylate	Weak antibacterial effect and increase mucosal prostaglandin synthesis

Table 1. Drugs used in prevention and treatment of gastric ulcer and their main mechanism(s) of action.

4.2 Non-conventional gastro-protective drugs

A number of drugs, other than traditional anti-ulcer medications, were investigated and showed an effect in prevention of gastric ulcer formation. Stress causing hypertension may concomitantly predispose to gastric ulcer. The effect of antihypertensive drugs, namely angiotensin II T$_1$ receptor blocker; telmisartan, was investigated for its effect as gastro-protective agent. The results showed that telmisartan and candesartan can prevent gastric ulcer formation, with higher potency of telmisartan than candesartan. Telmisartan's protection of gastric mucosa from non-steroidal anti-inflammatory drugs-induced ulceration is possibly through its anti-oxidant action and may also be ascribed, at least in part, to its peroxisome proliferator-activated receptor γ agonistic properties (Morsy et al., 2009).

Gastric ulcer is also commonly seen concurrently in type 2 diabetic patients. Moreover, peptic ulcers related to the diabetic state are more severe and are often associated with complications. The possible gastro-protective effects of insulin sensitizers thiazolidinediones; rosiglitazone and metformin were tested. Both drugs have the ability to ameliorate oxidative stress and inflammation, rendering them attractive candidates for the prevention of gastric ulcer in patients with type 2 diabetes. Both rosiglitazone and metformin prevented indomethacin-induced gastric ulcer in diabetic rats. Their gastro-protective effects were probably due to anti-secretory actions, enhanced mucosal protection and anti-oxidant activity. This was reflected on their ability to increase mucin concentrations and gastric mucosal nitric oxide levels. In addition, rosiglitazone increased gastric juice pH, providing superior gastro-protection to metformin (Morsy et al., 2010).

Other investigations tested the effect of another anti-diabetic drug; pioglitazone as a gastro-protective drug. Pioglitazone has an agonist of peroxisome proliferator-activated receptor γ and exerted strong effect in both preventing the formation of gastric ulcers and healing of already existing ones. This gastric ulcer preventing/healing effect of pioglitazone is, at least in part, mediated by endogenous nitric oxide. Astonishingly, under diabetic conditions, pioglitazone gastro-protective effect decreased. The attenuation of pioglitazone action is possibly due to reduction in nitric oxide, angiogenesis and increased expression and release of pro-inflammatory cytokines under diabetic conditions (Konturek et al., 2010).

Organoselenium compounds were tested in naproxen- and Helicobacter pylori-induced gastric ulcers and showed not only gastro-protective and ulcer healing effects, but also they possessed antibacterial effect against Helicobacter pylori (Santhosh et al., 2010). When tested on indomethacin-induced gastric ulcer in mice, melatonin demonstrated gastro-protective effects via having angiogenic properties through up-regulation of matrix metalloproteinase-2; an important regulator of angiogenesis (Ganguly et al., 2010).

5. Gastric protection by herbs

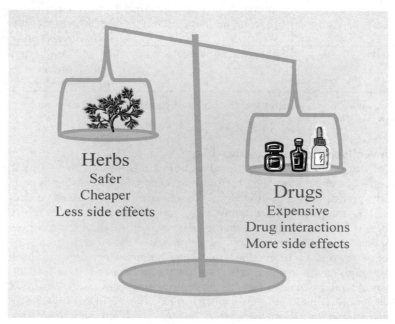

Fig. 4. Herbs, unlike traditional drugs are natural, safer, cheaper and with less side effects.

The need for more effective and cheaper management and prevention of gastric ulcer has attracted an increasing interest for herbal products because of their effectiveness, less side effects and relatively low costs (Fig. 4). For long, some herbal tea constituents and food additives have been known for their gastro-protective effects. For example, liquorice has been used as gastro-protective agent. Eugenol, a compound extracted from clove oil, has also protective effect against the formation of indomethacin-induced gastric ulcer. This effect was mediated by its anti-oxidant activity, decreasing acid-pepsin secretion and increasing mucus production (Morsy and Fouad, 2008).

Similarly, curcumin demonstrated protective effect against gastric ulcer via inhibiting gastric acid secretion, relieving oxidative stress and ameliorating apoptosis. A number of Chinese naturally occurring phytochemicals were reported to have gastro-protective action with potent anti-Helicobacter pylori effects (Li et al., 2005). Lysophosphatidic acid, which is a component of soybean lecithin and antyu-san, has a protective effect against gastric ulcer induction in an animal model, suggesting that daily intake of lysophosphatidic acid-rich foods or Chinese medicines may be beneficial for prevention of gastric ulcer in humans (Adachi et al., 2011). In the ongoing search for bioactive natural products of herbal origin that have ulcer protective activity, crude plant extracts and plant-derived compounds are tried in different experimental models.

5.1 Herbal extracts

Several studies on the gastro-protective effect of crude plant extracts have been undertaken. Although the pathogenesis of gastric ulcer is multi-factorial, secretion of gastric acid is still recognized as a central component of this disease; therefore the main therapeutic target is the control of this secretion using the anti-secretory drugs. On the other hand, many plant extracts, which significantly decrease the ulcer index in experimental animals, have no clinical effects owing to their deficient anti-secretory activity. Accordingly, a large number of studies have been addressing the relationship between plant extracts and their anti-secretory activity on animal experimental models.

We conducted a PubMed search to identify the most relevant articles to these crude plant extracts and focused on those related to the anti-secretory properties, published between January 2010 and December 2010. The number of articles retrieved in a search with such tight limitations reflected the increased scientific interest in using plant extracts in prevention and treatment of gastric ulcer. These natural herbal extracts that has gastro-protective effect include methanol extract of Abarema cochliacarpos bark, a plant that mainly grows in Brazil (da Silva et al., 2010). Another herb, celery (Apium graveolens), which is widely used as food additive worldwide, was also tested, and ethanol extracts of it showed anti-secretory properties (Al-Howiriny et al., 2010).

Extracts of herbs that mainly grow and are widely used in India were tested for their gastro-protective effects as aqueous extract of Pedalium murex leaves (Banji et al., 2010), methanol extract of Hedyotis puberula (Joseph et al., 2010), methanol extract of Punica granatum (Alam et al., 2010), aqueous extract of Myrtus communis (common myrtle) berries (Sumbul et al., 2010), extracts of Cinnamomum tamala leaves (Eswaran et al., 2010) and extracts of Xylocarpus granatum fruit (Lakshmi et al., 2010). Roxb (Ailanthus excelsa bark) (Melanchauski et al., 2010) and camelthorn (Alhagi maurorum) (Shaker et al., 2010) that are widely used in Egypt also showed gastro-protection against ulcers. Hot water extract of Trichosanthes cucumerina Linn that is mainly used in Sri Lanka also showed similar effects (Arawwawala et al., 2010).

5.2 Pure compounds

Purified compounds may have the privilege of specifying the exact compound that is exerting gastro-protective effects. Unlike total herbal extract, pure compounds may lack the presence of several combined components that may contradict each other's action or add an undesired adverse effect.

5.2.1 Flavonoids

Flavonoids represent a highly diverse class of secondary metabolites that constitute the largest and most important group of polyphenolic compounds in plants. The pleiotropic actions of natural compounds are important for developing new drugs for multifactorial diseases. This is particularly true with regards to flavonoids as they display several pharmacological properties in the gastro-protective area, acting as anti-secretory, cyto-protective and antioxidant agents. Besides their action as gastro-protective, flavonoids also can be alternatives for suppression or modulation of gastric ulcers associated with Helicobacter pylori. Flavonoid fraction extracted from Mouriri pusa leaves, a plant from Brazilian cerrado also known as manapuçá or jaboticaba do mato which is commonly used in the treatment of gastrointestinal disturbs in its native region, shows beneficial effects in prevention and reversal of gastric ulcer (Vasconcelos et al., 2010).

Quercetin has an anti-secretory mechanism of action. It has antihistaminic properties, therefore, decreases histamine levels, as well as preventing the release of histamine from gastric mast cells and inhibiting the gastric H^+/K^+ proton pump, diminishing acid gastric secretion. On the other hand, the gastro-protective effects of chalcones involve increasing the mucosal blood flow, stimulating the synthesis of mucus in the gastric mucosa and increasing prostaglandin levels. Nevertheless, the most important mechanism of action responsible for the anti-ulcer activity of flavonoids is their antioxidant properties, seen in garcinol, rutin and quercetin, which involve free radical scavenging, transition metal ions chelation, inhibition of oxidizing enzymes, increase of proteic and nonproteic antioxidants and reduction of lipid peroxidation. In addition, sofalcone (a chalcone) and quercetin (flavonol) have anti-Helicobacter pylori activity (Mota et al., 2009).

5.2.2 Alkaloids

Alkaloids represent a diverse group of low molecular weight nitrogen-containing secondary metabolites that have gastro-protective activity. For examples, the isoquinoline alkaloid isolated from Coptidis rhizome, coptisine; the quinolizidine alkaloid isolated from Sophora flavescens, matrine which decreases the acid secretion and inhibits the gastric motility; the piperidine alkaloid piperine, which protects the stomach against ulceration by decreasing the volume of gastric juice, gastric acidity and pepsin-A activity; the phenylakylamide alkaloid capsaicin, which inhibits the acid secretion, stimulates the alkali/mucus secretions and mainly increases the gastric mucosal blood flow; the steroidal alkaloid pachysandrine A obtained from Pachysandra terminalis; and the indole alkaloid nigakinone found in Picrasma quassioides, which decreases gastric acid/pepsin secretions and protects the mucous membrane (de Sousa et al., 2008).

5.2.3 Terpenoids

Terpenoids are a large and diverse class of naturally-occurring organic chemicals similar to terpenes. Gastro-protective terpenoids have been isolated from several plants, including sesquiterpenes from Artemisa douglasiana, triterpenes from Fabiana imbricate and carbenoxolone from Glycyrrhiza glabra. Most of the work on the gastro-protective activity has been focused on the clerodane diterpenes from Croton cajucara. Other diterpenes with anti-ulcerogenic effect include cordatin from Aparisthmium cordatum and trichorabdal A from Rabdosia trichocarpa (Schmeda-Hirschmann and Yesilada, 2005).

6. Conclusion

Gastric ulcer is a multi-factorial disease that has become a real socio-economic burden and opposes a great challenge in its treatment. Prevention is better than cure, as they say. Usage of medications designed for treatment of gastric ulcer as a means for its prevention is faced by several drawbacks; as limited effectiveness of these drugs in ulcer prevention, numerous side effects of available anti-ulcer drugs and the cost of gastric ulcer medications. Consequently, separate line of research has been devoted to investigate preventive measures of gastric ulcer. Despite of the size of investigations done on this subject, prevention of gastric ulcer is still a challenge especially in predisposed groups. Herbal compounds can provide an alternative preventive means for gastric ulcer as they are safer, cheaper and usually having limited, if any, side effects. For reaching the optimal remedy that can prevent gastric ulcer formation, more investigations are definitely still needed.

7. References

Abdiev, S.; Ahn, K.S.; Khadjibaev, A.; Malikov, Y.; Bahramov, S.; Rakhimov, B.; Sakamoto, J.; Kodera, Y.; Nakao, A. & Hamajima, N. (2010) Helicobacter pylori infection and cytokine gene polymorphisms in Uzbeks. *Nagoya J. Med. Sci.*, vol. 72, p.p. 167-172.

Aburaya, M.; Tanaka, K.; Hoshino, T.; Tsutsumi, S.; Suzuki, K.; Makise, M.; Akagi, R. & Mizushima, T. (2006). Heme oxygenase-1 protects gastric mucosal cells against non-steroidal anti-inflammatory drugs. *J. Biol. Chem.*, vol. 281, p.p. 33422-33432.

Adachi, M.; Horiuchi, G.; Ikematsu, N.; Tanaka, T.; Terao, J.; Satouchi, K. & Tokumura, A. (2011) Intragastrically Administered Lysophosphatidic Acids Protect Against Gastric Ulcer in Rats Under Water-Immersion Restraint Stress. *Dig. Dis. Sci.* [Epub ahead of print-PMID: 21298479].

Al-Howiriny, T.; Alsheikh, A.; Alqasoumi, S.; Al-Yahya, M.; ElTahir, K. & Rafatullah, S. (2010). Gastric antiulcer, antisecretory and cytoprotective properties of celery (Apium graveolens) in rats. *Pharm. Biol.*, vol. 48, p.p. 786-793.

Alam, M.S.; Alam, M.A.; Ahmad, S.; Najmi, A.K.; Asif, M. & Jahangir, T. (2010) Protective effects of Punica granatum in experimentally-induced gastric ulcers. *Toxicol. Mech. Methods*, vol. 20, p.p. 572-578.

Allen, A. & Flemstrom, G. (2005) Gastroduodenal mucus bicarbonate barrier: protection against acid and pepsin. *Am. J. Physiol Cell Physiol*, vol. 288, p.p. C1-19.

Alsarra, I.A.; Ahmed, M.O.; Alanazi, F.K.; Eltahir, K.E.; Alsheikh, A.M. & Neau, S.H. (2010). Influence of cyclodextrin complexation with NSAIDs on NSAID/cold stress-induced gastric ulceration in rats. *Int. J. Med. Sci.*, vol. 7, p.p. 232-239.

Arawwawala, M.; Thabrew, I.; Arambewela, L. & Handunnetti, S. (2010). Anti-inflammatory activity of Trichosanthes cucumerina Linn. in rats. *J. Ethnopharmacol.*, vol. 131, p.p. 538-543.

Banji, D.; Singh, J. & Banji, O.J. (2010). Scrutinizing the aqueous extract of leaves of pedalium murex for the antiulcer activity in rats. *Pak. J. Pharm. Sci.*, vol. 23, p.p. 295-299.

Chan, F.K. & Graham, D.Y. (2004). Review article: prevention of non-steroidal anti-inflammatory drug gastrointestinal complications--review and recommendations based on risk assessment. *Aliment. Pharmacol. Ther.*, vol. 19, p.p. 1051-1061.

Choi, S.R.; Lee, S.A.; Kim, Y.J.; Ok, C.Y.; Lee, H.J. & Hahm, K.B. (2009). Role of heat shock proteins in gastric inflammation and ulcer healing. *J. Physiol Pharmacol.*, vol. 60, Suppl. 7, p.p. 5-17.

da Silva, M.S.; de Almeida, A.C.; de Faria, F.M.; Luiz-Ferreira, A.; da Silva, M.A.; Vilegas, W.; Pellizzon, C.H. & Brito, A.R. (2010). Abarema cochliacarpos: gastroprotective and ulcer-healing activities. *J. Ethnopharmacol.*, vol. 132, p.p. 134-142.

de Sousa, F.H.; Leite, J.A.; Barbosa-Filho, J.M.; de Athayde-Filho, P.F.; de Oliveira Chaves, M.C.; Moura, M.D.; Ferreira, A.L.; de Almeida, A.B.; Souza-Brito, A.R.; de Fatima Formiga M.D. & Batista, L.M. (2008). Gastric and duodenal antiulcer activity of alkaloids: a review. *Molecules*, vol. 13, p.p. 3198-3223.

Eswaran, M.B.; Surendran, S.; Vijayakumar, M.; Ojha, S.K.; Rawat, A.K. & Rao, C. (2010). Gastroprotective activity of Cinnamomum tamala leaves on experimental gastric ulcers in rats. *J. Ethnopharmacol.*, vol. 128, p.p. 537-540.

Ganguly, K.; Sharma, A.V.; Reiter, R.J. & Swarnakar, S. (2010). Melatonin Promotes Angiogenesis During Protection and Healing of Indomethacin-Induced Gastric Ulcer: Role of Matrix Metaloproteinase-2. *J. Pineal Res.*, vol 49, p.p.130-140.

Graham, D.Y.; Javed, S.U.; Keihanian, S.; Abudayyeh, S. & Opekun, A.R. (2010). Dual proton pump inhibitor plus amoxicillin as an empiric anti-H. pylori therapy: studies from the United States. *J. Gastroenterol.*, vol. 45, p.p. 816-820.

Joseph, J.M.; Sowndhararajan, K. & Manian, S. (2010), Protective effects of methanolic extract of Hedyotis puberula (G. Don) R. Br. ex Arn. against experimentally induced gastric ulcers in rat. *J. Ethnopharmacol.*, vol. 131, p.p. 216-219.

Konturek, P.C.; Brzozowski, T.; Burnat, G.; Szlachcic, A.; Koziel, J.; Kwiecien, S.; Konturek, S.J. & Harsch, I.A. (2010). Gastric ulcer healing and stress-lesion preventive properties of pioglitazone are attenuated in diabetic rats. *J. Physiol Pharmacol.*, vol. 61, p.p. 429-436.

Lakshmi, V.; Singh, N.; Shrivastva, S.; Mishra, S.K.; Dharmani, P.; Mishra, V. & Palit, G. (2010). Gedunin and photogedunin of Xylocarpus granatum show significant anti-secretory effects and protect the gastric mucosa of peptic ulcer in rats. *Phytomedicine*, vol. 17, p.p. 569-574.

Lanas, A. (2008). Role of nitric oxide in the gastrointestinal tract. *Arthritis Res. Ther.*, vol. 10, Suppl. 2, p.p. S4.

Lanza, F.L.; Chan, F.K. & Quigley, E.M. (2009). Guidelines for prevention of NSAID-related ulcer complications. *Am. J. Gastroenterol.*, vol. 104, p.p. 728-738.

Lay, C.S. & Lin, C.J. (2010). Correlation of CYP2C19 genetic polymorphisms with helicobacter pylori eradication in patients with cirrhosis and peptic ulcer. *J. Chin Med. Assoc.*, vol. 73, p.p. 188-193.

Li, Y.; Xu, C.; Zhang, Q.; Liu, J.Y. & Tan, R.X. (2005). In vitro anti-Helicobacter pylori action of 30 Chinese herbal medicines used to treat ulcer diseases. *J. Ethnopharmacol.*, vol. 98, p.p. 329-333.

Lim, Y.J.; Lee, J.S.; Ku, Y.S. & Hahm, K.B. (2009). Rescue strategies against non-steroidal anti-inflammatory drug-induced gastroduodenal damage. *J. Gastroenterol. Hepatol.*, vol. 24, p.p. 1169-1178.

Majumdar, D.; Bebb, J. & Atherton, J. (2011). Helicobacter pylori infection and peptic ulcers. *Medicine*, vol. 39, p.p. 154-161.

Malfertheiner, P.; Chan, F.K. & McColl, K.E. (2009). Peptic ulcer disease. *Lancet*, vol. 374, p.p. 1449-1461.

Martin, G.R. & Wallace, J.L. (2006). Gastrointestinal inflammation: a central component of mucosal defense and repair. *Exp. Biol. Med. (Maywood)*, vol. 231, p.p. 130-137.

Melanchauski, L.S.; Broto, A.P.; Moraes, T.M.; Nasser, A.L.; Said, A.; Hawas, U.W.; Rashed, K.; Vilegas, W. & Hiruma-Lima, C.A. (2010). Gastroprotective and antisecretory effects of Ailanthus excelsa (Roxb). *J. Nat. Med.*, vol. 64, p.p. 109-113.

Morsy, M.; Ashour, O.; Amin, E. & Rofaeil, R. (2009). Gastroprotective effects of telmisartan on experimentally-induced gastric ulcers in rats. *Pharmazie*, vol. 64, p.p. 590-594.

Morsy, M.A.; Ashour, O.M.; Fouad, A.A. & Abdel-Gaber, S.A. (2010). Gastroprotective effects of the insulin sensitizers rosiglitazone and metformin against indomethacin-induced gastric ulcers in Type 2 diabetic rats. *Clin. Exp. Pharmacol. Physiol*, vol. 37, p.p. 173-177.

Morsy, M.A. & Fouad, A.A. (2008). Mechanisms of gastroprotective effect of eugenol in indomethacin-induced ulcer in rats. *Phytother. Res.*, vol. 22, p.p. 1361-1366.

Mota, K.S.; Dias, G.E.; Pinto, M.E.; Luiz-Ferreira, A.; Souza-Brito, A.R.; Hiruma-Lima, C.A.; Barbosa-Filho, J.M. & Batista, L.M. (2009). Flavonoids with gastroprotective activity. *Molecules.*, vol. 14, p.p. 979-1012.

Nakashima, S.; Ota, S.; Arai, S.; Yoshino, K.; Inao, M.; Ishikawa, K.; Nakayama, N.; Imai, Y.; Nagoshi, S. & Mochida, S. (2009). Usefulness of anti-ulcer drugs for the prevention and treatment of peptic ulcers induced by low doses of aspirin. *World J. Gastroenterol.*, vol. 15, p.p. 727-731.

Nayeb-Hashemi, H. & Kaunitz, J.D. (2009). Gastroduodenal mucosal defense. *Curr. Opin. Gastroenterol.*, vol. 25, p.p. 537-543.

Santhosh, K.B.; Tiwari, S.K.; Saikant, R.; Manoj, G.; Kunwar, A.; Sivaram, G.; Abid, Z.; Ahmad, A.; Priyadarsini, K.I. & Khan, A.A. (2010). Antibacterial and Ulcer Healing Effects of Organoselenium Compounds in Naproxen Induced and Helicobacter Pylori Infected Wistar Rat Model. *J. Trace Elem. Med. Biol.*, vol 24, p.p. 263-270.

Schmeda-Hirschmann, G. & Yesilada, E. (2005). Traditional medicine and gastroprotective crude drugs. *J. Ethnopharmacol.*, vol. 100, p.p. 61-66.

Shaker, E.; Mahmoud, H. & Mnaa, S. (2010). Anti-inflammatory and anti-ulcer activity of the extract from Alhagi maurorum (camelthorn). *Food Chem. Toxicol.*, vol. 48, p.p. 2785-2790.

Shoman, M.E.; Abdel-Aziz, M.; Aly, O.M.; Farag, H.H. & Morsy, M.A. (2009). Synthesis and investigation of anti-inflammatory activity and gastric ulcerogenicity of novel nitric oxide-donating pyrazoline derivatives. *Eur. J. Med. Chem.*, vol. 44, p.p. 3068-3076.

Sumbul, S.; Ahmad, M.A.; Asif, M.; Saud, I. & Akhtar, M. (2010). Evaluation of Myrtus communis Linn. berries (common myrtle) in experimental ulcer models in rats. *Hum. Exp. Toxicol.*, vol. 29, p.p. 935-944.

Sun, L.P.; Guo, X.L.; Zhang, Y.; Chen, W.; Bai, X.L.; Liu, J. & Yuan, Y. (2009). Impact of pepsinogen C polymorphism on individual susceptibility to gastric cancer and its precancerous conditions in a Northeast Chinese population. *J. Cancer Res. Clin. Oncol.*, vol. 135, p.p. 1033-1039.

Tahara, T.; Shibata, T.; Yamashita, H.; Hirata, I. & Arisawa, T. (2011). Influence of MDR1 polymorphism on H. pylori-related chronic gastritis. *Dig. Dis. Sci.*, vol. 56, p.p. 103-108.

Takeuchi, K. (2010). Prostaglandin EP receptors and their roles in mucosal protection and ulcer healing in the gastrointestinal tract. *Adv. Clin. Chem.*, vol. 51, p.p. 121-144.

Tomita, M.; Ando, T.; Minami, M.; Watanabe, O.; Ishiguro, K.; Hasegawa, M.; Miyake, N.; Kondo, S.; Kato, T.; Miyahara, R.; Ohmiya, N.; Niwa, Y. & Goto, H. (2009). Potential role for matrix metalloproteinase-3 in gastric ulcer healing. *Digestion,* vol. 79, p.p. 23-29.

Tulassay, Z. & Herszenyi, L. (2010). Gastric mucosal defense and cytoprotection. *Best. Pract. Res. Clin. Gastroenterol.*, vol. 24, p.p. 99-108.

University of Maryland Medical Center website. Accessed on 22 February, 2011. Available at http://www.umm.edu/patiented/articles/peptic_ulcers_000019.htm

Vasconcelos, P.C.; Andreo, M.A.; Vilegas, W.; Hiruma-Lima, C.A. & Pellizzon, C.H. (2010). Effect of Mouriri pusa tannins and flavonoids on prevention and treatment against experimental gastric ulcer. *J. Ethnopharmacol.*, vol. 131, p.p. 146-153.

Yoshida, N. & Yoshikawa, T. (2008). Basic and translational research on proteinase-activated receptors: implication of proteinase/proteinase-activated receptor in gastrointestinal inflammation. *J. Pharmacol. Sci.*, vol. 108, p.p. 415-421.

Zheng, Q.; Chen, W.J.; Lu, H.; Sun, Q.J. & Xiao, S.D. (2010). Comparison of the efficacy of triple versus quadruple therapy on the eradication of Helicobacter pylori and antibiotic resistance. *J. Dig. Dis.*, vol. 11, p.p. 313-318.

Part 3

Peptic Ulcer Management in Animals

12

Association Between Nonsteroidal Anti-Inflammatory Drugs and Gastric Ulceration in Horses and Ponies

Maria Verônica de Souza and José de Oliveira Pinto
Universidade Federal de Viçosa
Brazil

1. Introduction

Nonsteroidal anti-inflammatory drugs (NSAIDs) are widely employed in equine medicine to treat acute and chronic inflammation in tendon, ligament and musculoskeletal injuries, as well as after surgery (Cunningham & Lees, 1994; Lees et al., 2004; Dirikolu et al., 2008). These drugs are used because of their analgesic, anti-inflammatory, and anti-pyretic properties; they are also used as adjuvant therapy in the treatment of endotoxemia and to suppress platelet aggregation (Johnstone, 1983; MacAllister, 1994; MacAllister & Taylor-MacAllister, 1994; Mathews, 2002).

An ideal anti-inflammatory drug is potent and has few adverse effects. In fact, several of the commonly used NSAIDs have a narrow safety margin. It is imperative, therefore, to administer a correct dose at adequate intervals. Thus, use of these drugs for controlling pain in equine is recommended for well-hydrated animals aged over six weeks with normal oncotic pressure. Kidney and liver function should be normal, there should be no signs of gastric ulcers, and the animals should not be taking corticosteroids. Furthermore, two or more NSAIDs should not be given at the same time (Mathews, 2002).

It is essential to study in depth the adverse effects, the pharmacokinetics and pharmacodynamics of NSAIDs because of their side effects. The half-life of substances differs among species as a function of biotransformation pathways, drug metabolization time, associated disease (especially renal and hepatic conditions), age (younger animals have immature hepatic enzyme systems, whereas older animals have less efficient kidneys and livers), binding of NSAIDs to food components in the gastrointestinal tract, and association of NSAIDs with other drugs.

Studies on the relation between NSAIDs and gastric ulcers in equid species are complex because several factors may cause gastric injury: the physiological status of the stomach; a pH often below 2 (Murray, 1997, 1999); prolonged fasting (where the pH may be as low as 1.55) (Murray & Schusser, 1993); intense exercising in sports animals [which increases abdominal pressure, decreases stomach volume, and results in reflux of small intestine acids into the nonglandular mucosa (squamous mucosa) of the stomach] (Vatistas et al., 1999a; Lorenzo-Figueira & Merritt, 2002; McClure et al., 2005); diseases that cause loss of appetite or anorexia (Murray, 1999), and stress (confinement, administration of drugs, different environments, weaning), which may increase the level of circulating corticosteroids, in turn inhibiting the synthesis of prostaglandins and other chemical mediators, thereby generating favorable conditions for ulcers (MacKay et al., 1983; MacAllister et al., 1992; Andrews & Nadeau, 1999; Murray, 1999; Andrews et al., 2005; McClure et al., 2005; Pinto et al., 2009).

2. Types and mechanism of action of NSAIDs

There are several classifications of NSAIDs. These fall into five major chemical groups: carboxylic acid derivatives, enolic acid derivatives, specific cyclooxygenase 2 (COX-2) inhibitors, inhibitors of COX-2 with weak anti-inflammatory effect, and other nonsteroidal anti-inflammatory drugs. Carboxylic acid derivatives may be further subdivided into salicylic acids (e.g., aspirin and diflunisal), acetic acids (e.g., indomethacin, diclofenac, sulindac and eltenac), propionic acids (e.g., naproxen, ibuprofen, fenoprofen, flurbiprofen, ketoprofen and carprofen), aminonicotinic acids (e.g., flunixin meglumine), and fenamic acids (e.g., meclofenamic acid, sodium meclofenamate and mefenamic acid). Enolic acids may be subdivided into pyrazolones (e.g., phenylbutazone, monophenylbutazone, oxyphenbutazone, isopirin and apazone), and oxicam derivatives (e.g., piroxicam, droxicam, tenoxicam, and meloxicam). Selective COX-2 inhibitors are: celecoxib, etoricoxib, lumiracoxib, valdecoxib, parecoxib, firocoxib and nimesulide. Meloxicam and eltenac may be considered selective COX-2 inhibitors because of increased hepatic, renal and gastric tolerance in horses. Cyclooxygenase inhibitors with a weak anti-inflammatory effect include paracetamol and dipyrone. Other anti-inflammatory drugs not included in the above mentioned groups are dimethyl sulfoxide and glicosaminoglicans (Kore, 1990; Tasaka, 2006; Doucet et al., 2008; Burke et al., 2010).

After absorbing over 90% of NSAIDs bind to plasmatic proteins; the unbound fraction is biologically active (Tobin et al., 1986; Kore, 1990; Vicente, 2004). Most of these substances bind to albumin until saturation, at which point the concentration of the unbound fraction increases rapidly, which explains the relatively rapid onset of action of NSAIDs (Kore, 1990). According to Gerring et al. (1981), at least 98% of phenylbutazone is bound to plasma protein following administration at therapeutic doses.

Although NSAIDs are administered by several routes, they are generally metabolized by mixed function oxydase enzymes in the liver. A number of conjugated reactions are involved in eliminating these drugs. Excretion is primarily renal – glomerular filtration and tubular secretion – although some conjugates may be eliminated by the biliary tract. The excretion rate is often related with the pH; other weak acids may competitively inhibit secretory paths (Tobin et al., 1986; Kore, 1990; Vicente, 2004).

Effective plasmatic levels of NSAIDs administered orally are reached within an hour (Mathews, 2002). Several factors, however, may affect the absorption rate, such as the gastric pH, the presence of food, gastrointestinal motility, drug concentration, and the animal species (Kore, 1990; Mathews, 2002).

Phenylbutazone, an enolic acid pyrazolone derivative, is one of the most commonly used NSAIDs in equine medicine (Snow et al., 1979; Tobin et al., 1986; MacAllister et al., 1993; Kawcak, 2001; Dirikolu et al., 2008; Sabaté et al., 2009). This drug was synthesized by Stenzl in 1946 (Tasaka, 2006) and introduced into human medicine in 1949 for the treatment of rheumatoid arthritis, ankylosing spondylitis, and several other musculoskeletal conditions (Shearn, 1984). Because of its efficacy and low cost, it has been used mainly in horses since the 1950s (more specifically in 1952) for treating lameness caused by articular conditions, soft tissue diseases, and gastrointestinal colic (MacAllister et al., 1993; MacAllister, 1994; Vicente, 2004; Erkert et al., 2005; Tasaka, 2006). It is excreted unmetabolized in urine and as a metabolite of glucuronic acid oxidation and conjugation; the most relevant metabolites are oxyphenbutazone (active metabolite), γ-hydroxyphenylbutazone and γ-hydroxy-oxy-phenylbutazone (inactive metabolites) (MacAllister, 1994; Vicente, 2004; Igualada & Moragues, 2005).

Bioavailability studies have shown that the plasmatic kinetics of phenylbutazone is dose-dependent (Tobin et al., 1986). Sullivan & Snow (1982) compared in horses and ponies the intramuscular (2.5 mg/kg bwt) and enteral (5 mg/kg btw) routes for administering phenylbutazone and found that the absorption rate and bioavailability were slowed with intramuscular injections. These authors suggested that the drug precipitated in the neutral muscle pH. This property precludes intramuscular use because of binding to muscle proteins, which delays absorption and causes pain (Tasaka, 2006).

The plasmatic half-life of intravenously administered phenylbutazone in horses may range from 3.5 to 7.0 hours (Tobin et al., 1986; Lees et al., 1987; Vicente, 2004); it is about six hours in ponies (Snow et al., 1981). When administered orally, the phenylbutazone presents a variable, but longer half-life (3 to 10 h) (Tobin et al., 1986).

Regarding the mechanism of action of NSAIDs, it is known that following tissue damage (by trauma, hypoxia, toxins, endotoxins, etc.) short-chain fatty acids (such as arachidonic acid) are released from the cell membrane by phospholipase A_2 (Cunningham & Less, 1994; MacAllister, 1994; Lees et al., 2004, Tasaka, 2006). This enzyme works on cell membrane phospholipids to make arachidonic acid available for the enzymatic cascade involving cyclooxygenase or lipoxygenase in the cytoplasm (MacAllister, 1994; Tasaka, 2006). Cyclooxygenase 1 (COX-1) and COX-2 are the two cyclooxygenase isoforms that have been investigated in greater depth; there is an enzymatically active variant of the COX-1 gene named COX-3 (Smyth et al., 2010).

The COX-1 catalyzes the conversion of arachidonic acid into prostaglandins, which are involved in gastrointestinal, renal, and vascular physiological processes. COX-2 isoform produces an inflammatory response based on cytokines and inflammation mediators; the lipoxygenase cascade reaction yields primarily leukotrienes (Cunningham & Less, 1994; MacAllister, 1994; Jones & Blikslager, 2001; Lees et al., 2004; Tasaka, 2006; Smyth et al., 2010). COX-1 isoform is present in most tissues, and COX-2 is upregulated in monocytes, fibroblasts, synoviocytes, as well as chondrocytes in response to inflammatory stimuli (Johnston & Fox, 1997).

The majority of anti-inflammatory drugs block COX-1 and COX-2 to a greater or lesser extent (Tasaka, 2006; Burke et al., 2010). Studies have underlined the difficulty in separating the roles of COX-1 and COX-2 (Jones & Blikslager, 2001; Fitzpatrick et al., 2004); thus, the selectivity of these compounds is still controversial. Furthermore, some drugs may appear selective for an enzyme relative to another, but not potent. In fact truly selective or specific COX-2 inhibitors licensed for veterinary use are rare. Evidence suggests that phenylbutazone, flunixin meglumine and ketoprofen are not selective (Fitzpatrick et al., 2004; Burke et al., 2010; Pozzobon, 2010). Vicente (2004) has argued that phenylbutazone inhibit the COX-1 isoenzyme more than COX-2, where the inhibitory power of prostaglandin endoperoxide H synthase-1 (PGHS-1) is one to five times that of PGHS-2, resulting in adverse effects such as erosion or ulcers of the mucosa in the mouth and gastrointestinal tract, diffuse gastritis, hemorrhagic gastroenteritis, venous thrombosis, nephritis, and chronic renal injury, which have been widely discussed in the literature (Snow et al., 1981; MacAllister, 1983; Mathews, 2002; Fitzpatrick et al., 2004).

Price et al. (2002) argue that veterinarians working with small animals may be more concerned about the adverse effects of NSAIDs than those working with horses. The former prefer using carprofen and meloxicam, which appear to cause fewer side effects. These authors applied a questionnaire to 400 veterinary practitioners in the UK about pain management in horses. Of these 93 were used for data analysis; the data indicated that the four most frequently used analgesics in order of preference were: phenylbutazone (92%), flunixin meglumine (90%), butorphanol (89%), and dipyrone (75%). Phenylbutazone was preferred because of lower cost compared to other licensed NSAIDs. The analgesic potential was the most important criterion when choosing between NSAIDs or opioids.

Considering the analgesic potential of NSAIDs, the intravenous administration of single doses of phenylbutazone (4 mg/kg bwt), flunixin (1 mg/kg bwt) or carprofen (0.7 mg/kg bwt) to 63 horses for post-surgical pain was effective, but the mean required times for further analgesia were 8.4 h (phenylbutazone), 11.7 h (carprofen), and 12.8 h (flunixin) (Johnson et al., 1993). Erkert et al. (2005) compared the analgesic effect of phenylbutazone (4.4 mg/kg bwt at 24 h intervals) and flunixin meglumine (1.1 mg/kg bwt at 24 h intervals) in horses with the navicular syndrome and found similar responses among these drugs.

Sabaté et al. (2009) assessed the analgesic efficacy of suxibuzone and phenylbutazone for the treatment of pain caused by lameness in 155 horses aged from 2 to 25 years and body weight from 350 to 540 kg. All animals had acute or chronic nonspecific single limb lameness. The drugs were administered orally as follows: phenylbutazone (4.4 mg/kg bwt every 12 h) for 2 days, followed by phenylbutazone (2.2 mg/kg bwt every 12 h) for 6 days (n=79), and suxibuzone (6.6 mg/kg bwt every 12 h) for 2 days, followed by suxibuzone (3.3 mg/kg bwt every 12 h) for 6 days (n=76). The authors found no difference (P=0.113) between these treatments for pain relief in horses.

3. Gastric ulcers

Equine gastric ulceration is a highly prevalent multifactorial disease with vague and non-specific clinical signs. Abdominal pain, weight loss, and loss of performance may be seen. On the other hand, asymptomatic cases (Murray et al., 1987, MacAllister et al, 1992; MacAllister & Sangiab, 1993; Andrews & Nadeau, 1999; Murray et al., 2001; Murray & Pipers, 2001; Murray, 2002) diagnosed by gastroscopy have been described. Reports have shown a poor correlation between ulcer severity and clinical signs (Murray et al., 1987; MacAllister & Sangiab, 1993; Murray, 2002; Marqués, 2007; le Jeune et al., 2009); thus, animals with deeper lesions may have relatively mild signs, while others presenting with more significant abdominal discomfort may have only superficial erosions (Murray, 2002).

Murray et al. (2001) found asymptomatic gastric ulcers in 18 horses out of 209 animals that underwent gastroscopy. The practical experience of the authors of this chapter supports the above mentioned informations about clinical signs; monitoring ten ponies with untreated gastric ulcers (diffuse or localized hemorrhagic lesions), kept in free paddocks for eight months, revealed that 90% had no signs of bruxism, sialorrhea, decrease in appetite, rough hair-coat, diarrhea, abdominal discomfort, colic or any other sign of gastrointestinal tract involvement.

Studies have shown that foals may also develop gastric ulcers without apparent clinical manifestation (Murray et al., 1987; Marqués, 2007); thus, silent gastric ulceration is a common condition in these animals (Andrews & Nadeau, 1999). Léveillé et al. (1996) also reported a lack of clinical signs in three foals aged from 7 to 10 days that were given phenylbutazone 5 mg/kg bwt orally every 12 h during 7 days. On the other hand, necropsy revealed multifocal gastric ulcers.

Sports horses, such as performance and racehorses, have a high prevalence and severity of gastric ulcers (Hammond et al. 1986; Murray et al. 1989, 1996; Vatistas et al. 1999b; Pellegrini, 2005; Jonsson & Egenvall 2006; Orsini et al., 2009). A study conducted by Pellegrini (2005) showed that almost all performance horses have some kind of ulcer and that at least 60% of them have colonic ulcers. On the other hand, le Jeune et al. (2009) described the gastric ulceration syndrome in pregnant females (66.6%) and non-pregnant females (75.8%) kept free in irrigated pastures with alfalfa and grain supplements, but with no controlled physical activity. Luthersson et al. (2009) also reported this condition in nonracehorses.

Gastric ulcers may be found throughout the stomach of horses; the most commonly affected area is nonglandular mucosa – lined by stratified squamous epithelium – along the *margo plicatus* (Hammond et al., 1986; Murray et al., 1989, 1996; Andrews & Nadeau, 1999; Sandin et al., 2000; Ferrucci et al., 2003; Bruijn et al., 2009; le Jeune et al., 2009). The pathophysiology of ulcers consists of loss of equilibrium between aggressive factors (hydrochloric acid with or without synergistic action from volatile fatty acids, lactic acid, bile acids, and pepsin), and protective factors (mucus/bicarbonate barrier; prostaglandin E_2; adequate mucosal blood flow; cellullar restitution, and the epidermal growth factor) (Murray, 1992; Jeffrey et al., 2001; Andrews et al., 2005; Morrissey et al., 2008; Nadeau & Andrews, 2009).

Parietal cells produce a 10^6-times higher hydrogen ion concentration in gastric juices compared to plasma, a process that requires carbonic anhydrase, which catalyzes the reaction between water and carbon dioxide. Sodium bicarbonate – resulting from dissociated carbonic acid (H_2CO_3) – is transferred into the plasma from parietal cells; this process involves its exchange for chloride ions (Cl^-) by means of an HCO_3^-/Cl^- carrier protein in the basolateral membrane. The absorbed Cl^- moves to the apical membrane, exits through canaliculi, and enters the intestinal glands. Carbonic anhydrase-generated hydrogen ions are actively secreted by the membrane in apical cells into the lumen of the gland. This ion exchange process makes it possible for parietal cells to maintain a constant pH and at the same time a highly acid solution in the gastric lumen (Randall et al., 2000).

Gastrin, histamine (H_2 receptors), and acethycholine (vagus nerve) stimulate the H^+,K^+-ATPase enzyme, which in turn causes parietal cells in gastric glands to secrete chloridric acid (Andrews et al., 2005; Videla & Andrews, 2009). The stomach of adult horse secretes about 1.5 l/h of gastric juices, which contains 4–60 mMol of hydrochloric acid. The feeding regimen and the region of the stomach that is measured alter the pH of the gastric content (Luthersson et al., 2009). Andrews & Nadeau (1999) found that the pH was stratified, being neutral in the dorsal portion of the esophageal region, more acid (from 3 to 6) close to the *margo plicatus*, and even lower (from 1.5 to 4.0) close to the pylorus. The pH of the gastric content in continuously fed equines may remain around 3.1; in fasting animals, the pH may reach 1.6 (Murray & Schusser, 1993).

Studies have shown that freely grazing horses continuously produce large amounts of bicarbonate-rich saliva as a response to chewing, which has an important gastric acid buffering effect (Murray et al., 1996; Andrews & Nadeau, 1999; Andrews et al., 2005; le Jeune et al., 2009; Martineau et al., 2009; Videla & Andrews, 2009). On the other hand, the prevalence of ulcers did not differ significantly in full-time stabled horses, part-time stabled horses, or animals kept full-time on pastures (Bell et al., 2007).

Several ulcer-classifying systems based on the number and severity of lesions have been developed (Hammond et al., 1986; Murray et al., 1987; Johnson et al., 1994; Vatistas et al., 1994; Murray & Eichorn, 1996; MacAllister et al., 1997; Anon, 1999). Murray et al. (1987) characterized ulcers by location (nonglandular surface, *margo plicatus*, glandular surface) and severity. Lesions were graded from 0 to 4 (0=normal, 1=1-2 localized lesions, 2=3-5 localized ulcers or 1 diffuse lesion, 3=1-5 localized lesions with visible hemorrhage or multiple diffuse lesions with apparent mild to moderate loss of surface epithelium, and 4=greater than 5 localized ulcers or multiple diffuse lesions with apparent extensive loss of surface epithelium and/or hemorrhage).

Risk factors associated with this disease include diet, stress (moving horses from pasture to stall confinement, hospitalization, intense exercise, feed and water deprivation, among others), and administering NSAIDs (le Jeune et al., 2009, Luthersson et al., 2009; Nadeau & Andrews, 2009; Videla & Andrews, 2009) (the topic of this chapter). Reported factors related with disease prevalence in racehorses include a high-concentrate diet, low intake of hay, meal feeding, prolonged fasting, the type and intensity of training, as well as the use of NSAIDs (Vatistas et al., 1999a; Merritt, 2003; Roy et al., 2005; Jonsson & Egenvall, 2006). Studies on the relationship between NSAIDs and equine gastric ulcer are complex because of these many factors. Use of these drugs in human patients increases 3- and 5-fold the risk of peptic ulcers respectively in *H. pylori*-positive and *H. pylori*-negative patients (Voutilainen et al., 2001).

NSAID-induced gastric ulceration in horses was described in the late 1970s; phenylbutazone has been studied in greatest detail (Snow et al., 1979, Snow et al., 1981; MacAllister, 1983; Collins & Tyler, 1984; Tobin et al., 1986; Vicente, 2004). Studies describing the side effects of flunixin meglumine, ketoprofen and phenylbutazone started to be published in the 1980s (Trillo et al., 1984; MacAllister et al., 1992; MacAllister, 1994; MacAllister & Taylor-MacAllister, 1994). Other drugs, such as suxibuzone (a prophenylbutazone drug), firocoxib, monophenylbutazone (phenylbutazone-derivate), acetylsalicylic acid, eltenac, nimesulide and meloxicam, have also been studied (Prügner et al., 1991; Goodrich et al., 1998; Monreal et al., 2004; Villa et al., 2007; Andrews et al., 2009; Sabaté et al., 2009; Videla & Andrews, 2009; Pozzobon, 2010). Nevertheless, studies of phenylbutazone (or derivatives) have not been abandoned, possibly because of ulcerogenic effect and therapeutic efficacy (Vicente, 2004; Driessen, 2007). As mentioned previously, the nonsteroidal anti-inflammatory drugs are widely employed in equine clinical practice to treat acute and chronic inflammatory conditions, especially of the locomotor apparatus (Prügner et al., 1991; Jones & Blikslager, 2001; Sabaté et al., 2009; Videla & Andrews, 2009).

Gastric injury usually occurs when NSAIDs are given at high doses or prolonged treatments (Snow et al., 1979, 1981; MacAllister, 1983; MacKay et al., 1983); nevertheless, therapeutic doses have been known to cause ulcers in horses. The most widely accepted hypothesis for the association between NSAIDs and gastric ulcers is cyclooxygenase inhibition (See item 2 – Types and mechanism of actions of NSAIDs), in which conversion of arachidonic acid into prostaglandins is blocked (MacAllister, 1983; MacAllister et al., 1993; Murray, 1999). The physiologic vasodilating effect of prostaglandins (in particular PGE_2) on the stomach mucosa generates a bicarbonate buffering system that attenuates the corrosive action of hydrochloric acid contained in gastric secretions (Andrews & Nadeau, 1999; Murray, 1999; Morrissey et al., 2008). These substances increase gastric mucosa blood flow and mucus secretion, and reduce gastric acid production. They also facilitate basal cell migration towards the lumen for repairing the mucosa and maintaining the integrity of nonglandular and glandular mucosa; this takes place by stimulation of active surface-protecting phospholipid production. Inhibition of prostaglandin synthesis may give rise to ideal conditions for ulcers in the gastrointestinal tract (Andrews & Nadeau, 1999; Murray & Pipers, 2001; Andrews et al., 2005). According to Andrews et al. (2005), gastric mucosal ischemia may lead to hypoxia-induced cellular acidosis, and release of oxygen-free radicals, phospholipases and proteases, which may damage the cell membrane and result in necrosis.

As mentioned previously, the majority of NSAIDs are poorly selective, inhibiting COX-1 and COX-2 equally (Fitzpatrick et al., 2004; Vicente, 2004). Drugs that inhibit COX-1 are considered the main causative of stomach lesions, because this enzyme is generally – but not exclusively – responsible for the above mentioned adverse effects on the gastrointestinal tract (Jones & Blikslager, 2001; Lees et al., 2004; Videla & Andrews, 2009). Although the ulcer-causing potential may vary among NSAIDs, a study of rat stomachs with normal mucosa after acid challenge showed that inhibition of both cyclooxygenases causes gastrointestinal injury; however, inhibition of only one of these enzymes did not have this effect (Gretzer et al., 2001). Furthermore, administering NSAIDs on an empty stomach may result in local gastric irritation. Therefore, these drugs should be administered with food when given orally (Mathews, 2002; Lees et al., 2004; Monreal et al., 2004).

The site of NSAID-induced ulcers in the stomach of horses remains controversial. Some authors have stated that the glandular mucosa is more commonly affected (Carrick et al., 1989; Vatistas et al., 1999a; Monreal et al., 2004; Marqués, 2007; le Jeune et al., 2009), while others have argued that the nonglandular mucosa is affected more frequently (MacAllister et al., 1992; Andrews et al., 2005). According to Mokhber Dezfouli et al. (2009), Persian Arab horses with history of long term treatment with NSAIDs have high prevalence of the gastric ulcer in the glandular mucosa. In addition, it has been documented that phenylbutazone can cause severe ulceration of the glandular gastric mucosa following administration at high dosages for as short as a few days (Collins & Tyler, 1985; Lees, 2003). Moreover, according to Andrews et al. (2005), 80% of ulcers induced by phenylbutazone are located in the nonglandular mucosa.

MacAllister et al. concluded 1992 that flunixin meglumine (1.5 mg/kg bwt intramuscularly every 8 hours for 6 days) may result in ulcers of the nonglandular mucosa of ponies. In 1993, MacAllister et al. reported ulcers in the nonglandular and glandular mucosa of horses. The authors compared the adverse effects of phenylbutazone (4.4 mg/kg bwt), flunixin meglumine (1.1 mg/kg bwt) and ketoprofen (2.2 mg/kg bwt) given intravenously every 8 hours in horses during 12 days. The phenylbutazone presented the highest ulcerogenic potential of these three drugs. Other studies of horses and ponies revealed that the effect of NSAIDs on the nonglandular mucosa is less evident or undetected, and if there is pain, it is generally mild (Snow et al., 1979, 1981; MacKay et al., 1983).

The glandular region has adequate blood flow, cell restitution, mucus-bicarbonate layer, prostaglandin secretion, and growth factors (Murray, 1997; Andrews et al., 2005; Marqués, 2007; Nadeau & Andrews, 2009). The nonglandular mucosa has a thinner layer, no mucus-bicarbonate layer, and often desquamation in foals aged over 35 days, and may remain in the first month of life (MacAllister et al., 1992; Murray et al., 1987; Andrews & Nadeau, 1999; Andrews et al., 2005, Murray, 1997). This region is constantly exposed to chloridric acid, pepsin and bile acids (Andrews & Nadeau, 1999; Murray, 1999). Besides the stomach, the phenylbutazone-induced ulcers may occur in the intestine – with reports in the duodenum (Snow et al., 1979; Snow et al., 1981; MacAllister et al., 1993), ceco, colon and rectum (MacAllister, 1983, Ruoff et al., 1987, Boothe, 2001).

Meschter et al. (1984) has stated that the primary target of phenylbutazone intoxication in horses is the wall of smaller veins. Other changes (ulcers on the tongue, stomach and intestine, as well as renal necrosis and venous thrombosis) should be interpreted as being secondary to vein lesions. In 1990, Meschter et al. suggested that phenylbutazone-induced gastrointestinal ulceration results from direct toxic injury to endothelial cells within the microvasculature of the mucosa. Vascular tumefaction, stagnation and cessation of blood flow, formation of fibrin, perivascular extravasation with subsequent edema, thrombosis and necrosis of the mucosa occur; finally, the mucosal epithelium breaks down. These authors argued that vasoconstriction is not the primary cause of mucosal necrosis; once formed erosions and ulcers, they could persist because of other non-prostaglandin-mediated processes, such as bacterial invasion (Nadeau & Andrews, 2009). Murray (1999) added that NSAIDs appear to cause neutrophils to adhere to the vascular endothelium of the gastric mucosa, thereby reducing mucosal perfusion and releasing chemical mediators that add further damage. Doherty et al. (2003) have suggested that phenylbutazone does not alter the baseline secretion of gastric acid in horses; rather, it decreases lipopolysaccharide-induced effects on the volume of secretions and on sodium production, and concentration in parietal cells.

4. Some experimental studies of NSAIDs

After identifying the types and mechanisms of cyclooxygenases, several studies aimed to discover NSAIDs with appropriate analgesic, antipyretic and anti-inflammatory properties and minimal ulcer-generating effects (MacAllister et al., 1993; Cunningham & Lees, 1994; MacAllister, 1994). However, these drugs should currently be used with caution in horses, as animal studies have shown varying results. There are several risk factors – especially stress – associated with gastric ulceration; these factors may potentiate the ulcerogenic effect of NSAIDs during experiments. A description is given below of selected experimental studies showing associations, or lack thereof, between nonsteroidal anti-inflammatory drugs and gastric ulceration in equid species.

Snow et al. (1981) conducted an experiment with horses and ponies in which oral phenylbutazone (8.2 mg/kg bwt) was administered every 24 h during 13 days to six horses; also, the same drug at 10 to 12 mg/kg bwt every 24 h was administered to nine ponies during 6 to 8 days. All horses remained apparently healthy, but five ponies developed depression, hyporexia, weight loss, loose feces, and mouth ulcers; two ponies died. A biochemical analysis showed progressive decrease in total plasma proteins and albumin, a significant elevation of blood urea nitrogen, and a decrease in calcium and potassium concentrations. The authors suggested that ponies were more susceptible to the adverse effects of phenylbutazone.

The manufacturer's daily recommended dose of phenylbutazone for horses is 4.4 to 8.8 mg/kg bwt orally, and 2.2 to 4.4 mg/kg bwt intravenously (MacAllister, 1994). The risk of intoxication may increase when phenylbutazone is administered at daily doses above 8.8 mg/kg bwt for more than four days (MacKay et al., 1983). According to Hu et al. (2005), considering the toxicity of phenylbutazone, the higher dosage (8.8 mg/kg) may not be beneficial in chronically lame horses, because this dose was not associated with greater analgesic effects compared to 4.4 mg/kg dose in quarter horse-type breeding studied by Oklahoma State University (USA). In fact, the most commonly used analgesic dose for equine in the clinical setting is 2-4.4 mg/kg bwt given intravenously or orally every 12 h (Robinson & Sprayberry, 2009), for 5 to 7 days.

Although the dose of 4.4 mg phenylbutazone/kg bwt is considered safe to use in horses (Taylor et al., 1983; Tobin et al., 1986), the oral administration of this dosage every 12 h with concurrent intravenous administration of flunixin meglumine (1.1 mg/kg bwt every 12 h) for 5 days resulted in acute necrotizing colitis, with lesions most severe in the right dorsal colon in one of 29 adult horses (Keegan et al., 2008). According to the authors, considering that the drugs were lower than those that reportedly cause toxic effects, it is likely that it was the combination of NSAIDs, as well as the total increase in concentration irrespective of type, that was responsible for these abnormalities. On the other hand, neonatal foals (two days old) treated with recommended dosage of flunixin meglumine (1.1 mg/kg bwt/day) for five days, did not have clinicopathological or pathological differences compared to treatment with physiological saline, but the dose of 6.6 mg/kg/day increased total gastrointestinal ulceration, gastric ulceration and cecal petechiation (Carrick et al., 1989).

Administrating high doses of phenylbutazone (10 mg/kg btw) daily for ponies (Snow et al., 1979) and foals (Traub et al., 1983), and 8 mg/kg bwt daily for adult horses (Ruoff et al., 1987) resulted in ulcers in different parts of the gastrointestinal tract (from lips and tongue to the rectum), and marked edema and inflammation of the small intestine, colon, and rectum. In addition, MacAllister (1983) administered phenylbutazone 10 mg/kg bwt orally every 24 h to ten ponies during 14 days and found that seven animals were intoxicated, characterized by anorexia, oral ulcers, soft feces, and depression; six animals died, one of which by euthanasia. Necropsy revealed gastrointestinal ulcers, enteritis, necrotic colitis, peritonitis, and renal papillary necrosis.

Monreal et al. (2004) found ulcers on the glandular gastric mucosa in 100% of mix-breed horses (aged from 2 to 16 years, and body weight from 288 to 527 kg) treated with high doses of phenylbutazone (10.5 mg/kg bwt every 12 h, for two days, followed by 5.25 mg/kg bwt every 12 h, for 12 additional days); the same findings were present in only 40% of suxibuzone-treated animals (15 mg/kg bwt every 12 h, for two days, followed by 7.5 mg/kg bwt every 12 h, for another 12 days); the ulcers were significantly larger and deeper in the animals that were given phenylbutazone. Conversely, histopathology studies revealed similar inflammation when comparing these two drugs; there was severe neutrophilic inflammatory infiltration and signs of a healing reaction in both groups of animals. According to these authors, ulcers in the oral cavity, softened feces, anorexia, weight loss, hypoproteinemia and hypoalbuminemia, considered classical signs of phenylbutazone toxicosis, were seen in one horse only. Further, small mouth ulcers were encountered in two animals in the suxibuzone group.

Andrews et al. (2009) evaluated the gastric ulcerogenic effect of a top-dress formulation containing suxibuzone or phenylbutazone for 18 adult horses aged from 3 to 14 years and body weights ranging from 294 to 467 kg in study conducted at the Louisiane State University (USA). There were three groups: a control group, a group given phenylbutazone (2.6 mg/kg bwt), and a group given suxibuzone (3.5 mg/kg bwt), during 15 consecutive days. Gastric ulcers in the phenylbutazone-treated group were not more severe than those in the suxibuzone-treated group, suggesting that suxibuzone has no advantage over phenylbutazone in preventing gastric ulcers at recommended label doses.

Prügner et al. (1991) reported that intravenous administration of eltenac (1 mg/kg bwt at 24 h intervals) during three days was more effective (P<0.001) in reducing pain caused by lameness of several causes (tendinitis, pododermatitis, navicular disease, non-infectious arthritis, etc.) in 32 horses compared to placebo controls (n=32). Goodrich et al. (1998) studied this same drug in four groups of six horses given different doses (0.5, 1.5, 2.5 mg/kg bwt or sterile saline solution every 24 h for 15 days), and found that it was not toxic for the gastrointestinal tract at a dose of 0.5 mg/kg bwt; the authors concluded that eltenac might be beneficial for horses.

Videla & Andrews (2009) reviewed firocoxib, an NSAID approved for controlling pain and inflammation due to osteoarthritis in horses. This drug (0.1 mg/kg bwt orally every 24 hours, for 30 days) did not cause ulcers in the study sample. These authors suggested that the efficacy of firocoxib in horses with abdominal pain is unknown, and that it should not be administered to animals with abdominal discomfort and gastric reflux or dysphagia, as there is currently no systemic formulation of the drug. According to Doucet et al. (2008), firocoxib appears to be a safe alternative to the long-term use of phenylbutazone in horses.

Loew et al. (1985) stated that monophenylbutazone is five to six times less toxic than phenylbutazone, but it is less effective when given at the same dose. Pinto et al. (2009) studied whether monophenylbutazone was associated or not with gastric ulcers in ponies in a two-step experiment conducted at the Universidade Federal de Viçosa (Brazil). The first step consisted of three groups of two healthy ponies each, treated with daily intravenous doses (3, 4.5 or 6 mg/kg bwt during 12 days) of the drug. One pony in each group was given omeprazole (3 mg/kg bwt orally every day). The second step, conducted six month after the first, consisted of two groups, each with two healthy ponies; the first group was given monophenylbutazone 4.5 mg/kg bwt intravenous daily for 12 days, and the second group was given 5 mL of 0.9% NaCl intravenously. All ponies underwent endoscopy before and after the trial. At the end of the first step, endoscopy revealed nonglandular gastric mucosa ulcers along the *margo plicatus* (Fig. 1) only in the two animals that were given the highest dosage (6 mg/kg bwt) of the drug. However, the occurrence of ulcers was unrelated with the dose (P>0.05). The authors suggested that individual variation, confinement stress, daily handling, and administration itself of the drug, may have contributed to the number and severity of ulcers, a situation that has already been reported by other authors (MacAllister et al., 1992; Murray, 1999; Andrews et al., 2005). le Jeune et al. (2009) have suggested that stress may be a major contributing factor to ulcer development.

In the second step of Pinto et al.'s (2009) study, two animals developed gastric ulcers, one of which had been given monophenylbutazone (4.5 mg/kg bwt during 12 days) (Fig. 2); the

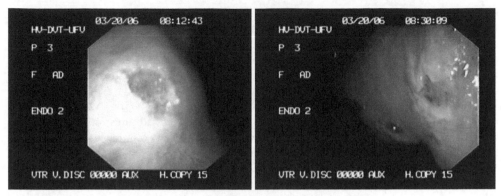

Fig. 1. Ulcers on the nonglandular gastric mucosa of a pony treated intravenously during 12 consecutive days with monophenylbutazone (6 mg/kg bwt every 24 h).

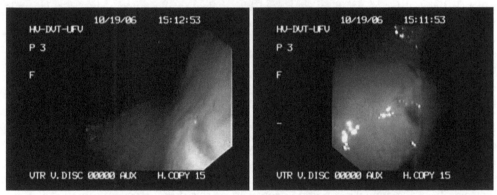

Fig. 2. Ulcers on the nonglandular gastric mucosa of a pony treated intravenously during 12 consecutive days with monophenylbutazone (4.5 mg/kg bwt every 24 h).

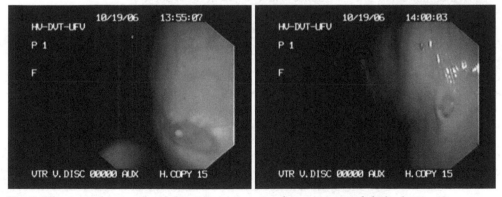

Fig. 3. Ulcers on the nonglandular gastric mucosa of a pony treated daily during 12 consecutive days with 5 mL of 0.9% NaCl intravenously.

other pony that presented gastric ulcers had been given only 5 mL of 0.9% NaCl intravenously, during 12 days (Fig. 3). Monophenylbutazone did not influence the occurrence of ulcers (P>0.05). The authors suggested that the discomfort associated with daily intravenous injections of saline solution may have generated enough stress to cause ulcers. MacAllister et al. (1992) also suggested an association between stress and application of medication, in a study where flunixin meglumine (1.5 mg/kg bwt every 8 h during 6 days) was given intramuscularly to ponies. MacAllister et al. (1993) encountered similar results when comparing the occurrence of ulcers following administration of flunixin meglumine and 0.9% NaCl to horses; there were no significant differences between these two groups.

Vatistas et al. (1999a) studied stress in thrirty mature Thoroughbred horses and suggested that the following situations could raise serum cortisol concentrations: road transport, exposure to a new environment, abrupt weaning in foals, physical restraint, anesthesia, nasogastric intubation, and diseases in general. Costa el al. (2007) have argued that the pathophysiology of stress-induced gastric mucosal injury remains controversial; the main suggested causal factor has been decreased blood flow in the mucosa due to splanchnic vasoconstriction associated with increased sympathetic tonus and an increased level of circulating catecholamines. Furthermore, increased endogenous corticosteroid concentrations during stress may inhibit prostaglandin synthesis. As mentioned previously, decreased prostaglandin levels result in loss of balance in mucosal protective factors; this is commonly stated as the primary cause of ulcers in foals and adult horses (Andrews & Nadeau, 1999; Andrews et al., 2005).

Villa et al. (2007) evaluated the pharmacokinetics and pharmacodynamics of nimesulide in 15 healthy horses aged from 3 to 6 years. The animals were divided into three groups. Group A was given nimesulide (1.5 mg/kg bwt) orally and intravenously; groups B and C were given nimesulide (1 mg/kg bwt) orally once. According to the authors, a 1.5 mg/kg bwt dose may yield the desired effects when administered every 12 or 24 h, depending on the severity of the animal's condition. However, as this dose exceeds the *in vitro* IC_{50} for cyclooxygenase 1 and 2 isoforms (see item 2 – Types and mechanism of action of NSAIDs), the selectivity is lost, which results in side effects due to COX-1 inhibition. Thus, the authors suggest that nimesulide should be used with caution in equid species.

Pozzobon (2010) assessed the side effects of meloxicam on the gastric mucosa and semen of six healthy ponies at the Universidade Federal de Santa Maria (Brazil). Two animals were treated with meloxicam (0.6 mg/kg bwt, orally) for 30 days, two were treated with ketoprofen (2.2 mg/kg bwt, orally) for 30 days, and two were not given anti-inflammatory drugs. The experiment was repeated three times, alternating the ponies per groups according to a Latin square design; thus, all animals were given all treatments. The study lasted 15 weeks, with a one-week interval between treatments. Gastroscopy done at the end of the study did not reveal gastric mucosal disease, even though the concentration of total prostaglandins in the seminal plasma was decreased (P<0.05) and the quality of semen was negatively affected; the findings suggested a physiological effect of COX-2 on the reproductive tissues of stallions.

Gastric ulcers have also been reported in donkeys from South West of England. Burden et al. (2009) examined at necropsy 426 non-working aged donkeys, and found that 41% of these animals had gastric ulcers. The mean age of the animals was 30.5 years; the study took two years. The majority (n=96; 49%) were medium-sized ulcers (> 2 cm^2; < 10 cm^2), located mainly on the nonglandular mucosa along the *margo plicatus* (n=155; 89%). Information on NSAID use (e.g., phenylbutazone, flunixin meglumine, meloxicam, etc.) was available for 418 animals (98%); 214 donkeys (50.2%) in the study had been given NSAIDs for at least 7 days immediately prior to death, and the majority of animals had been given these drugs for months or years. The authors, however, found no relation (P=0.9) between the risk of having gastric ulcers on the glandular mucosa and use of NSAIDs in these animals.

There is an ongoing search for new analgesic and anti-inflammatory drugs because of the adverse effects of NSAIDs. Videla & Andrews (2009) have recommended xylazine (0.2-0.4 mg/kg bwt) or detomidine (20-40 μg/kg btw) as alternatives to NSAIDs, since these drugs are good analgesics and have minimal effects on the gastrointestinal tract. However, these drugs have other side effects or may increase the cost of therapy. These same authors have suggested that the choice of NSAIDs for horses should take into account the following criteria: minimal side effects on the gastrointestinal tract, the minimal pain-controlling dose, and use of an anti-ulcer drug together with the anti-inflammatory medication.

Drugs for treating ulcers in equid species have been investigated; this is a complex topic, to be addressed in another chapter of this book. However, the authors of the current chapter believe it is important to report their study with omeprazole, a drug that binds irreversibly to the H$^+$, K$^+$-ATPase enzyme of gastric parietal cells (which secrete hydrogen ions into the stomach in exchange for K$^+$ ions), thereby inhibiting the production of chloridric acid. Omeprazole also selectively inhibits carbonic anhydrase, which adds to its acid suppressive properties (Daurio et al., 1999; MacAllister, 1999). Although this drug is considered the most effective inhibitor of gastric secretions (90% in 24 hour at 4 mg/kg bwt daily), it has a low bioavailability after oral intake (14-16%) (Andrews et al., 1992; Téllez et al., 2005). Murray et al. (1997) showed that the healing time of gastric ulcers was significantly shorter in horses given omeprazole (1.5 mg/kg bwt orally) daily during 28 days. MacAllister (1999) suggested that healing of ulcers using this drug appears to depend on the dose and duration of therapy; an oral dose of 4 mg/kg bwt daily during 28 days appears to have the highest success rate.

Pinto et al. (2008) administered omeprazole 4 mg/kg bwt orally for 31 consecutive days to verify its efficacy for healing gastric ulcers (score 1 to 4 in Murray et al., 1987) on the nonglandular mucosa of three ponies. Three other ponies with ulcers were controls, and were managed similarly except for therapy. At the end of the treatment, gastroscopy showed that the three controls no longer had ulcers, but two animals treated with omeprazole had marked granulomatous tissue over the ulcerated area (Figs. 4-5). Histopathology revealed tissue necrosis, fibrinous-leukocyte exudates, and exuberant granulation tissue. One of the fragments had hyperplastic squamous epithelium within the ulcer. In addition, filamentous structures similar to bacteria and spores of *Candida sp* were observed. The animals remained symptom-free throughout the treatment. Local *Candida sp* colonization may have been due to nearly complete omeprazole-induced inhibition of gastric acid secretion. Prim & Vila (2002) described a case of oropharyngeal candidiasis in a patient aged 65 years given omeprazole 20 mg daily. There are no reports of granulomas following the use of omeprazole in equid species, but findings suggesting enterochromaffin-like cell hyperplasia has been noted, and gastric carcinoid tumors has been observed in rats (Hoogerwerf & Pasricha, 2001). The exuberant granulomatous tissues were regressing gradually until complete disappearance from 60 to 100 days after their identification (Fig 6).

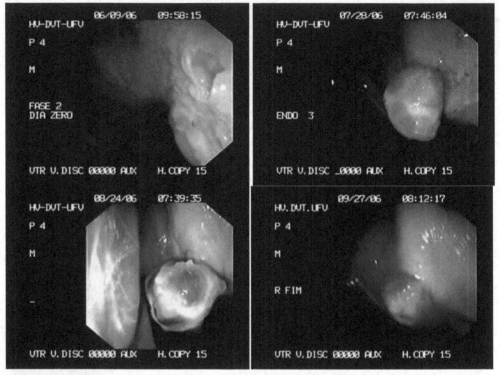

Fig. 4. Exuberant granulomatous tissue in a pony with gastric ulcers treated with omeprazole 4 mg/kg bwt orally for 31 days. The images show the monthly monitoring of the injury.

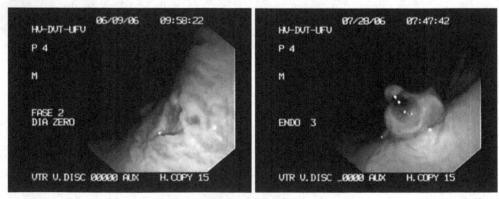

Fig. 5. Another granulomatous tissue at the ulcer on the nonglandular gastric mucosa, in pony treated with omeprazole (4 mg/kg bwt orally for 31 days).

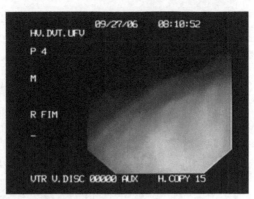

Fig. 6. Aspect of nonglandular gastric mucosa shown in Fig. 5, with complete disappearance of the granulomatous tissue about three months after its identification.

5. Conclusion

Nonsteroidal anti-inflammatory drugs are very useful for treating many clinical and surgical conditions in horses and ponies. Despite the significant amount of research, there is no single NSAID that is considered completely safe. Therefore, while the ideal drug is not discovered, careful measures (dose, application interval, and duration of treatment) should be taken when using these drugs, which are considered relevant risk factors for the gastric ulceration syndrome.

6. References

Andrews, F.M., Buchanan, B.R., Elliot, S.B., Clariday, N.A. & Edwards, L.H. (2005). Gastric ulcers in horses. *Journal of Animal Science*, Suppl.83, November, pp.8-21, ISSN: 0021-8812.

Andrews, F.M., Jenkins, C.C., Blackford, J.T., Frazier, D.L., Olovsson, S.G. & Mattsson, H. (1992). Effect of oral omeprazole on basal and pentagastrin-stimulated gastric secretion in young female horse. *Equine Veterinary Journal*, Suppl.13, August, pp.80-83, ISSN: 0425-1644.

Andrews, F.M. & Nadeau, J.A. (1999). Clinical syndromes of gastric ulceration in foals and mature horses. *Equine Veterinary Journal*, Vol.31, No.29, April, pp.30-33, ISSN: 0425-1644.

Andrews, F.M., Reinemeyer, C.R. & Longhofer, S.I. (2009). Effects of top-dress formulations of suxibuzone and phenylbutazone on development of gastric ulcers in horses. *Veterinary Therapeutics*, Vol.10, No.3, pp.113-120, ISSN: 1528-3593.

Anon (1999). The equine gastric ulcer concil: Recommendations for the diagnosis and treatment of equine gastric ulcer syndrome (EGUS). *Equine Veterinary Education*, Vol.11, No.5, October, pp.262-272, ISSN: 0957-7734.

Bell, R.J., Mogg, T.D. & Kingston, J.K. (2007). Equine gastric ulcer syndrome in adult horses: a review. New Zealand Veterinary Journal, Vol.55, No.1, February, pp.1-12, ISSN: 0048-0169.

Boothe, D.M. (2001). The analgesic, antipyretic, anti-inflammatory drugs, In: Veterinary Pharmacology and Therapeutics, Adams, H.R., pp. 433-451, Iowa State University Press, ISBN: 0-8138-1743-9, Iowa, USA.

Bruijn, C.M., Schutrups, A.H. & Seesing, E.H.A. (2009). Prevalence of equine gastric ulceration syndrome in Standardbreds. Veterinary Record, Vol.164, No.26, pp.814-815, ISSN: 0042-4900.

Burden, F.A., Gallagher, J., Thiemann, A.K. & Trawford, A.F. (2009). Necropsy survey of gastric ulcers in a population of aged donkeys: prevalence, lesion description and risk factors. Animal, Vol.3, No.2, February, pp.287-293, ISSN: 1751-7311.

Burke, A., Smyth, E.M. & FitzGerald, G.A. (2010). Analgésicos-antipiréticos farmacoterapia da gota, In: Goodman & Gilman. As Bases Farmacológicas da Terapêutica, Lazo, J.S. & Parker, K.L., pp.601-638, AMGH Editora Ltda, ISBN: 0-07-142280-3, São Paulo, Brazil.

Carrick, J.B., Papich, M.G., Middleton, D.M., Naylor, J.M. & Townsend, H.G.G. (1989). Clinical and pathological effects of flunixin meglumine administration to neonatal foals. Canadian Journal of Veterinary Research, Vol.53, No.2, April, pp.195-201. ISSN: 0830-9000.

Collins, L.G. & Tyler, D.E. (1984). Phenylbutazone toxicosis in the horse: a clinical study. Journal of American of Veterinary Medical Association, Vol.184, No.6, March, pp.699-703, ISSN: 0003-1488.

Collins L.G. & Tyler, D.E. (1985). Experimentally induced phenylbutazone toxicosis in ponies: description of the syndrome and its prevention with synthetic prostaglandin E2. American Journal of Veterinary Research, Vol.46, No.8, August, pp.1605-1615, ISSN: 0002-9645.

Costa, P.R.S., Araújo, R.B., Costa, M.C. & Maia, R.E.N. (2007). Endoscopia gastroduodenal após administração de nimesulida, monofenilbutazona e meloxicam em cães. Arquivo Brasileiro de Medicina Veterinária e Zootecnia, Vol.59, No.4, August, pp.903-909, ISSN: 0102-0935.

Cunningham, F.M. & Lees, P. (1994). Advances in anti-inflammatory therapy. British Veterinary Journal, Vol.150, No.2, March-April, pp.115-134, ISSN: 1413-9596.

Daurio, C.P., Holste, J.E., Andrews, F.M., Merritt, A.M., Blackford, J.T., Dolz, F. & Thompson, D.R. (1999). Effect of omeprazole paste on gastric acid secretion in horses. Equine Veterinary Journal, Vol.31, No.S9, April, pp.59-62, ISSN: 0425-1644.

Dirikolu, L., Woods, W.E., Boyles, J., Lehner, A.F., Harkins, J.D., Fisher, M., Schaeffer, D.J. & Tobin, T. (2008). Nonsteroidal anti-inflammatory agents and musculoskeletal injuries in Thoroughbred racehorses in Kentucky. Journal of Veterinary Pharmacology and Therapy, Vol.32, No.3, June, pp.271-279, ISSN: 1365-2885.

Doherty, T.J., Andrews, F.M., Blackford, J.T., Rohrbach, B.W., Sandin, A. & Saxton, A.M. (2003). Effects of lipopolysacchride and phenylbutazone on gastric contents in the horse. Equine Veterinary Journal, Vol.5, No.35, July, pp.472-745, ISSN: 0425-1644.

Doucet, M.Y., Bertone, A.L., Hendrickson, D., Hughes, F., MacAllister, C., McClure, S., Reinemeyer, C., Rossier, Y., Sifferman, R., Vrins, A.A., White, G., Kunkle, B., Alva, R., Romano, D. & Hanson, P.D. (2008). Comparison of efficacy and safety of paste formulation of firocoxib and phenylbutazone in horses with naturally occurring osteoarthritis. *Journal of American of Veterinary Medical Association*, Vol.232, No.1, January, pp.91-97, ISSN: 0003-1488.

Driessen, B. (2007). Pain: systemic and local/regional drug therapy. *Clinical Techniques in Equine Practice*, Vol.6, No.2, June, pp.135-144, ISSN: 1534-7516.

Erkert, R.S., MacAllister, C.G., Payton, M.E. & Clarke, C.R. (2005). Use of force analysis to compare the analgesic effects of intravenous administration of phenylbutazone and flunixin meglumine in horses with navicular syndrome. *American Journal of Veterinary Research*, Vol.2, No.66, February, pp.284-288, ISSN: 0002-9645.

Ferrucci, F., Zucca, E., Di Fabio, V., Croci, C. & Tradati, F. (2003). Gastroscopic findings in 63 Standardbred racehorses in training. *Veterinary Research Communications*, Vol.27, Suppl.1, September, pp.759-762, ISSN: 0165-7380.

Fitzpatrick, J.L., Nolan, A.M., Lees, P. & May, S.A. (2004). Inflammation and pain, In: *Bovine Medicine Diseases and Husandry of Cattle*, Andrews, A.H., Blowey, R.W., Boyd, H. & Eddy, R.G., pp.1045-1066, Blackwell Science, ISBN: 0-632-05596-0, Iowa, USA.

Gerring, E.L., Lees, P. & Taylor, J.B. (1981). Pharmacokinetics of phenylbutazone and its metabolites in the horse. *Equine Veterinary Journal*, Vol.13, No.3, July, pp.152-157, ISSN: 0425-1644.

Goodrich, L.R., Furr, M.O., Robertson, J.L. & Warnick, L.D. (1998). A toxicity study of eltenac, a nonsteroidal anti-inflammatory drug, in horses. *Journal of Veterinary Pharmacology and therapeutics*, Vol.21, No.1, February, pp.24-33, ISSN: 0140-7783.

Gretzer, B., Maricic, N., Respondek, M., Schuligoi, R. & Peskar, B.M. (2001). Effects of specific inhibition of cyclo-oxygenase-1 and cyclo-oxygenase-2 in the rat stomach with normal mucosa and after acid challenge. *British Journal of Pharmacology*, Vol. 132, No.7, January, pp.1565-1573, ISSN: 0007-1188.

Hammond, C.J., Mason, K.L. & Watkins, K.L. (1986). Gastric ulceration in mature Thoroughbred horses. *Equine Veterinary Journal*, Vol.18, No.4, July, pp.284-287, ISSN: 0425-1644.

Hoogerwerf, W.A. & Pasricha, P.J. (2001). Agents used for control of gastric acidity and treatment of peptic ulcers and gastroesophageal reflux disease, In: *The Pharmacological Basis of Therapeutics*, Gilman, A.G., Limbird, L.E. & Hardman, J.G., pp.1005-1020, Mc Graw-Hill, ISBN: 0-07-135469-7, New York, USA.

Hu, H.H., MacAllister, C.G., Payton, M.E. & Erkert, R. (2005). Evaluation of the analgesic effects of phenylbutazone administered at a high or low dosage in horses with chronic lameness. *Journal of American Veterinary Medical Association*, Vol.226, No.3, February, pp.414-417, ISSN: 0003-1488.

Igualada, C. & Moragues, F. (2005). Determination of phenylbutazone and oxyphenbutazone in animal urine by ion trap liquid chromatography-mass spectrometry. *Analytica Chimica Acta*, Vol.529, No.1/2, January, pp.235-238, ISSN: 0003-2670.

Jeffrey, S.C., Murray, M.J. & Eichorn, E.S. (2001). Distribution of epidermal growth factor receptor (EGFr) in normal and acute peptic-injured equine gastric squamous epithelium. *Equine Veterinary Journal*, Vol.33, No.6, November, pp.562-569, ISSN: 0425-1644.

Johnson, B., Carlson, G.P., Vatistas, N., Snyder, J.R., Lloyd, K.L. & Koobs, J. (1994). Investigation of the number and location of gastric ulceration in horses in race training submitted to the California racehorse *post-mortem* program. *Proceedings of the 40th Annual Convention of the American Association of Equine Practitioners*, Vancouver, British Columbia, Canada, December, pp.123-124.

Johnson, C.B., Taylor, P.M., Young, S.S. & Brearley, J.C. (1993). Post-operative analgesia using phenylbutazone, flunixin or carprofen in horses. *Veterinary Record*, Vol.133, No.14, October, pp.336-8, ISSN: 0042-4900.

Johnston, S.A. & Fox, S.M. (1997). Mechanisms of action of anti-inflammatory medications used for the treatment of osteoarthritis. *Journal of the American Veterinary Medical Association*, Vol.210, No.10, May, pp.1486-1492, ISSN: 0003-1488.

Johnstone, I.B. (1983). Comparative effects of phenylbutazone, naproxen and flunixin meglumine on equine platelet aggregation and platelet factor 3 availability *in vitro*. *Canadian Journal of Comparative Medicine*, Vol.47, No.2, April, pp.172-179, ISSN: 0846-8389.

Jones, S.,L. & Blikslager, A. (2001). The future of antiinflammatory therapy. *Veterinary clinics of North America: Equine Practice*, Vol.17, No.2, August, pp.245-262, ISSN: 0749-0739.

Jonsson, H. & Egenvall, A. (2006). Prevalence of gastric ulceration in Swedish Standardbreds in race-training. *Equine Veterinary Journal*, Vol.38, No.3, May, pp. 209-213, ISSN: 0425-1644.

Kawcak, C.E. (2001). Ortopedia, In: *Segredos em Medicina de Equinos*, Savage, C.J., pp.218-232, Artmed, ISBN: 85-7307-702-6, Porto Alegre , Brazil.

Keegan, K.G., Messer, N.T., Reed, S.K., Wilson, D.A. & Kramer, J. (2008). Effectiveness of administration of phenylbutazone alone or concurrent administration of phenylbutazone and flunixin meglumine to alleviate lameness in horses. *American Journal of Veterinary Research*, Vol.69, No.2, February, pp.1670-173, ISSN: 0002-9645.

Kore, A.M. (1990). Toxicology of nonsteroidal anti-inflammatory drugs. *Veterinary Clinics of North America: Small Animal Practice*, Vol.20, No.2, March, pp.419-30, ISSN: 0195-5616.

Lees, P. (2003). Pharmacology of drugs used to treat osteoarthritis in veterinary practice. *Inflammopharmacology*, Vol.11, No.4-6, pp.385-399, ISSN: 0925-4692.

Lees, P., Landoni, M.F., Giraudel, J. & Toutain, P.L. (2004). Pharmacodynamics and pharmacokinetics of nonsteroidal anti-inflammatory drugs in species of veterinary interest. *Journal of Veterinary Pharmacology and Therapeutics*, Vol.27, No.6, December, pp.479-490, ISSN: 0140-7783.

Lees, P., Taylor, J.B., Maitho, T.E., Millar, J.D. & Higgins, A.J. (1987). Metabolism, excretion, pharmacokinetics, and tissue residues of phenylbutazone in the horse. *Cornell Veterinarian*, Vol.77, No.2, April, pp.192-211, INSS: 0010-8901.

le Jeune, S.S., Nieto, J.E., Dechant, J.E. & Snyder, J.R. (2009). Prevalence of gastric ulcers in Thoroughbred broodmares in pasture: a preliminary report. *Veterinary Journal,* Vol.181, No.3, June, pp.251-255, ISSN: 1090-0233.

Léveillé, R., Miyabayashi,T., Weisbrode, S.E., Biller, D.S., Takiguchi, M. & Williams, J.F. (1996). Ultrasonographic renal changes associated with phenylbutazone administration in three foals. *Canadian Veterinary Journal,* Vol.37, No.4, April, pp.235-236, ISSN: 0008-5286.

Loew, D., Schuster, O., Knoell, H.E. & Graul, E.H. (1985). Pharmacology, toxicology and pharmacokinetics of mofebutazone. *Zeitschrift für Rheumatologie,* Vol.44, No.4, July-August, pp.186-192, ISSN: 0340-1855.

Lorenzo-Figueras, M. & Merritt, A.M. (2002). Effects of exercise on gastric volume and pH in the proximal portion of the stomach of horses. *American Journal of Veterinary Research,* Vol.63, No.11, November, pp.1481-1487, ISSN: 1413-9596.

Luthersson, N., Nielsen, K.H., Harris, P. & Parkin, T.D. (2009). Risk factors associated with equine ulceration syndrome (EGUS) in 201 horses in Denmark. *Equine Veterinary Journal,* Vol.41, No.7, September, pp.625-630, ISSN: 2042-3306.

MacAllister, C.G. (1983). Effects of toxic doses of phenylbutazone in ponies. *American Journal of Veterinary Research,* Vol. 44, No.12, December, pp.2277-2279, ISSN: 1413-9596.

MacAllister, C.G. (1994). Nonsteroidal anti-inflammatory drugs: their mechanism of action and clinical uses in horses. *Veterinary Medicine,* Vol.89, No.3, March, 1994, pp.237-240, ISSN: 1041-7826.

MacAllister, C.G. (1999). A review of medical treatment for peptic ulcer disease. *Equine Veterinary Journal,* Suppl.29, April, pp.45-49, ISSN: 2042-3306.

MacAllister, C.G., Andrews, F.M., Deegan, E., Ruoff, W. & Olovson, S.G. (1997). A scoring system for gastric ulcers in the horse. *Equine Veterinary Journal,* Vol.29, No.6, November, pp.430-433, ISSN: 2042-3306.

MacAllister, C.G., Morgan, S.J.; Borne, A.T. & Pollet, R.A. (1993). Comparison of adverse effects of phenylbutazone, flunixin meglumine, and ketoprofen in horses. *Journal of American of Veterinary Medical Association,* Vol.202, No.1, January, pp.71-77, ISSN: 0003-1488.

MacAllister, C.G. & Sangiah, S. (1993). Effect of ranitidine on healing of experimentally induced gastric ulcers in ponies. *American Journal of Veterinary Research,* Vol.54, No.7, July, pp.1103-1107, ISSN: 1413-9596.

MacAllister, C.G., Sangiah, S. & Mauromounstakos, A. (1992). Effect of a histamine H2 type receptor antagonist (WY 45, 727) on the healing of gastric ulcers in ponies. *Journal of Veterinary Internal Medicine,* Vol.6, No.5, September-October, pp.271-275, ISSN: 0891-6640.

MacAllister, C.G. & Taylor-MacAllister, C. (1994). Treating and preventing the adverse effects of nonsteroidal anti-inflamatory drugs in horses. *Veterinary Medicine,* Vol.89, No.3, March, pp.241-246, ISSN: 1041-7826.

MacKay, R.J., French, T.W., Nguyen, H.T. & Mayhew, I.G. (1983). Effects of large doses of phenylbutazone administration to horses. *American Journal of Veterinary Research,* Vol.44, No.5, May, pp.774-780, ISSN: 1413-9596.

Marqués, J.F. (2007). Equine gastric ulcer syndrome. *Large Animal Veterinary Rounds,* Vol.7, No.3, March, pp.1-6.

Martineau, H., Thompson, H. & Taylor, D. (2009). Pathology of gastritis and gastric ulceration in the horse. Part 1: Range of lesions present in 21 mature individuals. *Equine Veterinary Journal,* Vol.41, No.7, May, pp.638-644, ISSN: 2042-3306.

Mathews, K.A. (2002). Non-steroidal anti-inflammatory analgesics: a review of current practice. *Journal of Veterinary Emergency and Critical Care,* Vol.12, No.2, June, pp.89-97, ISSN: 1476-4431.

McClure, S.R., Carithers, D.S., Gross, S.J. & Murray, M.J. (2005). Gastric ulcer development in horses in a simulated show or training environment. *Journal of American Veterinary Medical Association,* Vol.22, No.5, September, pp.775-777, ISSN: 0003-1488.

Merritt, A.M. (2003). The equine stomach: A personal perspective. *Proceedings of the 49th Annual Convention of the American Association of Equine Practitioners,* New Orleans, Louisiana, USA, November, pp.75-102.

Meschter, C.L., Gilbert, M., Krook, G., Maylin, G. & Corradiono, R. (1990). The effects of phenylbutazone on the intestinal mucosa of the horse: a morphological, ultrastructural and biochemical study. *Equine Veterinary Journal,* Vol.22, July, pp.255-263, ISSN: 0425-1644.

Meschter, C.L.; Maylin, G.A. & Krook, L. (1984). Vascular pathology in phenylbutazone intoxicated horses. *Cornell Veterinarian,* Vol.74, No.3, July, pp.282-297, ISSN: 0010-8901.

Mokhber Dezdouli, M.R., Hassanpour, A., Nadalian, M.Gh. & Seifi, H.A. (2009). Gastric ulceration in Persian Arab horses in Iran: frequency, haematology and biochemistry. *Iranian Journal of Veterinary Research,* Vol.10, No.2, September, pp.146-151, ISSN: 1728-1997.

Monreal, L., Sabaté, D., Segura, D., Mayós, I. & Homedes, J. (2004). Lower gastric ulcerogenic effect of suxibuzone compared to phenylbutazone when administered orally to horses. *Research in Veterinary Science,* Vol.76, No.2, April, pp.145-149, ISSN: 0034-5288.

Morrissey, N.K., Bellenger, C.R. & Baird, A.W. (2008). Bradykinin stimulates prostaglandin E2 production and cyclooxygenase activity in equine nonglandular and glandular gastric mucosa *in vitro. Equine Veterinary Journal,* Vol.40, No.4, June, pp.332-336, ISSN: 0425-1644.

Murray, M.J. (1992). Aetiopathogenesis and treatment of peptic ulcer in the horse: a comparative review. *Equine Veterinary Journal,* Vol.13, Suppl.13, August, pp.63-74, ISSN: 0425-1644.

Murray, M.J. (1997). Overview of equine gastroduodenal ulceration. *Proceedings of the 43th Annual Convention of the American Association of Equine Practitioners,* Phoenix, Arizona, USA, December, pp.382-387.

Murray, M.J. (1999). Pathophysiology of peptic disorders in foals and horses: a review. *Equine Veterinary Journal,* Suppl.29, April, pp.14-18, ISSN: 0425-1644.

Murray, M.J. (2002). Disease of the stomach, In: *Manual of Equine Gastroenterology*, Mair, T., Divers, T. & Ducharme, N., pp.241-248, W.B. Saunders, ISBN: 0-7020-2486-4, Chatham, UK.

Murray, M.J. & Eichorn B.S. (1996). Effects of intermittent feed deprivation, intermittent feed deprivation with ranitidine administration, and stall confinement with *ad libitum* access to hay on gastric ulceration in horses. *American Journal of Veterinary Research*, Vol.57, No.11, November, pp.1599-1603, ISSN: 0002-9645.

Murray, M.J., Grodinsky, C., Anderson, C.W., Radue, P.F. & Schmidt, G.R. (1989). Gastric ulcers in horses: A comparison of endoscopic findings in horses with and without clinical signs. *Equine Veterinary Journal*, No.S7, June, pp.68-72, ISSN: 0425-1644.

Murray, M.J., Hart, J. & Parker, G.A. (1987). Equine gastric ulcer syndrome: endoscopic survey of asymptomatic foals. *Proceedings of the 33th Annual Convention of the American Association of Equine Practitioners*, New Orleans, Louisiana, USA, November-December, pp.769-776.

Murray, M.J., Haven, M.L.; Eichorn, E.S., Zhang, D., Eagleson, J. & Hickey, G.J. (1997). Effects of omeprazole on healing of naturally-occurring gastric ulcers in Thoroughbred racehorses. *Equine Veterinary Journal*, Vol.29, No.6, November, pp.425-429, ISSN: 0425-1644.

Murray, M.J., Nout, Y.S. & Ward, D.L. (2001). Endoscopic finding of the gastric antrum and pylorus in horses: 162 cases (1996-2000). *Journal of Veterinary Internal Medicine*, Vol.15, No.4, July, pp.401-406, ISSN: 0891-6640.

Murray, M.J. & Pipers, F. (2001). *A Clinician's Guide to Equine Gastrointestinal Endoscopy*, Merial, Duluth, Georgia, USA.

Murray, M.J. & Schusser, G.F. (1993). Measurement of 24-h gastric pH using an indwelling pH electrode in horses unfed, fed and treated with ranitidine. *Equine Veterinary Journal*, Vol.25, No.5, September, pp.417-421, ISSN: 0425-1644.

Murray, M.J., Schusser, G.F., Pipers, F.S. & Gross, S.J. (1996). Factors associated with gastric lesions in Thoroughbred horses. *EquineVeterinary Journal*, Vol.28, No.5, September, pp.368-374, ISSN: 0425-1644.

Nadeau, J.A. & Andrews, F.M. (2009). Equine gastric ulcer syndrome: the continuing conundrum. *Equine Veterinary Journal*, Vol.41, No.7, September, pp.611-615, ISSN: 2042-3306.

Orsini, J.A., Hackett, E.S. & Grenager, N. (2009). The effect of exercise on equine gastric ulcer syndrome in the Throughbred and Standardbred Athlete. *Journal of Equine Veterinary Science*, Vol.29, No.3, March, pp.167-171, ISSN: 0737-0806.

Pelligrini, F.L. (2005). Results of a large-scale necroscopic study of equine colonic ulcers. *Journal of Equine Veterinary Science*, Vol.25, No.3, March, pp.113-117, ISSN: 0737-0806.

Pinto, J.O., Souza, M.V., Costa, P.R.S., Ribeiro Júnior, J.I., Maia, L. & Monteiro, G.M. (2009). Influência da monofenilbutazona associada ou não ao omeprazol sobre o sitema digestório e renal de pôneis hígidos. *Ciência Rural*, Vol.39, No.1, January-February, pp.96-103, ISSN: 0103-8478.

Pinto, J.O., Souza, M.V., Costa, P.R.S., Ribeiro Júnior, J.I. & Moreira, J.C.L. (2008). Tecido de granulação exuberante com presença de Candida sp no estômago de pôneis tratados com omeprazol. *Veterinária e Zootecnia*, Vol.15, No.3, December, pp.449-455, ISSN: 0102-5716.

Pozzobon, R. (2010). *Avaliação Farmacocinética, Hematológica e Espermática de Pôneis Tratados com Meloxicam.* Thesis, Universidade Federal de Santa Maria, Brazil.

Prim, F.J.P. &Vila, I. (2002). Tratamiento continuado com omeprazol y aparición de candidiasis orofaríngea. *Atención Primária*, Vol.30, No.10, December, pp.663-664, ISSN: 0212-6567.

Price, J., Marques, J.M., Welsh, E.M. & Waran, N.K. (2002). Pilot epidemiological study of attitudes towards pain in horses. *Veterinary record*, Vol.151, November, pp.570-575, ISSN: 0042-4900.

Prügner, W., Huber, R. & Lühmann, R. (1991). Eltenac, a new anti-inflammatory and analgesic drug for horses: clinical aspects. *Journal of Veterinary Pharmacology and therapeutics*, Vol.14, No.2, June, pp.193-199, ISSN: 0140-7783.

Randall, D., Burggren, W. & French, K. (2000). Adquirindo energia: ingestão de alimentos, digestão e metabolismo, In: *Fisiologia Animal: Mecanismos e Adaptações*, pp.582-618, Editora Guanabara Koogan, ISBN: 97-885-770594-3, Rio de Janeiro, Brazil.

Robinson, N.E. & Sprayberry, K.A. (2009). *Current Therapy in Equine Medicine 6*, Appendix 1, pp.951, Saunders, ISBN: 978-1-4160-5475-7, Missouri, USA.

Roy, M.A., Vrins, A., Beauchamp, G. & Doucet, M.Y. (2005). Prevalence of ulcers of the squamous gastric mucosa in Standardbred horses. *Journal of Veterinary Internal Medicine*, Vol.19, No.5, September, pp.744-750, ISSN: 1939-1676.

Ruoff, W.W., Read, W.K. & Cargile, J.L. (1987). An equine gasric ulcer model to test H-2 antagonists. *Proceedings of the 68th Annual Meeting of the Conference of Research Workers in Animal Diseases*, Chicago, IL, USA, November, pp.58.

Sabaté, D., Homedes, J., Salichs, M., Sust, M. & Monreal, L. (2009). Multicentre, controlled, randomised and blinded field study comparing efficacy of suxibuzone and phenylbutazone in lame horses. *Equine Veterinary Journal*, Vol.41, No.7, June, pp.700-705, ISSN: 0425-1644.

Sandin, A., Skidell, J., Haggstrom, J., Girma, K. & Nilsson, G. (2000). Post mortem findings of gastric ulcers in Swedish horses older than age one year: a retrospective study of 3715 horses (1924-1996). *Equine Veterinary Journal*, Vol.32, No.1, January, pp.36-42, ISSN: 2042-3306.

Shearn, M.A. (1984). Agentes antiinflamatórios não-esteróides, analgésicos não-opiáceos, drogas utilizadas na gota, In: *Farmacologia Básica e Clínica*, Katzung, B.G., pp.452-471, Editora Guanabara, ISBN: 85-226-0139-9, Rio de Janeiro, Brazil.

Smyth, E.M., Burke, A. & FitzGerald, G.A. (2010). Autacóides derivados de lipídios: eicosanóides e fator de ativação das plaquetas, In: *Goodman & Gilman. As Bases Farmacológicas da Terapêutica*, Lazo, J.S., Parker, K.L., pp.585-600, AMGH Editora Ltda, ISBN: 0-07-142280-3, São Paulo, Brazil.

Snow, D.H., Bogan, J.A., Douglas, T.A. & Thompson, H. (1979). Phenylbutazone toxicity in ponies. *Veterinary Record*, Vol.105, No.2, July, pp.26-30, ISSN: 0042-4900.

Snow, D.H., Douglas, T.A., Thompson, H., Parkins, J.J. & Holmes, P.H. (1981). Phenylbutazone toxicosis in equidae: a biochemical and pathophysiologic study.

American Journal of Veterinary Research, Vol.42, No.10, October, pp.1754-1759, ISSN: 1413-9596.

Sullivan, M. & Snow, D.H. (1982). Factors affecting absorption of non-steroidal anti-inflammatory agents in the horse. *Veterinary Record*, Vo.110, No.24, pp.554-558, ISSN: 0042-4900

Tasaka, A.C. (2006). Antiinflamatórios não-esteroidais, In: *Farmacologia Aplicada à Medicina Veterinária*, Spinosa, H.S., Górniak, S.L. & Bernardi, M.M., pp.256-272, Guanabara Koogan, ISBN: 9788527711807, Rio de Janeiro, Brazil.

Taylor, J.B., Walland, A., Lees, P., Gerring, E.L., Maitho, T.E. & Millar, J.D. (1983). Biochemical and haematological effects of a revised dosage schedule of phenylbutazone in horses. *Veterinary Record*, Vol.112, No.26, June, pp.599-602, ISSN: 0042-4900.

Téllez, E., Ocampo, L., Bernad, M. & Sumano, H. (2005). Pharmacodynamic study of a long-acting parenteral formulation of omeprazole in horses. *Journal of Veterinary Pharmacology and Therapeutics*, Vol.28, No.6, December, pp.587-589, ISSN: 0140-7783.

Tobin, T., Chay, S., Kamerling, S., Woods, W.E., Weckman, T.J., Blake, J.W. & Lees, P. (1986). Phenylbutazone in horse: a review. *Journal of Veterinary Pharmacology and Therapeutics*, Vol.9, No.1, March, pp.1-25, ISSN: 0140-7783.

Traub J.L., Gallina, A.M., Grant, B.D., Reed, S.M., Gavin, P.R. & Paulsen, L.M. (1983). Phenylbutazone toxicosis in the foal. *American Journal of Veterinary Research*, Vol.44, No.8, August, pp.1410-1418, ISSN: 1413-9596.

Trillo, M.A., Soto, G. & Gunson, D.E. (1984). Flunixin toxicity in a pony. *Equine Practice*, Vol.6, No.3, March, pp.21-30, ISSN: 0162-8941.

Vatistas, N.J., Sifferman, R.L., Holste, J., Cox, J.L., Pinalto, G. & Schultz, K.T. (1999a). Induction and maintenance of gastric ulceration in horses in simulated race training. *Equine Veterinary Journal*, Suppl. 29, April, pp.40-44, ISSN: 0425-1644.

Vatistas, N.J., Snyder, J.R., Carlson, G., Johnson, B., Arthur, R.M., Thurmond, M. & Lloyd, K.C.K. (1994). Epidemiological study of gastric ulceration in the Thoroughbred race horse: 202 horses 1992-1993. *Proceedings of the 40th Annual Convention of the American Association of Equine Practitioners*, Vancouver, British Columbia, Canada, December, pp.125-126.

Vatistas, N.J., Snyder, J.R., Carlson, G., Johnson, B., Arthur, R.M., Thurmond, M., Zhou, H. & Lloyd, K.L.K. (1999b). Cross sectional study of gastric ulcers of the squamous mucosa in Thoroughbred racehorses. *Equine Veterinary Journal*, No.S29, April, pp.34-39, ISSN: 0425-1644.

Vicente, C.B. (2004). *Farmacoterapia Comparada de la Fenilbutazona en Diferentes Especies Animales: Estudio Alométrico*. Thesis, Universidad Complutense de Madrid, Spain.

Videla, R. & Andrews, F.M. (2009). New perspectives in equine gastric ulcer syndrome. *Veterinary Clinics of North America: Equine Practice*, Vol.25, No.2, August, pp.283-301, ISSN: 1558-4224.

Villa, R., Cagnardi, P., Belloli, C., Zonca, A., Zizzadoro, C., Ferro, E. & Carli, S. (2007). Oral and intravenous administration of nimesulide in the horse: rational dosage regimen from pharmacokinetic and pharmacodynamic data. *Equine Veterinary Journal*, Vol.39, No.2, March, pp.136-142, ISSN: 2042-3306.

Voutilainen, M., Mäntynen, T., Fäkkilä, M., Juhola, M. & Sipponen, P. (2001). Impact of non-steroidal anti-inflammatory drug and aspirin use on the prevalence of dyspepsia and uncomplicated peptic ulcer disease. *Scandinavian Journal Gastroenterology*, Vol.38, No.8, August, pp.817-821, ISSN: 0036-5521.

Permissions

The contributors of this book come from diverse backgrounds, making this book a truly international effort. This book will bring forth new frontiers with its revolutionizing research information and detailed analysis of the nascent developments around the world.

We would like to thank Jianyuan Chai, Ph.D, for lending his expertise to make the book truly unique. He has played a crucial role in the development of this book. Without his invaluable contribution this book wouldn't have been possible. He has made vital efforts to compile up to date information on the varied aspects of this subject to make this book a valuable addition to the collection of many professionals and students.

This book was conceptualized with the vision of imparting up-to-date information and advanced data in this field. To ensure the same, a matchless editorial board was set up. Every individual on the board went through rigorous rounds of assessment to prove their worth. After which they invested a large part of their time researching and compiling the most relevant data for our readers. Conferences and sessions were held from time to time between the editorial board and the contributing authors to present the data in the most comprehensible form. The editorial team has worked tirelessly to provide valuable and valid information to help people across the globe.

Every chapter published in this book has been scrutinized by our experts. Their significance has been extensively debated. The topics covered herein carry significant findings which will fuel the growth of the discipline. They may even be implemented as practical applications or may be referred to as a beginning point for another development. Chapters in this book were first published by InTech; hereby published with permission under the Creative Commons Attribution License or equivalent.

The editorial board has been involved in producing this book since its inception. They have spent rigorous hours researching and exploring the diverse topics which have resulted in the successful publishing of this book. They have passed on their knowledge of decades through this book. To expedite this challenging task, the publisher supported the team at every step. A small team of assistant editors was also appointed to further simplify the editing procedure and attain best results for the readers.

Our editorial team has been hand-picked from every corner of the world. Their multi-ethnicity adds dynamic inputs to the discussions which result in innovative outcomes. These outcomes are then further discussed with the researchers and contributors who give their valuable feedback and opinion regarding the same. The feedback is then collaborated with the researches and they are edited in a comprehensive manner to aid the understanding of the subject.

Apart from the editorial board, the designing team has also invested a significant amount of their time in understanding the subject and creating the most relevant covers. They scrutinized every image to scout for the most suitable representation of the subject and create an appropriate cover for the book.

The publishing team has been involved in this book since its early stages. They were actively engaged in every process, be it collecting the data, connecting with the contributors or procuring relevant information. The team has been an ardent support to the editorial, designing and production team. Their endless efforts to recruit the best for this project, has resulted in the accomplishment of this book. They are a veteran in the field of academics and their pool of knowledge is as vast as their experience in printing. Their expertise and guidance has proved useful at every step. Their uncompromising quality standards have made this book an exceptional effort. Their encouragement from time to time has been an inspiration for everyone.

The publisher and the editorial board hope that this book will prove to be a valuable piece of knowledge for researchers, students, practitioners and scholars across the globe.

List of Contributors

Aly Saber
Port-Fouad general hospital, Port-Fouad, Port-Said, Egypt

Christo van Rensburg and Monique Marais
Stellenbosch University, South Africa

Nathalie Salles
Pôle de Gérontologie Clinique, Hôpital Xavier Arnozan, France

Karl E. Peace
Jiann-Ping Hsu College of Public Health, Georgia Southern University Statesboro, USA

Işık Özgüney
Department of Pharmaceutical Technology, Faculty of Pharmacy, University of Ege, Turkey

Rômulo Dias Novaes and João Paulo Viana Leite
Federal University of Viçosa, Brazil

Ibrahim Abdulkarim Al Mofleh
College of Medicine, King Saud University, Kingdom of Saudi Arabia

Khaled A. Abdel-Sater
Al-Azhar University Assiut branch, Assiut, Department of Physiology, Faculty of Medicine for Boys, Egypt
King Abdul-Aziz University Rabigh branch, Rabigh, Department of Physiology, Faculty of Medicine for Boys, KSA

Maria do Carmo Souza
Federal University of Mato Grosso, Brazil

Yasunori Hamauzu
Shinshu University, Japan

Mohamed Morsy and Azza El-Sheikh
Pharmacology Department, Minia University, Egypt

Maria Verônica de Souza and José de Oliveira Pinto
Universidade Federal de Viçosa, Brazil

Printed in the USA
CPSIA information can be obtained
at www.ICGtesting.com
JSHW011428221024
72173JS00004B/718